FORCED EXIT

Other Books by Wesley J. Smith

The Lawyer Book: A Nuts and Bolts Guide to Client Survival

The Doctor Book: A Nuts and Bolts Guide to Patient Power

The Senior Citizen's Handbook: A Nuts and Bolts Guide to More Comfortable Living

Winning the Insurance Game (co-authored with Ralph Nader)

The Frugal Shopper (co-authored with Ralph Nader)

Collision Course: The Truth about Airline Safety (co-authored with Ralph Nader)

No Contest: Corporate Lawyers and the Perversion of Justice in America (co-authored with Ralph Nader)

Culture of Death: The Assault on Medical Ethics in America

Power over Pain: How to Get the Pain Control You Need (co-authored with Eric M. Chevlen, M.D.)

Consumer's Guide to a Brave New World

FORCED EXIT

EUTHANASIA,
ASSISTED SUICIDE, AND THE NEW
DUTY TO DIE

WESLEY J. SMITH

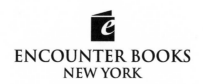

ENCOUNTER BOOKS
NEW YORK

Paperback edition published in 2006 by Encounter Books, an activity of Encounter for Culture and Education, Inc., a nonprofit, tax exempt corporation.

Encounter Books website address: www.encounterbooks.com

Manufactured in the United States and printed on acid-free paper.

The paper used in this publication meets the minimum requirements of ANSI/NISOZ39.48-1992 (R 1997)(*Permanence of Paper*).

Library of Congress Cataloging-in-Publication Data

Smith, Wesley J.
    Forced Exit/ Wesley J. Smith.
        p. cm.
        Includes bibliographical references and index.
    ISBN 1-59403-119-3 (alk. paper)
1. 2. 3. 4. I. Title.

R726 .S576 2005
179.7 22–dc 22
2005021499

10   9   8   7   6   5   4   3   2   1

DEDICATION

*To my father, Wesley L. Smith, who faced his
own death with such courage and fortitude,
and to my mother, Leona Smith,
who loved him, and loves me, so well.*

Contents

INTRODUCTION

THE SEEDS FOR THIS BOOK, AND FOR MY efforts as an anti-euthanasia activist, were sown on November 1, 1992. On that day, a Sunday, my friend Frances went to a hotel, checked in, got into bed, took some sleeping pills, pulled a plastic bag over her head, and died.

Frances's suicide was not an act born of impulse or momentary despair. She had been planning it for years. Indeed, almost from the moment I met her in Los Angeles in 1988, she had spoken enthusiastically about how empowering and ennobling it would be for her to take her own life. In her mind's eye, she saw herself beginning to experience the debilitations of age. Rather than endure a slow decline and become a "burden" to her friends, Frances would say, "I'm going to hold a going-away party," where she hoped her many friends would surround her as she lay on a couch, tell her how much she meant to them, hold her hands and stroke her brow as she swallowed the drugs from her "hoard of pills," and where she would slowly and quietly transform from living friend to deeply treasured memory.

Most of us were appalled by her suicide fixation, and each in our own way tried to convince her not to do it. We told her repeatedly that we valued her presence among us. We tried to assure her that growing old did not make one less valuable as a human being, and that illness or disability did not make one a burden. We urged her to seek counseling, hoping that if she put as much energy and effort into living as she seemed to be putting into plans for dying, she could find renewed meaning and joy from a life that clearly did not satisfy her. We worried about her continually and wondered where on earth she had picked up all the euphemisms for self-destruction that sprinkled her vocabulary, such as "deliverance" and "final passage."

It is important to note that in the first two years of our friendship, as Frances fantasized about her future death, she was not ill. She was, however, very unhappy. She had divorced years before, and her ex-husband had then married a younger woman, a fact of Frances's life that humiliated and embittered her. The divorce had also hit her hard in the pocketbook, removing her from a thoroughly enjoyed life of upper-middle-class ease and gentility and forcing her to count pennies from her rent-controlled one-bedroom apartment. Meanwhile, the fact that her successor and her ex (who was ill with Alzheimer's) continued to live well was a constant wound that ate at Frances with every sparse alimony check she cashed, money she genuinely needed and at the same time deeply resented.

Frances had other emotional burdens. One of her two sons was cognitively and emotionally disabled from injuries sustained in an auto accident. The accident had come just as the young man was making a big breakthrough in the screenwriting trade and had cut him off from a dream come true. Frances never stopped worrying about him, and she despaired about his future once she was gone. Even more painful, Frances was so estranged from her other son that it would be an exaggeration to call their interaction a relationship.

Frances's talk about her future suicide would wax during her more unhappy times and wane during the times she felt productive and useful—surely no coincidence. She was very active in local community clubs and was always thinking about how she could help her friends with business ideas, introducing them to others in her stable of associates and acquaintances who she felt could provide sage advice, opportunity or help with ideas. Her female friends told me that hers was a great shoulder to cry on, especially for pals who had relationship difficulties. She definitely helped me and she knew it. She took great pride in being the inspiration for my book *The Senior Citizen's Handbook: A Nuts and Bolts Guide to More Comfortable Living*.

Unfortunately, Frances's happy times were generally short-lived, and thoughts about suicide would again tug at her as relent-lessly as gravity. It was like some perverse dance. She would plan the thing, we would change her mind, and then, for no apparent reason, she would announce she was planning it again.

At one point we all became convinced that Frances wasn't just talking anymore, that she was about to do it. Interventions were held. We pleaded and cajoled, doing everything we could think of to help her keep a firm grip on life—all to no avail. It would take a miracle, it seemed, to dissuade her.

Then, a miracle of sorts did happen. But it was nothing super-natural: Her alimony was cut off. Suddenly, Frances had a cause! The suicide was forgotten as Frances headed for court on a full head of steam, acting as her own attorney to force resumption of her payments, and she succeeded. Clearly, here was a woman who, despite all her romanticized talk of her warm and fuzzy "deliver-ance," desperately needed a reason to live. But her triumph did not satisfy her for long. As the glow of her court victory wore off, Frances again spoke of suicide. At about this time she was diag-nosed with treatable lymphatic leukemia. She developed a neuropathy (a degenerative state of the nervous system), from which she experienced a distressing burning sensation on her skin. (Frances would complain bitterly that her HMO doctors did not take her pain seriously, yet she refused to take the pain medication prescribed for her.) She was also a candidate for a hip replacement. And underneath it all was the abiding sadness about her life's many disappointments.

By this time I had moved to San Francisco, so I had less per-sonal contact with Frances than in previous years, although we kept up a lively interaction over the phone. Then, one day, one of her friends called, very upset, telling me, "Frances is planning to die next week, on her birthday." I called Frances immediately. I implored her at least to see a psychiatrist before doing it. She refused, saying, "He might give me a pill that would make me not want to kill myself."

I was later told that she invited her friends in Los Angeles to her long-planned going-away party. All of them refused to attend. They loved her. They did not want her to kill herself. They would not support this chosen action.

Frances then told everyone the suicide was off. She even

called my mother, who had also become her friend, and said that a "divine intervention" had saved her life. We all breathed a sigh of relief.

Frances was lying. Secretly, she paid a distant cousin five thousand dollars to go with her to a hotel, where her only baggage was a stash of pills and a plastic bag. Two days afterward, I and her other friends received her photocopied suicide note (the return address was simply "Frances"); in it she spoke of herself as being "in control" and stated that the "act is not one of 'suicide'—I consider that [it] is my final passage."

Frances's death was not noble and uplifting, as she had fantasized. We miss Frances and mourn her loss, but she has not left behind the sweet garden of memory she fervently believed (hoped) her death would create. None of her friends appreciated the morbid experience of receiving photocopies of her suicide letter in the mail after she was gone, and most of us felt angry, betrayed and empty in the wake of her self-destruction.

MORE THAN THIRTY THOUSAND PEOPLE die by their own hand each year in the United States, more than are murdered and only about ten thousand fewer than are killed in auto accidents. Suicide is the second leading cause of death among college students and the third leading cause of death among young people ages 15 to 24. The suicide rate for children ages 10 to 14 has more than doubled in the last ten years. The elderly, like Frances, are also particularly susceptible to self-destruction.

Usually after a suicide, those who were close to the deceased person wonder why it happened, they grieve, and finally they go on with their lives. But I had a queasy feeling that there was more to Frances's death than appeared on the surface. It was as if she had somehow been *encouraged* to pursue death, although her friends had all tried to persuade her to embrace life. I attempted to set this feeling aside but it would not go away. My unease was abstract, yet it was very real. I reminded myself of a character in a Stephen King novel who can sense, yet cannot see, the darkness that lurks behind a façade of normality.

I decided to investigate. Frances was one of the most organized women I have ever met. She kept a file on everything. I called the executrix of her will and asked her to look through Frances's papers to see whether she had kept a suicide file and, if so, to please send it to me.

A week later, the file arrived. It wasn't very thick. There were some news clippings that put a positive spin on suicide and a smattering of poetry. But most of the material was from an organization I had paid scant attention to before: the Hemlock Society. Specifically, Frances had collected several issues of the organization's newsletter, the *Hemlock Quarterly*. That these writings had a major influence on Frances there can be little doubt. She had highlighted much of the text with a yellow marking pen. Several issues were dog-eared from frequent reading.

As I read the material, my jaw dropped. The documents seemed scurrilous to me—nothing less than pro-suicide propaganda extolling self-destruction as a morally correct and empowering experience. Most of the newsletters had stories in them—allegedly letters from satisfied readers—of warm and successful suicides, and/or advocacy pieces by euthanasia proponents. The articles had an almost religious tone that made me feel as if I were reading tracts from some bizarre death cult.

The January 1988 issue of the *Hemlock Quarterly* caught my eye because it was especially well worn.[1] One of the stories inside, entitled "A Peaceful Passing" and signed by "A New Member in California" (supposedly a grief counselor), told in glowing terms of the suicide of Sam, allegedly a terminal cancer patient. Frances had underscored these words from the story:

> Believe it or not, we laughed and giggled and [Sam] seemed to relish the experience. I think for Sam it was finally taking control again after ten years of being at the mercy of a disease and medical protocols demanded by that disease.

Suicide promoted as uplifting, enjoyable fun sickened me.

This wasn't the only disturbing passage. Sam's suicide was described as peaceful and calm, and the reader was assured that "all went smoothly" through the suicide, funeral and burial. The writer even extolled the act of assisting the death as "very profound in my life," one that "has changed me and grown me."[2] In other words, the suicide was empowering and beneficial, not only for the deceased but for the "helper."

Another story in the newsletter, called "Planning Made Death Peaceful," written by a "loving family member," described the author's "instant" agreement to assist the "self-deliverance" of a relative with an "uncurable [sic], debilitating and hideous illness." (Note: "incurable" is not a synonym for "terminal." After all, arthritis is incurable.) The story described how the author over time collected the drugs to be used (just as Frances had done) and how the relative died "in complete peace within 15 or 20 minutes at most." The last paragraph had caught Frances's attention, as evidenced by the yellow highlighting:

> It was indeed a good deliverance; much of it was due to foresight and planning. We had the necessary medications and the necessary knowledge. But I will always believe that most of it was due to the steadfast will and soul of my family member, who made a decision for self-deliverance and fully accepted it.[3]

In other words, this "good deliverance" occurred because the ill person had the moral fortitude to go through with it, seeming to imply that those who don't have such courage are somehow not "steadfast" or that they lack "soul."

Other articles in the issue explained how to commit suicide. One provided a listing of the drugs that were good for suicide, describing the relative toxicity and the amount of each drug required to constitute a lethal dose ("Drug Dosage Table").[4] Frances had underscored the names of the drugs with the highest toxicity levels.

In "Self-Deliverance with Certainty," the reader was instructed on the proper use of a plastic bag, described as a death method that is "less than perfect but...not very much less than perfect."[5] Chills ran up my spine. It was as if I had an exact description of Frances's death, so closely had she followed these instructions.

There was a disclaimer of sorts in the article on drug dosages that read, "Only for information of members of the National Hemlock Society for possible self-deliverance from a future terminal illness and used in conjunction with material found in the book, *Let Me Die Before I Wake*."[6] The entire message of the newsletter was so positive and supportive of suicide as an answer to life's difficulties that this caveat seemed to mean absolutely nothing. Frances, who was *not* terminally ill, had not underscored the warning passage.

The more I thought about the Hemlock Society propaganda and its direct connection with Frances's death, the angrier I grew. Who were these people to push a pro-suicide message on the depressed and vulnerable, people looking desperately for some way to be in control of their unhappy lives? They didn't even know Frances. Yet they had given her the moral support to kill herself and had taught her how to do it. Although Frances was without question responsible for her own self-destruction, I felt that the Hemlock Society had fostered her romanticism about suicide. As I saw it, morally they had much to answer for.

As it turned out, I was not alone in believing that the euthanasia movement, in which the Hemlock Society plays an active part, has influenced the rise of suicide rates in our country, at least among the elderly. For example, Barbara Haight, who directs a program at the Medical University of South Carolina's College of Nursing to prevent suicide among the elderly, believes that the rise in euthanasia advocacy over the last ten years, the publicity surrounding Jack ("Dr. Death") Kevorkian, and other related events have "made suicide more acceptable to people who once would not have considered it because of religious and family concerns. They see it as a solution to their problems."[7] Frances is a case in point.

In my anger, I wrote an article about Frances for the "My Turn" section of *Newsweek* called "The Whispers of Strangers," which was meant to be a wake-up call about the dangers of the euthanasia movement and the message it sends to weak and vulnerable people.[8] My article touched people, but not in the way I had expected. I received about 150 letters. A few were supportive, thanking me for warning about the euthanasia movement and commiserating about the pain that suicide causes survivors. But the vast majority of my correspondents were outraged that I had criticized euthanasia. They did not believe it can destroy moral concepts, or that "the preservation of human life is our highest moral ideal," or that "a principal purpose of government" is to protect human life, or that "those who fight to stay alive in the face of terminal illness," such as the actor Michael Landon, are "powerful uplifters of the human experience."[9]

These sentiments enraged my detractors. I was lectured that the idea of human life as "sacred...is no longer tenable."[10] I was accused of wanting "the pleasure of seeing her [Frances] as an incontinent living corpse ravaged by pain and drugs."[11] My thoughts about protecting life were seen as proof that "Wesley Smith lacks genuine compassion."[12] Another writer accused me of "self-righteous arrogance" because I disapproved of Frances's act to "advance slightly the date on which...she must inevitably shuffle off this mortal coil."[13] An especially harsh critic compared me to "Torquiemada [sic] of the Spanish Inquisition who devised fiendish tortures because our highest moral ideal was to get infidels to adapt [sic] Christianity."[14] And more than one correspondent echoed the hope expressed by "M.B." that I should "live a long and suffering life."[15] Many correspondents expressed views that can only be described as pro-suicide. "This is the 90s, and suicide IS an alternative to life," one letter writer advised me.[16] "I congratulate Frances," another reader wrote, "on her decision to end her life when and how she wanted."[17] R.K. thought that "we as a society will come to see the day we view suicide (and euthanasia) as acceptable and even good."[18] L.M.S. was moved to proclaim that "suicide, as the act is called—for a person without responsibilities, or with a chronic disease—*is* a noble act" (italics in original).[19]

I was genuinely surprised. Were my correspondents outside the cultural mainstream, or was I? If I was, when had the values that not so long ago were deemed self-evident truths changed so dramatically? And where was I when this changed occurred?

The next paragraph in my article also attracted attention and criticism. I had written:

> Of greater concern to me is the moral trickledown effect that could result should society ever come to agree with Frances. Life is action and reaction, the proverbial pebble thrown into the pond. We don't get to Brave New World in one giant leap. Rather, the descent to depravity is reached by small steps. First, suicide is promoted as a virtue. Vulnerable people like Frances become early casualties. Then follows mercy killing of the terminally ill. From there, it is a hop, skip, and a jump to killing people who don't have a good "quality" of life, perhaps with the prospect of organ harvesting thrown in as a plum to society.[20]

Every reader who commented on this passage, both supporters and detractors of my point of view, was convinced that I was overreacting. Each believed that such a progression was unthinkable in the United States, that as a humane people we would never allow ourselves to engage in such inhumane conduct. I was advised earnestly to have a bit more faith in people.

Unfortunately, I wasn't being paranoid or alarmist. As this book will detail, my fears about "moral trickledown" (more commonly known as the "slippery slope," to which I will frequently refer)—and more—are justified either by events already happening or by proposals put forward seriously by mainstream opinion setters, by the medical intelligentsia, and by public policy makers. For example:

- In the United States, several courts have ruled that laws prohibiting assisted suicide are unconstitutional. One state, Oregon, has passed a law (Measure 16) that would specifically permit doctors to prescribe lethal drugs to patients diagnosed as having six months or less to live.

- Advocacy in favor of assisted suicide "only" for the terminally ill is already passé among euthanasia advocates. Legalizing hastened death is now promoted for the "hopelessly ill" or "desperately ill," as well as the dying. The "hopelessly ill" are disabled people, those with chronic illnesses, the frail elderly. Some "rational suicide" proponents advocate including those with severe mental or emotional problems who have no physical illness.

- Ann Landers has endorsed the establishment of death clinics where the elderly could go to be put to death rather than receive long-term care, calling the notion "a sane, sensible, civilized alternative to existing in a nursing home, draining family resources, and hoping the end will come soon. Too bad it's against the law...."[21]

- Some people are already being killed on the basis of quality-of-life considerations, specifically the cognitively disabled, both unconscious and conscious, by having their feeding tubes removed in order to cause their deaths. Tube feeding has in fact been classified as a medical procedure, to permit the practice of withholding it in such cases.

- The American Medical Council on Ethics and Judicial Affairs for a short period of time advocated that vital organs be harvested from anencephalic babies (born with parts of the brain missing) while they are still alive. The council was forced by opposition from the American Medical Association to retract this opinion, pending further study. But it is highly likely that the issue will return in the near future. If such a policy were ever implemented, it would mark the first time in the United States since the end of slavery that the bodies of living human beings could be legally exploited as a natural resource without their explicit consent.

And these items represent just the tip of the iceberg.

IN THE NEARLY TEN YEARS SINCE this book was first published, much has happened in the international cultural struggle over euthanasia and assisted suicide. In the original edition, I worried deeply about cases in the Ninth and Second United States Circuit Courts of Appeals that had declared a constitutional right to assisted suicide. Happily, the Supreme Court of the United States disagreed. Its 1997 unanimous ruling that assisted suicide is not a constitutional right prevented the euthanasia death agenda from being imposed upon the nation via judicial fiat. The supreme courts of two states separated geographically by thousands of miles, Alaska and Florida, have similarly ruled in subsequent decisions (1997 Florida and 2001 Alaska) that their respective state constitutions do not guarantee a right to privacy that requires the legalization of assisted suicide.

In Europe, litigation to permit assisted suicide also failed. In 2001 a British woman, Diane Pretty, sued in an English court for a ruling to prevent her husband from being prosecuted for assisting her suicide. Pretty, who was terminally ill with amyotrophic lateral sclerosis—called motor neuron disease in England—achieved much public sympathy and became the talk of Great Britain. When she lost in the trial court, she took her case to the House of Lords. After the British high court also turned her down, she appealed to the European Union Court on Human Rights, claiming, among other allegations, that the British law against assisted suicide violated her EU right to be treated with dignity. The EU court, however, rightly noted that the law was not the cause of Pretty's difficulties; her disease was. The case was the equivalent in Europe of the United States Supreme Court's ruling against a constitutional right to assisted suicide. (Diane Pretty died naturally of her disease in May 2002.)

(The one exception to judicial restraint occurred in Colombia, where euthanasia was imposed on Colombians by court order. That ruling is not yet in effect, awaiting the promulgation of death regulations to govern how and when doctors will be allowed to kill patients.)

With courts internationally refusing to impose assisted suicide upon free people—and it is distinctly arguable whether the Colombians are free people—the issue is now, quite literally, up to us. If the door is going to be opened wide to the death culture, in a free country *we* will be the ones opening it. And if we do invite the wolf inside, we will have only ourselves to blame when we suffer the consequences of our own foolishness.

When this book first came out in 1997, many worried that the euthanasia movement's success in passing Oregon's Measure 16 would be repeated throughout the nation, indeed, that the death culture would sweep the country. The threat still remains, but it hasn't happened yet—although not for lack of effort by euthanasia advocates.

There have been two assisted suicide legalization initiatives on state ballots since the original publication of *Forced Exit*. In 1998, voters in Michigan, who had the most intimate knowledge of the death agenda thanks to Michigander Jack Kevorkian, rejected legalization by a whopping 71-29 percent. In 2000, Maine also refused to approve assisted suicide, albeit by a narrow 51-49 percent margin. As I write these words in February 2005, there appears to be no state whose voters will, in the immediate future, be asked via initiative to legalize assisted suicide.

Stymied by voters, assisted suicide advocates have introduced legalization bills in several state legislatures each year. So far, these efforts have all been for naught. But in May 2002, out of the blue, Hawaii came within a whisker of legalizing assisted suicide— nearly passing legislation patterned after Oregon's law. Strongly pushed by Governor Benjamin Cayetano, an assisted suicide enthusiast, the legislation passed the Hawaii House of Representatives by

30-20 and then passed a preliminary state senate vote by 13-12. After much pressure was brought to bear on state senators by Hawaiian voters in a very short time, the senate two days later refused to legalize assisted suicide by a narrow 14-11 vote.

Still, proponents of assisted suicide had much to cheer. For the first time in history, one house of a state legislature had voted to legalize medicalized killing. With Hawaii proving itself to be a "weak link" in defense of the equality-of-human-life ethic, we can expect that beautiful state to become the front line of the international euthanasia debate for many years to come. Meanwhile, in 2005, Vermont, Arizona and California all have assisted suicide legalization bills pending in their legislatures.

When *Forced Exit* was first published, Jack Kevorkian seemed unstoppable. Juries had refused repeatedly to convict him of assisted suicide and he seemed able to prey upon disabled and dying people at will. Then, Kevorkian videotaped himself lethally injecting ALS patient Thomas Youk, and he narcissistically brought the tape to euthanasia proponent Mike Wallace for airing on *60 Minutes*. This time Kevorkian had gone too far. The public ruckus that resulted from a televised murder literally forced the Oakland County prosecutor—who had won his elective office on a plank of leaving Kevorkian alone—to prosecute him. A jury convicted Kevorkian of second-degree murder; the judge told him to "consider yourself stopped"; and he is now in state prison where he belongs.

Meanwhile, the sparsely populated Northern Territory of Australia legalized euthanasia, albeit briefly. This legislation did not sit well with the Australian Parliament, which acted quickly to overturn the territorial law. Tragically, before the parliament could act, four people had been poisoned to death using a computer program designed by the "Australian Kevorkian," Philip Nitschke.

Still, despite their many defeats, proponents of euthanasia and assisted suicide have achieved more than perhaps even they would have imagined was possible only ten years ago. Oregon's assisted suicide law has gone into effect and more than two hundred people (that we know of) have had their lives extinguished by poison that doctors legally prescribed. Former attorney general Janet Reno granted Oregon doctors a waiver to the usual requirement of the

Controlled Substances Act that federally controlled drugs not be used to kill. When a new attorney general, John Ashcroft, sought to undo Reno's waiver, he was enjoined from doing so by an Oregon-based federal judge determined to protect that state's assisted suicide law, a ruling upheld by the Ninth Circuit Court of Appeals in a 2-1 vote. Advocates for euthanasia applauded the decision as a matter of upholding "states' rights." Yet a great irony went unnoted in media reports about the court's ruling: Some of the very same euthanasia advocates who now championed states' rights so fervently had, only a few years previously, sought to destroy the states' ability to legislate against assisted suicide by pushing or supporting the case to create a constitutional right to assisted suicide. But then, consistency is not the point of the euthanasia movement; legalizing mercy killing is. (As these words are written, the case is being appealed to the Supreme Court of the United States by the U.S. government.)

Despite the ongoing scandals associated with euthanasia in the Netherlands, which have only accelerated in the years since this book first appeared, that country has now formally legalized the practice, in the process doing away with the one remaining impediment to euthanasia: the technical illegality of mercy killing. Proving that emotions rather than facts too often matter most in this debate, the well-documented horrors in the Netherlands did nothing to dissuade lawmakers in Belgium from legalizing Dutch-style euthanasia in May 2002. There are also strong and ongoing attempts to legalize euthanasia in France, South Africa, Australia and Switzerland (where informal assisted suicide is already so well tolerated that "suicide tourism" is a reality there).

Meanwhile, the problem of "futile care theory" has grown more dangerous than when I described it in the first edition of this book. Futile care theory holds that when a doctor believes that the quality of a patient's life is not worth living (or spending resources upon), the doctor can unilaterally refuse *wanted* medical treatment. When I first warned about the subject in *Forced Exit*, futile care impositions tended to be ad hoc and hence easier to thwart in court—as the parents of Baby Ryan did in Spokane. Today, there is a systematic, nationwide attempt by many in the bioethics movement to impose futile care theory upon the populace via formal hospital protocols that give anonymous hospital ethics committees the power to turn thumbs up or thumbs down to wanted medical treatment deemed "inappropriate" after the case has gone through a bureaucratic process. Indeed, as the expanded discussion of the topic of futile care in this edition of *Forced Exit* will demonstrate, these protocols are designed explicitly—at least in part—to stack the legal deck *against* the patient and family seeking treatment that the doctor or hospital wishes to refuse. Will these protocols work, opening the door to explicit health care rationing? Only time will tell, but there can be little doubt that futile care theory presents an acute and rising threat to the equality-of-human-life ethic.

The attempt by the bioethics movement to permit the dehydration of conscious, cognitively disabled people who require feeding tubes to stay alive, such as people discussed in the first edition of this book like Robert Wendland and Michael Martin, has not yet succeeded. Indeed, so long as family members disagree, the courts still protect conscious patients by requiring a high level of proof before allowing feeding tubes to be removed. That is the good news. The bad news is that those deemed permanently unconscious have fewer protections even though that diagnosis is often wrong. Indeed, in the Robert Wendland case, the California Supreme Court seemed to state that unconscious people do not have the same constitutional rights as the conscious. If my reading of this decision is correct, it marks a terrible precedent, creating a dual system of rights that could strip the weakest and most vulnerable among us of their legal personhood. Meanwhile, the Terri Schiavo tragedy in Florida demonstrated the lengths to which some courts will go to justify removing food and fluids from profoundly cognitively disabled people.

THE EUTHANASIA STRUGGLE IS ONE THAT remains eminently winnable. But if a permanent victory is to be won, it won't be easy or quick. Indeed, the struggle to maintain morality in medicine and protect the inherent equality of sick and disabled people is the challenge of our times. It is my hope that this second revised edition of *Forced Exit* will help its readers pierce the emotionalism, fear mongering and euphemism that are the standard fare of the euthanasia/assisted suicide movement and achieve a greater understanding of the issue and the importance of the stakes involved. Since the more people learn about euthanasia the less they tend to like it, such education is vital if we are to maintain a moral health care delivery system.

Finally, it is important to reemphasize that we must do much more than merely say no to killing. Our ill, elderly, disabled and despairing brothers and sisters deserve to have their suffering taken seriously and addressed. We must commit ourselves to the task of resolving the problems that may give rise to a desire to commit suicide: the undertreatment of pain and depression, isolation and marginalization, worries about being a burden on loved ones and society. These are tasks that require our time, attention and, above all, love. If we truly want to be compassionate, we will reject euthanasia and assisted suicide and do our part as individuals and as a society to ensure that each of us, regardless of age, state of health, or physical and mental abilities, has access to life with dignity. If we succeed in doing this, the battle will be won and the euthanasia movement will simply fade away.

Wesley J. Smith
Castro Valley, California
May 2005

A Word about Terminology

Before we begin our discussion of euthanasia, I would like to clarify the terminology employed in this book. Many different terms are used by different sources for the acts of killing that will be discussed within these pages: *Active voluntary euthanasia, nonvoluntary euthanasia, involuntary euthanasia, passive euthanasia, good death, death with dignity, planned death, assisted death, aid in dying,* and so on. These terms and phrases, which may have great meaning in the ivory tower of academia or among assisted suicide ideologues, are of little use in a book designed for a general audience; in this context, the would only be confusing (as sometimes they are meant to be).

I will generally use the terms *kill, euthanasia,* and/or *assisted suicide.* I use the word *kill* because it is accurate and descriptive of what euthanasia and assisted suicide are about: "to deprive of…or put an end to life." Some may object to this word because it elicits a strong emotional reaction—and well it should. But killing is precisely what we are discussing here. The subject is too serious, in my view, to accept the fuzzy words and euphemisms preferred by euthanasia advocates as the spoonful of sugar that helps the hemlock go down.

By *euthanasia* I mean the killing of one person by another (usually but not always a doctor) because the person killed has a serious disease or injury, is disabled, is emotionally or mentally disturbed, is anguished, or is elderly. *Euthanasia* means, literally, "good death." While it was not coined originally to describe mercy killing, by now it is so much a part of the language that no usable alternative exists.

Assisted suicide, for my purposes, means self-killing for the same rea-sons that euthanasia is undertaken. It differs from suicide in that it is not a solitary action but rather a joint effort. Another person actively participates, assists in, and/or facilitates the termination of life. Thus, if a doctor injects a patient with a sedative followed by curare (a lethal poison)—the usual practice in the Netherlands—that is euthanasia. If a doctor knowingly prescribes drugs for another to use in a suicide, or someone mixes a lethal dose of drugs in liquid form for another knowingly to drink, those are examples of assisted suicide.

In my view, the practical distinctions between euthanasia and assisted suicide are about as substantial as the differences between the actions of the left and the right leg in walking: One step naturally follows the other.

ONE

DEATH FUNDAMENTALISM

O N OCTOBER 23, 1991, FIFTY-EIGHT-YEAR-OLD Marjorie Wantz and forty-three-year-old Sherry Miller kept their appointment at a cabin in a park near Detroit with an unemployed pathologist named Jack Kevorkian. Although he was then still relatively unknown, Kevorkian had made headlines more than a year earlier after hooking up Janet Adkins, who had early-stage Alzheimer's disease, to a suicide machine of his own design that killed her by way of intravenously administered barbiturates and poison when she flipped a switch. (Adkins died well before her disease became debilitating, a good ten years prior to the point when it could have been expected to end her life.) Now Wantz and Miller wanted to die.

Neither was terminally ill. According to later court testimony, both were suffering from depression. Miller was disabled by multiple sclerosis. A few years prior to her death, just when Miller's disease had begun to worsen and restrict her activities, her husband left her, taking custody of their children. Miller was forced by the divorce to live with her elderly parents, and she worried about being a burden to them.[1] She claimed that her disgust with her own disabilities was her reason for wanting to die. Yet Miller, forty-three, might eventually have adapted to her disability—as so many people disabled later in life do—as well as to the loss of her family, and she might have created a new life for herself.

After benign growths had been removed from Wantz's vagina, she began to complain bitterly of severe pelvic pain. Many doctors

tried to discover the cause through various means, including surgery. None was found. Indeed, her autopsy would show that she
had no organic disease whatsoever. Not coincidentally, Wantz suffered from a depressive disorder, had been treated in mental
hospitals and, according to an article in the *Detroit News,* had been
using a sleep aid called Halcion in higher-than-recommended doses
because of insomnia.[2] (Halcion, if abused, can cause the side effect
of suicidal impulses.)

Entering the cabin, the women lay down on cots. Kevorkian
hooked Wantz up to his suicide machine, and soon she was no
more. But he couldn't find a vein in Miller's emaciated arms.
Always a tinkerer, he improvised. He rushed out and obtained a
canister of carbon monoxide and a facemask and jury-rigged
another suicide machine. Soon Miller was dead too. Their bodies
would later be found amid dozens of burning candles.

On May 10, 1996, a jury acquitted Kevorkian of the common-
law crime of assisting the suicides of Wantz and Miller, despite its
being undisputed that he had done just that.* (He was never
charged in the Adkins case.) Much ado was made in the media
about the jury's swallowing Kevorkian's specious claim that he did
not intend for the women to die and merely wanted to alleviate suffering. In all of the commentary, perhaps the most important point
was missed: the statement by some jury members to reporters after
the trial that it did not matter to them that Miller and Wantz were
not terminally ill. That incontrovertible aspect of the case simply
was not significant in their decision-making processes. (Of the 130
or so people Kevorkian helped kill, approximately 70 percent were
not terminally ill. Five had no diagnosable illness upon autopsy.)[3]

Although he would be imprisoned for murder in 1999,
Kevorkian's acquittal in the deaths of Wantz and Miller was a
watershed event in the history of euthanasia in the United States.
The proposal to give doctors the legal right to kill certain patients
was no longer unthinkable, but rather, distinctly possible.

The acquittals also exposed the often-avoided truth about the

---

*At the time of the Wantz and Miller killings, Michigan did not prohibit assisted sui-
cide by statute. On the basis of previous court rulings, the Michigan Supreme Court
later ruled that assisted suicide was a crime.

so-called "right to die" movement. The shrug of the shoulders by the jury and by the nation over the tragic deaths of Wantz and Miller—one disabled, the other deeply emotionally disturbed—demonstrates that euthanasia is not about allowing the "terminally ill" who are in "unrelievable pain" and on the brink of death to "die with dignity," as the issue is usually described in the media. Rather, as the more candid proponents of euthanasia acknowledge, it is about creating a culture and a medical system that accept assisted suicide not only for the terminally ill but for anyone suffering a "hopeless illness" (a term that I will define shortly), a beneficence for suffering individuals and a good for society as a whole that will reduce health-care costs and the burdens of care on society and families.

This is a truly radical idea. If we accept it, we will have moved away from being a society that promotes improved medical and psychological care and emotional support as the proper and humane response to a patient's desire to die, to being one that condones killing as both appropriate and somehow compassionate. To state it dramatically but accurately, if euthanasia is legalized, doctors will be given a license to kill some of their patients and these patients will be given a legally enforceable right to be killed.

What makes this proposition so extraordinary is that protecting human life is the central purpose of organized society. Consequently, intentional killing by private persons is profoundly disfavored and severely restricted, being legally allowed only in exceptionally limited circumstances—acts of legitimate self-defense or defense of others, and even then only when deadly force is reasonably necessary to protect human life. The state, too, has severe restrictions on killing. Police may kill only when necessary to protect themselves, other officers or the public. A soldier can kill if following legal orders in a combat situation. The death penalty is permitted in most states, but only after the condemned is accorded a fair trial and multiple appeals often taking many years.

Legalized euthanasia would dismantle this venerable tradition. Allowing killing in the commonplace circumstances of terminal illness, chronic illness and pain, disability or prolonged mental illness, including depression—as is currently advocated by many in the euthanasia movement—would render the ethical, moral and legal foundations of society unrecognizable. Legalization would shake the physician-patient relationship to its core. For one thing, the essential bond of trust between doctor and patient would likely be torn asunder. A recent survey of cancer patients found that if their physician were to raise the issue of assisted suicide with them, they would lose trust in the doctor. Moreover, the cancer patients stated they would change doctors if they discovered that their physician had helped kill another patient.[4] Add the changing economics of health care to the distrust equation, in which doctors actually lose money if they provide patients with "too much" care (doctors' conflicts of interest are discussed in Chapter 6), and the potential for estrangement between patient and doctor is made manifest.

Losing Our Way

What is driving people to abandon traditional moral standards and embrace the death culture? The Canadian newspaper columnist Andrew Coyne, reacting to the widespread public support of Robert Latimer, who murdered his twelve-year-old daughter because she was disabled by cerebral palsy (discussed further in Chapter 7), said it most eloquently and succinctly when he wrote: "A society that believes in nothing can offer no argument even against death. A culture that has lost its faith in life cannot comprehend why it should be endured."[5]

Seen in this light, support for euthanasia is not a cause but rather a symptom of the broad breakdown of community and the ongoing unraveling of our mutual interconnectedness. The consequences of this moral Balkanization can be seen all around us: in the disintegration of family cohesiveness; in the growing nihilism among young people, leading to a rise in suicides, drug use and other destructive behaviors; in the growing belief that the lives of sick, disabled and dying people are so meaningless and unimportant that killing them—or helping them kill themselves—can be countenanced and even encouraged.

But there is more to this story than passive cultural decay. There are several interrelated and interconnected cultural themes that have combined to produce the euthanasia juggernaut. The most visible is a new and radical notion of individualism that elevates personal autonomy above all other cultural values. Not that there is anything wrong with a broad and healthy respect for the rights of individual expression and freedom of conduct. Individualism is an inherent American trait, as natural to us as building dams is to beavers. But unbridled individualism leads to social anarchy that asphyxiates true freedom. That is why self-determination, while very important, is but one of several equally important and sometimes conflicting values that add up to the dynamic concept that the Founders called "ordered liberty." One such competing value—let's call it "community"—promotes mutual interpersonal care, concern and support. Government and society promote community when they prevent harm to the weak and vulnerable—for example, by stopping suicides—not as some loathsome act of paternalism but as a human obligation to protect, care for and love one another.

Ordered liberty protects and defends the forest and the trees, the society as well as the individual. Individual freedom is certainly valued and encouraged, but if the greater good is to be protected, it cannot be absolute: It is properly limited when individual acts are unduly harmful to self, to others or to the whole, even if the harm is indirect. Thus, the community prevents individuals from injecting heroin because drug addiction harms both the person who is abusing the drug and the overall society. People are forbidden to sell their vital organs, even if they want to, in order to prevent individual harm and to ensure that the poor will not be exploited. Likewise, the law absolutely prohibits adult siblings from marrying, even if they are deeply in romantic love, because of the adverse societal consequences that would follow from allowing open sexuality between close blood relatives. In these and many more examples that could be given, individual self-expression and fulfillment are subordinated to other vital community concerns.

This mix of competing and complementary values has created a nuanced public policy around issues of death and suicide. On the one hand, it criminalizes euthanasia and assisted suicide in order to protect suffering individuals by reducing the danger that the dying and chronically ill will be exploited or coerced into an early death.

Such laws also protect society from the moral harm that would result should the killing of the dying, the sick and the disabled become routine.[6] At the same time, we properly allow people to refuse unwanted medical treatment, even if that choice might lead to death. (The vital distinctions between being killed and refusing medical treatment are discussed in later chapters.) Suicide, in and of itself, however, is not considered a crime in any state, being viewed as a cry for help rather than a violation of law. Even so, there has heretofore never been a "right" to self-destruction. Police generally are empowered to use nonlethal force to prevent a suicide and are authorized, if necessary, to bring the self-destructive person to a psychiatric facility for observation. Moreover, if the patient is found beyond a reasonable doubt to present a danger to his or her own safety, he or she can be hospitalized for treatment until the threat passes. A multitude of once suicidal people who are happy to be alive today would have been dead had "society" not cared enough to protect them from themselves during their time of despair.

Euthanasia proponents deem such policies paternalistic, at least as they relate to ill, disabled and chronically mentally distraught individuals. They urge us to accept a relatively new concept known as "rational suicide," which views self-destruction as the result of a rational decision and thus appropriate when one's personal circumstances become particularly difficult. According to proponents of this view, if suicide is a rational choice, as opposed to an irrational urge, then it should not only be accepted but also be facilitated upon repeated request. To many of these advocates, committing physician-facilitated rational suicide is, in the words of the Hemlock Society's cofounder Derek Humphry, the "ultimate civil liberty."[7]

Who should have the right to such a hastened death? Early on in euthanasia advocacy, proponents swore that it was to be reserved only for those who were terminally ill when nothing else could be done to relieve pain and suffering. But once entered, the slippery slope grows progressively steep. Now, even before euthanasia has been widely legalized, many advocates have upped the ante, arguing that euthanasia should be available for those suffering from "desperate," "incurable" or "hopeless" illness.

These terms are cleverly designed to fool the listener into

believing that the reference is still to terminal disease. In reality, rational-suicide advocates are opening the door for physician-assisted suicide for almost anyone who has a sustained desire to die. For example, "hopeless illness," the preferred term of the moment, is generally defined in psychiatric literature as including but not being limited to:

> terminal illnesses, [maladies causing] severe physical and/or psychological pain, physically or mentally debilitating and/or deteriorating conditions, and circumstances where [the] quality of life [is] no longer acceptable to the individual.[8]

This definition is wide enough to drive a hearse through. A condition causing severe physical or psychological pain could be virtually any illness, injury, or emotional malady, from incontinence to migraine headache, from clinical depression to diabetes, from arthritis to cancer. Moreover, by definition, a person only wants to commit suicide because he or she, at the time, believes that "life is no longer acceptable." Thus, the concept of "hopeless illness" is a prescription for abandoning depressed and suffering people to a policy of death on demand.

This kind of thinking has advanced so far that proposed guidelines have been published under which mental health professionals could participate in their client's/patient's decision "to suicide." (Some advocates of "rational suicide" now use the word as a verb.) Among these guidelines, a mental health counselor could "validate the client's decision to commit suicide," should become "knowledgeable about the various methods of self-administration, including types of drugs, lethality of dosages, and efficacy of methods," and if objecting to rational suicide would be required to refer "the client to a qualified counselor who does not have any conscientious objection" to suicide.[9]

Legalized euthanasia would not occur in a vacuum. The abandoning and anti-community values it represents would undoubtedly ripple throughout our culture and be adopted by the many structures of society, and would likely usher in a new era in which exercising personal autonomy and maximizing self-determination would become the culture's overriding purpose, rather than an important *part* of a broad mix of values that make up a healthy, balanced and free society. Our duties and responsibilities to community and to each other would be eclipsed, sacrificed on the altar of individual fulfillment. We would become so many islands, interacting but isolated, individuals placed side by side with few mutual commitments. Woe betide the unfortunates who "can't keep up," even if they self-destruct. They can do with their bodies what they want, and we will shrug as an increasing number of despairing individuals "choose" to end their lives.

The bioethicist Arthur Caplan fears we may already be on the precipice of this runaway self-determinism. He writes of the sad case of Thomas W. Passmore, a man with a history of mental illness, who, thinking he saw the sign of the devil on his right hand, cut it off with a circular saw. He was taken to a hospital, where, according to Caplan, things took a "crazy turn." Upon being told by the surgeon that his hand could be saved, Passmore refused treatment, still believing that his hand carried the sign of evil. A psychiatrist interviewed Passmore; lawyers were consulted; a judge refused to intervene. In the end, no one would decide that Passmore was incompetent to make his own medical decisions, and his hand was permanently lost.

This was a profound abandonment of a mentally ill, self-destructive man in desperate need of help. Thanks to the increasingly extreme view of self-determination, those who should have assisted Passmore were instead morally paralyzed. So distorted were their perceptions of their responsibility to Passmore, so stunted were their facilities to engage in critical thinking, that they allowed a hallucinating man to dismember himself because of a sign of evil that was not there. As Caplan so aptly put it, "A nation that has created a health-care system in which doctors, nurses and administrators are not sure whether it is the right thing to do to sew a mentally ill man's severed hand back onto his arm is a society gone over the edge regarding autonomy."[10]

What happened to Passmore's hand will happen to people's lives if this trend continues. Euthanasia and assisted suicide represent the ultimate abandonment of people made vulnerable by physical or mental illness, inadequate medical care, or depression. Legalization would lead to a moral and ethical catastrophe in which those least able to defend themselves would be victimized.

It is also interesting to observe that those most vocal in pushing the death agenda seem to be those least likely to be victimized by it. Jack Kevorkian aside, most leaders of the euthanasia movement—such as the author and journalist Betty Rollin; Barbara Coombs Lee, head of Compassion & Choices (a new euthanasia advocacy organization formed when the Compassion in Dying Federation merged with the Hemlock Society); Faye Girsh, former president of the Hemlock Society; and Dr. Timothy Quill, a physician and euthanasia advocate—are people of the "overclass": well-off whites with a strong and supportive family or social structure who never believe they could be victimized or pressured into an early death. They want what they want (to be able to die) when and how they want it. They downplay the harm that will follow for the poor, the uneducated, those without access to medical care, or the disabled, many of whom, as will be detailed later, view themselves as being in the crosshairs on this issue. Not to worry, these death culture leaders breezily assert, "protective guidelines" will fix everything.

Euthanasia is being promoted by its advocates through a very sophisticated political campaign, funded in the millions by several foundations, such as multi-billionaire George Soros's Open Society.[11] Proponents use all the tools of the political trade. Focus groups and polls have told them that people respond negatively to words such as "euthanasia," and so they resort to euphemisms such as "aid in dying," "deliverance" and "gentle landing" to describe killing. Their research also shows that arguments appealing to traditional notions of freedom resonate with people. Thus, like a boxer repeatedly jabbing at an open cut on an opponent's face, they pepper their advocacy with the lexicon of freedom and elicit an emotional response in the listener, especially with that buzz word of all buzz words, "choice." They argue that legalizing physician-assisted suicide is about personal autonomy, the right to be left alone. Appealing to our traditional distrust of government, advocates self-righteously assert that legalization of physician-hastened death would deny the state "any right to compel innocent, competent adults to needlessly suffer," as if laws prohibiting killing were some fiendish authorization for torture.[12] Some even compare the "right to die" campaign to the civil rights movement. Martin Luther King Jr. must be turning over in his grave.

Claiming the civil-liberties high ground for the idea of "choosing the manner and timing of one's death" serves another polemic purpose. It keeps the discussion on a theoretical level and allows suicide proponents to avoid an in-depth analysis of the dysfunctional context within which the "choices to die" would be exercised. But successfully deflecting discussion of these context issues does not make them any less important. As Matthew Rothschild, the editor of *Progressive* magazine and a strong civil libertarian, puts it, "I think a lot of people are persuaded by the civil liberties cloak that has falsely been placed around this issue. But the reality is quite the opposite. Euthanasia is not a 'choice' issue at all. Rather, choices to die would be made by others for people who are powerless and who are weak, whose right to live would be taken out of their own hands."[13]

Another driving force behind the euthanasia movement is the issue of "control." At the same time that they hoist high the banner of hastened death as a liberty, proponents exploit people's fear of death and the suffering that can accompany the dying process, promising that choosing the time and manner of death will somehow tame the Grim Reaper. In this atmosphere, dying naturally is increasingly promoted as a "bad death" if it involves discomfort or time, and hastened death is presented as empowering, courageous and somehow noble.

For some suicide advocates, controlling death has become a fixation. One cannot seriously engage the issue for long without hearing certain terms: good death, planned death, assisted death, death with dignity, rational death, deliverance, gentle landing, soft landing—the list goes on and on.

The Dutch physician Dr. I. van der Sluis, who has opposed his country's slide down euthanasia's slippery slope for more than twenty years, has observed the same phenomenon in the Netherlands. "I have studied [euthanasia proponents'] mentality," he told me. "They are like a little church, a cult of death. The subject fascinates them. They are always obsessing on dying and the suffering that may be a part of dying."[14] The disability rights activist and college professor Paul Longmore, who resists legalized euthanasia as a form of bigotry against the disabled, agrees. "Some of these people can only be described as 'death fundamentalists,'" he says. "They are so fixated on death and their ideology, that the facts of the debate have little meaning for them."[15]

Death fundamentalism, an apt description, may be contagious. My friend Frances was a death fundamentalist; so fixated was she on her own self-destruction, even before she became ill, that no appeal to reason or emotion could dissuade her from her chosen course or convince her to search for a different answer to her problems. When the suicide guru Derek Humphry published his how-to-commit-suicide book, *Final Exit,* in August 1991, it made the *New York Times* bestseller list. A few years ago, 175 people attended a "self-deliverance" course taught by Humphry, in which people were instructed on how to commit suicide by using a plastic bag. He has since run "how to commit suicide" shows on cable access television. For those who missed the course, Humphry's current organization, ERGO (Euthanasia Research and Guidance Organization), sells illustrated instructions (ingredients: a plastic bag, two elastic bands, a paper painter's mask and an ice bag).

Suicide has become something of a cottage industry. Conventions are held in which manufacturers of suicide contraptions display their wares. One such device is the "debreather," a mask through which air is recycled and oxygen is removed.[16] Another popular item is the "Exit Bag," which the Right to Die Network of Canada advertises in the following breathless terms:

> The customized EXIT BAG is made of **clear** strong industrial plastic. It has an adjustable collar (with elastic sewn in back and a six-inch Velcro strip in front) for snug but *comfortable* fit. It is extra large (22x36") to reduce heat build-up. It comes with flannelette lining inside the collar so that the plastic won't irritate sensitive skin. AND it comes with an optional separate *terry-cloth neckband* to create a "turtleneck" for added comfort and snugness of fit. [Emphasis in the original.][17]

I was able to purchase an Exit Bag along with instructions for suicide for $44, no questions asked.

Meanwhile, Philip Nitschke, an Australian pro-euthanasia physician, topped Jack Kevorkian's suicide machine by creating a computer program to allow people to commit assisted suicide at the push of a button; the program has been posted on the Internet. (The first PC-facilitated death occurred on September 26, 1996.) For several years he was funded by the Hemlock Society to develop a suicide formula made from everyday household items, the so-called "peaceful pill." Nitschke caused a furor in Australia when it was publicized that he stated in an on-line magazine interview that he intended his research to be made available to "the troubled teen."[18] He later justified his assertion on the basis that "we seem to think 18 year-olds are old enough to go and kill people in war."[19]

Before his imprisonment, Jack Kevorkian made himself into an iconic figure, a high priest of death fundamentalism. According to *Newsweek*, Kevorkian, while in medical school in the 1950s, "made regular visits to terminally ill patients and peered deeply into their eyes. His objective was to pinpoint when the precise moment of death occurred."[20] Kevorkian is a ghoulish artist who paints grotesque pictures, such as one of "a child eating the flesh off a decomposing corpse."[21] He has long been fascinated with the mechanics of capital punishment.[22] He even transfused blood from corpses into living human beings without testing the procedure on animals to make sure it was safe.[23]

Kevorkian is so death-obsessed that he proposes the nauseating prospect of performing experiments on people as they are being killed in order to learn more about human death, a procedure he named "obitiatry." He used to call assisted suicide "medicide" but now labels it "patholysis." In his own words, from his book *Prescription Medicide:*

> If we are ever to penetrate the mystery of death—even superficially—it will have to be through obitiatry. Research using cultured cells and tissues and live animals may yield objective biological data...but knowledge about the essence of human death will of necessity require insight into the nature of the unique awareness or consciousness that characterizes human *life*. That is possible only through obiatric [*sic*] research on living human bodies. [Emphasis in the original.][24]

Indeed, the primary motivation behind Kevorkian's death crusade was to pave the way for live human experiments on those being killed, not to ease suffering. Again, from *Prescription Medicide:* "[Assisted suicide] is not simply to help doomed persons kill themselves—that is merely the first step, an early distasteful professional obligation...... [W]hat I find most satisfying is the prospect of making possible the performance of invaluable experiments or other beneficial medical acts under conditions that this first unpleasant step can help establish."[25]

The increase in the popularity of legalized euthanasia is also a vote of no confidence in the medical profession. (This is supremely ironic, since the same advocates who don't trust doctors to care for them properly want to empower physicians to hasten their deaths.) Not having caught up with how recent changes in the economics of health care have begun to radically alter the ethics of medicine, some assisted suicide supporters embrace medicalized killing as a safeguard of sorts against being hooked up to medical machines against their will and forced to suffer as cash cows, lingering in an agonizing limbo until they die or their health insurance runs out—whichever comes first. Thus, even though the hospital intensive care unit is now often a money drain on hospitals instead of a profit center, making it increasingly difficult for patients to obtain the life-sustaining treatment they *want*, euthanasia is still sold in some quarters as a guarantee of sorts against having invasive medical procedures forced upon the unwilling.

While the ongoing changes in health-care financing make it more likely that patients will receive too little care than too much, the terror of being forced into a lingering death is not irrational. In years past, too many people saw their loved ones writhing in pain that could have been relieved; too many had their own suffering ignored; too many were treated impersonally and dismissively by health-care professionals. As one study into the euthanasia issue put it, "Public perceptions about...assisted suicide and euthanasia are determined by many issues, including fears of intolerable suffering at the end of life, and a perception that the healing professions have paid inadequate attention to relieving suffering when a cure is not possible. This perception may well be right."[26]

Paradoxically, the very people who support euthanasia because they don't trust the medical profession, or fear they will be victimized by unwanted care or medical neglect of their suffering, nevertheless accept the idea that doctors should be relied on to engage in medicalized killing. Yet these same doctors, it is widely recognized, are generally undertrained in treating pain and do a terrible job of diagnosing clinical depression in their chronically ill and dying patients.

Then there is the issue of compassion, which euthanasia advocates claim as their primary motivation. Some speak as if they have a monopoly on this virtue, while casting euthanasia opponents as people who care more about legalism than about relieving suffering. It's not true, of course. The root meaning of the word compassion is to "suffer with." Killing as a medical treatment is many things, but "suffering with" is not one of them. Moreover, truly dignified, compassionate and effective means exist today to reduce or eliminate pain and suffering without eliminating the patient, such as pain control, treatment for depression, independent-living assistance for people with disabilities, hospice and other care opportunities. Unfortunately, these measures receive only a fraction of the media visibility and publicity that attend the drive to legalize killing. For example, most people don't even know what hospice care is, much less how to obtain it. This is tragic, because these underutilized and underfunded programs can make all the difference in the lives of people who are suffering, and often can change a desire to die into a determination to live.

Finally, there is a less visible but perhaps ultimately the most influential and dangerous force driving the euthanasia juggernaut: money. Our health-care system is quickly being transformed from a fee-for-service system, where medical professionals earn money by treating people, to a system dominated by for-profit health maintenance organizations (HMOs), in which health insurance companies make money primarily by reducing costs. In an HMO, a penny saved is literally a penny earned. That is why legalized euthanasia would be especially profitable to the fast-growing for-profit HMO industry. Just imagine the money that can be saved—and thus earned—in not treating AIDS patients because their deaths have been hastened by euthanasia, in not treating cancer patients because their deaths have been hastened through euthanasia, in not treating people with physical disabilities because their lives were ended by euthanasia. To put it bluntly, the day doctors are legally allowed to kill patients, Wall Street investors in for-profit HMOs will be dancing in the streets.

Derek Humphry of the Hemlock Society made this point explicitly in a chapter entitled "The Unspoken Argument" in his book *Freedom to Die: People, Politics, and the Right to Die Movement.* Pointing out that "Elders or otherwise incurable people are often aware of the burdens—financial and otherwise—of their care," Humphry and his co-author, Mary Clement write:

> A rational argument can be made for allowing PAS [physician-assisted suicide] in order to offset the amount society and family spend on the ill, as long as it is the voluntary wish of the mentally competent terminally ill and incurable adult. There will likely come a time when PAS becomes a commonplace occurrence for individuals who want to die and feel it is the right thing to do by their loved ones. There is no contradicting the fact that since the largest medical expenses are incurred in the final days and weeks of life, the hastened demise of people with only a short time left would free resources for others. Hundreds of billions of dollars could benefit those patients who not only can be cured but who also want to live.[27]

Money imperatives often help shape our values and ethics. If promoting certain behavior can make fortunes, rationalizations to justify the conduct will soon be found, even if it is inherently immoral. One reason that slavery became so entrenched in the Old South was that the peculiarities of the Southern economy made human bondage profitable for those in power. Similarly, the genocide of Native Americans was often stimulated by the expectation that there was money to be made from taking their lands. For a modern equivalent of putting dollars ahead of human lives, just look at the activities of the tobacco industry, which has been accused, among other moral wrongs, of promoting tobacco use by young people despite knowing its profound health dangers.

It may not be a coincidence, then, that the ethics regarding end-of-life medical care are changing just as the money imperative in medical practice has reversed itself. When the system was primarily fee-for-service, the prevailing medical ethic was to keep patients alive at all costs, or at least until the health insurance ran out. But now that managed care has supplanted fee-for-service, we hear much talk about "good death" and "death with dignity," about how patients should be more willing to give up the ghost and refuse end-of-life medical treatment. Then there is the worrying prospect that doctors may soon be empowered to refuse *wanted* life-sustaining treatment in order to save medical resources.

Legitimizing the Euthanasia Consciousness

Most people, of course, don't think about public policy in such philosophical terms. More often, public attitudes and perceptions are a product of cultural currents driven by television, music, movies, magazines, talk shows, and the manner in which news events are reported, as well as the general moral beliefs of the citizenry. So, too, with euthanasia.

Most people are not activists either for or against euthanasia, paying little attention to the issue except in passing. Consequently, what many believe and think they know about the issue is often the result of attitudes seeping unnoticed into their consciousness from the society around them. It is here, among the uninvolved, that organs of the popular culture have for years been quietly altering public perceptions about death and dying without people's conscious awareness that it is happening.

People with certain mindsets dominate the popular culture. These attitudes are reflected in our entertainment, particularly Hollywood-made movies, where euthanasia is deemed politically correct. Television shows often deal with the issue, almost always presenting hastened deaths in a sympathetic light as the "only" choice available to alleviate a desperate patient's suffering. Popular television series such as *ER, Homicide, Chicago Hope, Star Trek—Deep Space Nine, Star Trek Voyager* (in which we learn that Vulcans like Mr. Spock practice ritual suicide in old age), and *Law and Order,* just to name a few, have all aired episodes dealing positively with the theme of hastened death. Motion pictures have also implicitly supported the assisted suicide mindset, sometimes to great public acclaim. The most recent example of this phenomenon is *Million Dollar Baby,* which received the Academy Award for Best Picture of the Year, 2004. Directed by and starring Clint Eastwood, the film was promoted publicly as being something like a female version of the classic boxing film *Rocky.* But rather than climaxing with a dramatic championship match, *Million Dollar Baby* ends with euthanasia, when Clint Eastwood's character (Frankie) kills his boxing protégé Maggie (played by Hillary Swank) because she doesn't want to go on living as a quadriplegic after being injured in a match.

It isn't just the disability that leads to Maggie's suicidal desire. In the world of the script, she is plunged headlong from triumph to utter hopelessness. Indeed, by having Maggie's situation go quickly from bad to very much worse, the scriptwriters manipulate the audience emotionally into thinking, "Of course she wants to die. Given the same situation, who wouldn't?"

First, Maggie becomes a ventilator-dependent quadriplegic. After a life of triumphant physicality, this would be difficult to adjust to even under ideal circumstances. But Maggie's life as a disabled woman is anything but ideal. Despite supposedly receiving the best care, she soon develops bed sores so serious that one of her legs is amputated. Then her venal and uncaring family pressures her into signing over control of her assets. Finally, after trying to kill herself in a terribly painful way—by nearly biting her tongue off—she is force-sedated to prevent further suicide attempts.

Frankie is in anguish over his friend's plight and concludes that he is actually killing Maggie by letting her live. So, his love for her overcomes his Catholic guilt and he ends her life by removing the respirator and injecting her with an overdose of adrenalin. The intent of the scriptwriters, of course, is to leave not a dry eye in the house.

Clint Eastwood stated adamantly, in the face of intense criticism of *Million Dollar Baby* led by leaders of the disability rights movement, that he did not intend his movie to push euthanasia as an acceptable public policy. Still, it is striking and disturbing how similar the plotline of *Million Dollar Baby* is to the notorious pro-euthanasia plotline of a 1939 German propaganda movie *I Accuse* (*Ich Klage An*), a film explicitly made "to persuade the German public to accept the idea of 'euthanasia.'"[28]

In both films, the tragic and doomed heroine is a very talented and independent woman; a boxer and a brilliant pianist, respectively. In both, the heroine becomes seriously disabled and can no longer pursue her life's dream. (In *I Accuse*, the heroine contracts multiple sclerosis and loses her ability to play piano; she also fears becoming a quadriplegic. In *Million Dollar Baby*, the heroine's neck is broken, resulting in quadriplegia.). Both heroines beg their primary male companions (the husband in *I Accuse* and the surrogate father in *Million Dollar Baby*) to put them out of their misery. Both men initially, and weakly, resist, but eventually come to see that killing their beloved is the only way to spare her pointless suffering.

The primary difference between the two movies is that *I Accuse* ends with the husband righteously defending himself in the dock against criminal charges, pointing an accusing finger at the camera and proclaiming "I accuse!" at society for not permitting the compassionate and purely voluntary ending of lives no longer worth living. In *Million Dollar Baby*, Frankie is apparently devastated by what he has done and he disappears, never to be heard from again. Nevertheless, the message of the rightness of mercy killing is more than implied: Frankie's act is depicted as heroic by the film's narrator, played by Morgan Freeman. No wonder the noted disability rights activist Steve Drake castigated *Million Dollar Baby* as a "melodramatic assault on people with disabilities" that "plays out killing as a romantic fantasy and gives emotional life to the 'better dead than disabled' mindset."[29] (For more on *I Accuse*, see Chapter 3.)

Nor is it just the movies and television. Popular magazines also drive public perceptions about important social issues such as assisted suicide. Not surprisingly, articles that depict assisted suicide as right, caring and compassionate are ubiquitous, typified by an article in the *New Yorker* some years ago in which the writer extols his mother's assisted suicide. He concludes, "Having seen the simple logic of euthanasia in action and witnessed the comfort of that control, what astonishes me is how many people die by other means."[30] Similarly, the January 1997 *Ladies' Home Journal* had a "special report" on assisted suicide consisting of a "round table" discussion. Amazingly, no opponents of legalization were presented in the entire article.

This is powerful stuff. When a popular television program depicts a courageous and handsome doctor killing a patient as the "only way" to relieve unremitting suffering, or the sympathetic and beautiful homicide inspector winking at a mercy killing because she would have done the same thing in the suspect's place, the audience gives no thought to the false premises that underlie the drama or to the consequences of making such acts routine. When famous talk-show hosts bring families on television to justify the hastened deaths of their loved ones, it is difficult to see past our sympathy for the plight of the deceased or the grief of his or her family to the broader issues; consequently, viewers tend to come away from these programs and reports thinking favorably of "the right to die." When the biggest movie stars win Academy Awards for movies that put a positive spin on euthanasia, the idea of killing as an answer to the problem of human suffering becomes easier to accept. And when popular magazines and newspaper stories almost invariably concentrate with laserlike intensity on a suffering individual who "just wants to die," while failing to train an equally penetrating light on the many ways of relieving suffering without killing or on the potential for coercion or abuse that are inherent in legitimized euthanasia, it is not surprising that viewers and readers tend to develop pro-euthanasia attitudes.

Most of the stories written about the Kevorkian reign of assisted killings were cases in point. One example was the reporting about the death of Jack Leatherman, who had pancreatic cancer, on September 3, 1996. The story in the *Boston Globe* was typical: it told about the man's death at seventy-three and the nature of his illness, and it reported the allegation by one of Kevorkian's representatives that "no amount of pain relief could control the pain that he was suffering."

That assertion was not questioned or investigated. Had it been, reporters would have discovered that morphine pills are very effective in controlling the pain associated with pancreatic cancer. Moreover, according to the board-certified oncologist and pain-control specialist Dr. Eric Chevlen, in the rare event in which opioids are insufficient to control pancreatic cancer pain adequately, a medical procedure can be performed to numb the nerve that transmits pain stimuli from the abdomen to the spinal cord and the brain, thereby eliminating all pain caused by the cancer.[31] Yet that story, which would have given cancer victims and their families so much hope, was never reported.

With a few exceptions, stories that highlight the reasons to oppose legalization of euthanasia generally do not receive equivalent coverage. If reported, these stories typically are not presented with the same level of notional intensity or drama. A story of hospice care helping someone die a natural death in comfort and surrounded by a loving family is not news at all unless the person is famous. It is no big deal if a cancer patient is no longer suicidal because he received effective pain control. It's the proverbial dog-bites-man story—happens every day.

Also contributing mightily to the growing acceptance of euthanasia is a form of pervasive cultural decay that I call "terminal nonjudgmentalism" (TNJ). Our society has become so steeped in relativism, so unable to distinguish right from wrong, that it increasingly fails to react to or criticize truly reprehensible concepts or conduct. When destructive ideas and practices are not condemned, it is effectively a form of praise. That which is not seen as wrong must be right. As the winds of the death culture blow with increasing velocity, the vitality of the equality-of-life ethic withers.

A good example of TNJ in action—or, better, inaction—can be seen in the pro-euthanasia book *A Chosen Death,* by Lonny Shavelson, and the reaction of critics to its contents.[32] Shavelson, described on the book jacket as an emergency room physician and a photojournalist, writes about five assisted suicides he observed or participated in during the book's preparation. One case, that of "Gene," stands out in its heartlessness and brutality.

As depicted by Shavelson, Gene is a depressed, lonely widower with a pronounced alcohol problem. Twice previously he has tried to commit suicide. The first attempt occurred before he had two strokes that left him moderately impaired—but definitely not terminally ill.

Gene wants to end it all. He contacts a chapter of the Hemlock Society and asks its head, a woman given the pseudonym "Sarah," to assist in his death. According to Shavelson, Sarah has experience in this dark business, having previously assisted a close friend to commit suicide. Sarah found her first killing experience tremendously satisfying and powerful, "the most intimate experience you can share with a person.... More than sex. More than birth...more than anything," including being present for "the deliveries of my four grandchildren."[33] A committed death fundamentalist, Sarah wants again to enjoy the intense rush she experienced facilitating her friend's death, and so she jumps at the chance to help kill Gene.

Gene hems and haws, avoiding suicide and seemingly relishing the newfound companionship of Sarah and Shavelson that his suicide wish has provided him. Then, one night, he decides the time has come to die. He calls Shavelson and Sarah to his home for his suicide. Shavelson watches as Sarah mixes a poisonous brew and gives it to Gene, saying, "O.K., toots, here you go," as if she were handing him a beer.[34]

Gene drinks the liquid and begins to fall asleep, with Sarah holding his head on her lap. As he begins to snore, Sarah places a plastic bag over his head and begins to croon, "See the light. Go to the light."[35] (Sarah apparently had seen the movie *Poltergeist* once too often.)

But then, suddenly, faced with the prospect of immediate death, Gene changes his mind. He screams out "I'm cold!" and tries to rip the bag off his face. But Sarah won't allow it. From Shavelson's account:

> His good hand flew up to tear off the plastic bag. Sarah's hand caught Gene's wrist and held it. His body thrust upwards. She pulled his arm away and lay across Gene's shoulders. Sarah rocked back and forth, pinning him down, her fingers twisting the bag to seal it tight at his neck as she repeated, 'the light, Gene, go toward the light.' Gene's body pushed against Sarah's. Then be stopped moving."[36]

If Shavelson's depiction of the event is accurate, there is a word that describes what happened to Gene, and that word is *murder*.

The right, proper, ethical and humane thing for Shavelson to do as he watched Sarah asphyxiate Gene would have been to knock Sarah off the helpless man and then quickly dial 911 for an ambulance and the police. But Shavelson did nothing:

> "Stop, Sarah" raced through my mind. For whose sake, I thought—Gene's, so intent on killing himself? The weight of unanswered questions kept me glued to my corner. Was this a suicide, Gene's right finally to succeed and die? Or was this a needless death encouraged by Sarah's desire to act? Had Gene's decision to have me there, to tell me his story, given me the right to stop what was happening—

or, equally powerful, the responsibility not to interfere? Or was I
obliged by my very presence as a fellow human being, to jump up
and stop the craziness? Was it craziness?[37]

Sarah is holding Gene down, preventing him from tearing off the
plastic bag. But Shavelson, unable to distinguish right from wrong,
is paralyzed and merely watches the struggle that culminates in
Gene's death.

I interviewed Lonny Shavelson about all this. How could he
watch a woman snuff the life out of a man clearly struggling to stay
alive? Did he agree that Gene's death was a murder? I reminded
Shavelson that when he and I had met previously, in a radio station
greenroom before a debate, I had asked him why he hadn't tried to
stop Sarah. His response at the time was "I am a journalist."[38]
Shavelson now acknowledged saying this, but he correctly noted
that our conversation about the issue at that time was brief and not
conducive to a more detailed response. (Nor, in fairness to Shavelson, was it a conversation geared toward inclusion in a book,
although I did mention I would want to interview him about the
issue for this one.) So I asked him to clarify his statement or comment further. Shavelson demurred, saying that his answer would be
too complex for a "sound-bite response."[39] He did, however, point
out the section in his book where he is about to describe Gene's
asphyxiation as containing the reason why he did not act. In that
section Shavelson wrote, "Events suddenly moved faster than my
thoughts."[40] In other words, he was claiming that it all happened
too quickly. Yet Shavelson is an emergency room physician; surely
he should be equipped to deal with fast-moving events.

I then asked Shavelson whether he thought Gene's death fell
within the guidelines that are being proposed to regulate and limit
legalized assisted suicide. He said that he believed Gene's condition
to be "outside" the acceptable reasons for assisted suicide in any
guidelines he supported or knew of, and added that regulating
assisted suicide would mean that such deaths as Gene's could be
prevented because legalization would "clarify what is and is not
acceptable."[41] However, he agreed that nothing in any guidelines
would prevent a death cultist like Sarah from acting outside the
guidelines, just as her killing of Gene was clearly outside any
acceptable conduct under the law as it exists today. In fact, I con-

tend that Gene could easily have been labeled "hopelessly ill," and thus would have fallen within some proposed "guidelines."

The point that Shavelson and other death fundamentalists miss is that so-called protective guidelines are meaningless; they provide only a veneer of respectability. They don't close the door to deaths outside their parameters. Rather, they break the doors of hastened death wide open by destroying the existing locks. Once killing is deemed an appropriate response to suffering, the threshold dividing "acceptable" killing from "unacceptable" killing will be continually under siege. But the fiction of control, essential to the public's acceptance of euthanasia, will have to be maintained, so the definition of what will be seen as "legitimate" killing will be expanded continually, as has occurred in the Netherlands (see Chapter 4).

What about the reviewers of Shavelson's book? Surely they shared my horror at Gene's murder and Shavelson's passivity in the face of it. Not a chance. The *San Francisco Chronicle* review was typical. The reviewer, Steve Heilig, a bioethicist and co-editor of the *Cambridge Quarterly of Healthcare Ethics*, didn't condemn Shavelson for allowing a murder to take place, unimpeded, under his very nose. Nor did he demand that Shavelson reveal the identity of Sarah and Gene so that the death could be appropriately subjected to a criminal inquiry. Rather, the review merely recounts that Shavelson is "appalled" at Sarah's "unregulated secretive approach" (not "appalled" enough to protect Gene, however) and opines that "the book superbly tackles this most difficult of ethical issues." What we don't condemn, we allow.

Another recent pro-euthanasia book that has been praised with faint condemnation is *Rethinking Life and Death: The Collapse of Our Traditional Ethics* by Peter Singer.[42] *Rethinking Life and Death* can fairly be called the *Mein Kampf* of the euthanasia movement, in that it drops many of the euphemisms common to pro-euthanasia writing and acknowledges euthanasia for what it is: killing. Indeed, Singer is straightforward about how pervasive these death practices have become in our society and, unlike his fellow death fundamentalists, is quite candid about their destructiveness to the concept that all human life is inherently equal, a degeneration he celebrates and I condemn. Indeed, what makes Singer's book noteworthy is that he takes the step that most euthanasia proponents avoid for tactical reasons: He specifically advocates the outright destruction of the equality-of-human-life ethic that has undergirded Western civilization for two thousand years.

Singer advocates what he calls a "quality-of-life ethic." Under the quality-of-life ethic, being human is not a crucial determinant of one's inherent rights because, Singer believes, human lives do not all have an inherently equal moral value. Rather, being a *person* is what counts to Singer, and only persons enjoy the right to life.

Most of us think "person" and "human" are synonymous. Not Singer. He elevates some "nonhuman animals" (such as dogs, elephants and pigs) to the status of persons, on the basis of his contention that they are self-aware. At the same time, he strips some human beings of personhood, specifically those with cognitive disabilities and all newborn infants, because of their lack of the "relevant characteristics" of self-awareness over time and the ability to reason. (Singer is far from alone in this advocacy. The odious notion of the born human nonperson pervades current bioethics thinking.)[43]

The practical application of these theories? Singer specifically embraces infanticide. Since, according to the author, an infant has no inherent right to life, a baby can be killed ethically if parents and doctors decide this is for the best. Speaking specifically of Down syndrome babies, Singer writes:

> We may not want a child to start on life's uncertain voyage if the prospects are clouded. When this can be known at a very early stage in the voyage, we may still have a chance to make a fresh start. This means detaching ourselves from the infant who bas been born, cutting ourselves free before the ties that have already begun to bind us to our child have become irresistible. Instead of going forward and putting all our efforts into making the best of the situation, we can still say no, and start again from the beginning.[44]

In other words, according to Singer an acceptable answer to the difficulties of having a baby born with Down syndrome or another birth defect is to kill the child, an option that Singer muses should be available to parents for the first twenty-eight days of an infant's life.

Singer has been making such proposals for years. That he is nevertheless *respected* internationally as a "philosopher" and "bioethicist" is proof enough of rampant TNJ.

Further proof is the book review in the *New York Times*, May 7, 1995, by Daniel J. Kevles of the California Institute of Technology. The closest Kevles comes to criticizing Singer's thesis is to suggest that some of his opinions are "highly debatable." Indeed, the review states that *Rethinking Life and Death* "is analytically rich on the moral rights of newborns compared with those of unborn fetuses, and how we treat anyone who is so physically or cerebrally degraded that they have no chance of a life of reasonable fulfillment."[45] In other words, that the right to live often depends on the values and attitudes of those who possess the power to kill is of no serious concern.

The death-fundamentalist community expressed nothing but kudos for the book. A book review in *Hemlock TimeLines*, the successor to the *Hemlock Quarterly* as the official newsletter of the Hemlock Society, applauds: "The true message of this book is one of reason and responsibility."[46] The comments of Ralph Mero, former director of Compassion in Dying, an offshoot of Hemlock created to actively assist the suicides of the terminally ill, reveals a similar death-cult mindset: "*Rethinking Life and Death*...should be required reading for physicians, legislators and judges. The new medical ethics being forged today will revolutionize our attitudes toward everything from fertilized zygotes to comatose bodies. Out of it should come a heightened respect for *persons and personhood* and just in time" (italics in original).[47] Derek Humphry, cofounder of the Hemlock Society, donated a book-jacket blurb that states in part, "Brilliantly debunks old concepts and introduces honesty to modern medical ethics."

It is a sad and frightening day when a noted author writes a book advocating infanticide and involuntary euthanasia of the cognitively disabled, when a major New York publishing company publishes it, and when it is received to the sound of general applause. (Singer has, however, been severely criticized and demonstrated against in Germany, a country with an acute memory of the horrors that can result from adopting such values as his. See

Chapter 3.) And Singer is far from being a fringe character. Indeed, he may be one of the most famous philosophers in the world today, a man who enjoys an international following not only for his advocacy of infanticide but as the inspiration for the "animal rights" movement. Incredibly, even as he argued that parents and doctors should have the right to kill unwanted babies, Singer received the ultimate symbol of respect in 1999 when Princeton University named him the first Ira W. De Camp Professor in Bioethics at its Center for Human Values.

Exploring Hidden Premises

The abuse and exploitation inherent in the euthanasia consciousness are rarely discussed explicitly but are often readily apparent, even in pieces that promote the practice. A prominent article published in a major magazine typifies the kind of euthanasia promotion that is so depressingly common throughout the media.

On November 14, 1993, the cover story of the *New York Times Magazine* was "There's No Such Thing as a Simple Suicide" (hereafter cited as "No Simple Suicide").[48] The story details the sad saga of a dying woman, "Louise," who killed herself with the active assistance and moral support of Ralph Mero, a Unitarian minister and the cofounder of the pro-euthanasia group Compassion in Dying. An offshoot of the Hemlock Society, Compassion in Dying actively counsels dying people who express a desire to commit suicide and assists in their self-killing.

Mero insists that he eschews publicity and is acting only out of selfless compassion. Yet he and his "work" have somehow managed to be featured in an Ann Landers advice column (complete with mailing address), in the major article in the *New York Times Magazine,* and in many national print and television newsmagazine pieces and documentaries.[49]

Lisa Belkin, a former *New York Times* reporter and author of *First Do No Harm,* a book about medicine and ethics, wrote the "No Simple Suicide" story. This excellently written piece presents Louise's story as melodrama, taking the reader on an emotionally wrenching roller-coaster ride of her assisted suicide, complete with a cast of heroes and villains and a gripping life-and-death plot. To make matters more compelling, we are told that the tale is true, with only the dying woman's name changed to protect her family's privacy.

The Story

"There's No Such Thing as a Simple Suicide" chronicles the last few months of Louise's life. We learn early on that Louise suffers from an unidentified degenerative brain condition. Her doctor, described as "a warm, down-to-earth woman," informs Louise that she has only months, perhaps weeks, to live. Louise is afraid of dying in a hospital, hospice or other "facility," a scenario her doctor bluntly tells her is quite likely to occur. Louise tells her doctor that rather than die in a cold, impersonal facility, she would rather kill herself. The doctor almost leaps at the chance to prescribe the drugs for Louise to take.

We are told that the doctor had previously "cooperated" with another patient's suicide, but that there had been difficulties, so she contacts Ralph Mero at Compassion in Dying to solicit his help and active assistance in facilitating Louise's death. The doctor later tells Belkin, "I was ecstatic to find someone who's doing what [Mero is] doing. I loved the fact that there were guidelines. It made so much sense. This was a human being who could help, not some book."[50]

A few days later Mero visits Louise, who lives with her mother. He tells Belkin that Louise appeared relieved when he didn't flinch or judge her desire to kill herself and that she asked him to be with her when she died. Mero agreed, stating that the decision was hers.

Louise asked her friends to attend her suicide, but none would. When a medical assistant of one of her doctors hears that Louise's "trusted friends" have refused to sanction her suicide, she befriends and supports the ill woman.

Mero, the medical assistant, Louise and her mother become a cohesive group with one firm goal: Louise's assisted suicide. They meet to discuss how the self-termination will be performed. The deadly drugs will be mixed with a small amount of food and anti-nausea medication so they can be kept down. Louise is to be monitored as she dies, and the assistant is to administer anti-pain medication if Louise seems to be suffering. After the death, the doctor will report to the authorities that the deceased was terminally ill and that the death was from natural causes after a prolonged illness, so no autopsy will be conducted. The doctor is also to falsify the death certificate as to the actual cause of death.

Weeks pass. Louise grows ever weaker. Yet the frail woman does not kill herself. Mero becomes alarmed. He calls Belkin to inform her that he and the group have been told by the doctor that time is running out. It is feared that the disease may soon render Louise mentally incompetent. Mero worries that Louise's "window of opportunity will slam shut" because Compassion in Dying will assist suicides only for persons who are mentally competent. He also worries that if Louise waits much longer she will be unable to self-administer the deadly drugs.

Lisa Belkin drops everything and flies to Seattle to speak with Louise, who tells the reporter that she wishes to conclude some business and spend some more time with her mother before killing herself. This upsets Belkin, who blurts out the doctor's prognosis: Louise does not have much time within which she will be capable of killing herself.

Yet, for all of her stated desire to commit assisted suicide, Louise still does not act. Some time later, the medical-assistant-turned-friend tells the group that she will talk to Louise to see if she can get the suicide back on track. She asks the dying woman, "I kind of want to get an idea of what your time line is. Where do we stand?" Louise's eyes brim with tears and she tells the medical assistant that she does not want to talk about it. The woman apologizes. Louise justifies her delay by saying that she wants to wait until Mero returns from out of town to get his opinion of her condition. The medical assistant replies that is a "bad idea" because Mero might not notice subtle changes in her condition.

Still Louise does not kill herself. Mero withdraws, checking in by phone but keeping the conversations short. He tells Belkin that he wants to remain in the background so as not to influence the outcome.

Then Mero gets a message. Louise is finally ready. The group assembles. Louise eats poisoned ice cream and applesauce that have been prepared pursuant to Mero's previous instructions and immediately falls asleep on the couch, clutching a teddy bear.

Hours pass as Louise sleeps. The group waits for her to die. She does not. Mero worries that he might have to help the process with a plastic bag. Finally, Louise's breathing slows and she expires. Mero contacts the funeral director and leaves.

As the article concludes, we are informed that Louise's death was not listed as a suicide and that her friends and relatives were told that she "died in her sleep with her mother at her side, as she had wanted."

The Propaganda

On its face, the article appears to be an objective piece of journalism: Belkin does not praise or criticize the people involved or the events, nor does she give her personal opinion on the merits of Mero's cause. Go a bit deeper, however, and the piece can be seen as an advertisement for legalizing and legitimizing assisted suicide and euthanasia.

What leads to this conclusion? First is the manner in which the article came to be written. Belkin didn't find the story; the story found her. As Belkin appropriately reveals, the board of directors of Compassion in Dying contacted her, inviting her to observe their usually secret suicide-assistance activities.

There is nothing illegal, immoral or unusual about a reporter being contacted about story material. Stories are often found in this manner. However, it is safe to assume that Mero and the board had more in mind than merely illustrating the emotional difficulties surrounding terminal illness. Surely they hoped to further their cause through the article. That being so, it is likely they would carefully choose a writer in the hope of finding one who could be expected to take a positive view of their work. In fact, Belkin uncritically accepts the methods and motives of Mero, the doctor and the friend.

Whether or not Belkin approached her work with a bias in favor of assisted suicide, a more important matter is the powerful message communicated by "No Simple Suicide." Bluntly stated, whether Belkin intended it or not, the article promotes the euthanasia cause by seeking to persuade the reader that assisted suicide is an acceptable act. Proponents of legalizing assisted suicide and euthanasia are ever about the task of proselytizing the public, seeking converts to their cause. The more we are exposed to depictions of assisted suicide, the more commonplace it will seem and, then, the more acceptable. Through this process we become desensitized. Practices that we once found abhorrent begin to seem like a normal part of life—or, more precisely, death. "No Simple Suicide" serves this purpose in several ways:

1. *It implements the either/or strategy.* One of the tools used by pro-euthanasia advocates when arguing for legalization is to create a false premise: Either we provide "deliverance" to suffering people, or they will be forced into cruel and unnecessary anguish. Either they die peacefully and painlessly now, or they die in agony later.

"No Simple Suicide" similarly casts Louise's plight as a forced choice between two horrible options: assisted suicide or an out-of-control death at a "facility." Not once is the reader (or Louise, as far as we know) informed that hospice and palliative care could probably have mitigated most if not all of her pain and discomfort. As reported, not once is the reader told that the hospice experience is designed to provide love, comfort, and support for the patient and the family, supplied by medical and mental health professionals and volunteers. Not once is the reader told that hospice care can be supplied *in the home*—clearly a major issue for the dying woman. Not once is the reader told that the very purpose of hospice care is to facilitate a gentle and peaceful transition from life to whatever comes next. The fact that the truly compassionate option was virtually unexplored, from what is reported, speaks volumes about the doctor's agenda and that of Mero and perhaps the friend.

It is also notable that Louise's doctor treats her patient's suicidal desire as expected, rather than as a cry for help. Yet studies prove that the vast majority of dying people do not exhibit suicidal tendencies. When dying patients do ask for suicide, they are almost always clinically depressed, just as are suicidal people who are not terminally ill. Depression is a treatable condition. Unfortunately, most doctors are not adept at recognizing depression in their dying patients. Thus, whether through ignorance or arrogance, Louise's doctor probably abandoned her patient to the throes of depression, which could well have been overcome.

It is also assumed by all involved in the young woman's

assisted suicide that she will not change her mind. Yet medical studies have shown that this is often not true. Indeed, the "will to live" among terminally ill people "shows substantial fluctuation."[51] In other words, one day a patient may request suicide, but the next week be very glad to be still alive. And that seems to have been the case here. Louise did not have an unremitting desire to self-destruct. The only people with an unyielding death agenda were those who surrounded her.

2. *It creates the impression that euthanasia is a loving rather than a violent act.* The suspicion that there was an unspoken agenda behind "No Simple Suicide" is supported by the striking artwork that illustrates many of the scenes described in the text. While Belkin undoubtedly had little or nothing to do with their creation, the pictures, which appear to be oil or watercolor paintings, are powerful and moving. The article doesn't tell us Louise's actual age or what she looked like, but the pictures depict Louise as a woman in her late twenties, her youth and delicate beauty adding to the tragedy of her condition. In one picture, Louise is curled up peacefully asleep on a couch after eating the poisoned ice cream. She is holding a teddy bear as her gray-haired mother sits beside her, the older woman's hand resting lightly upon her dying daughter's leg. In another picture, we see Louise and Mero in a counseling session. He is a strong presence, solid and dependable with his white beard and black suit, a striking contrast to the frail Louise, who has a blanket wrapped around her shoulders. In another picture, Louise's mother is pictured leaning over her daughter, who is so weak that the older woman can barely hear her speak.

The paintings have been created in the warm colors of autumn so as to invite us in to linger, as if we were standing in front of a crackling fire—indeed, to enter and become intimate participants in the unfolding drama. The paintings grab our hearts and rivet our attention solely and exclusively and in extreme close-up on the suffering of the dying woman. Thus we are made less likely to think critically, to look beyond Louise's personal tragedy to the broader implications of what is being done to her. And because the scenes appear gentle and warm, we are far less likely to recoil in horror at the actual events.

3. *It creates the impression that Louise's assisted suicide was a*

necessary choice. Belkin's prose conveys the idea that Mero and the others are compassionate pioneers leading the country toward an enlightened view of facing and overcoming the ravages of terminal illness. In fact, according to Belkin, that is how the group viewed themselves, writing that each saw Louise's pending assisted suicide as a "poetic expression of control, a triumph over the indignities of disease." That is a typical view held by death fundamentalists and no doubt is the view Mero hoped would be accepted by the reader.

Belkin came to a less romantic but equally erroneous conclusion about the affair. The only time she expresses a personal opinion in the article, she describes Louise's assisted suicide as a "second choice" to not being sick, and as the "most acceptable" of the dying woman's "unacceptable options." But that is a distinction without a difference. Whether euthanasia is pushed as a heroic statement of control or a rational choice between the lesser of two evils, the result is the same: legitimization of that which ultimately is profoundly destructive to individuals, the health-care system and society.

Whether motivated by the death-fundamentalist notions of Mero, the "pragmatic choice" view of Belkin, the participants' genuine desire to serve Louise, or a combination of these factors, Louise was pushed by those around her into suicide because that was the death they wanted her to have. As the psychiatrist Dr. Herbert Hendin, director of the American Foundation for Suicide Prevention, has written about the case: "Like many people in extreme situations, Louise...expressed two conflicting wishes—to live and to die—and found support only for the latter."[52] One wonders what the outcome would have been had someone—*anyone*—supported Louise's oft-expressed desire to live and stayed with her to the natural end of her life. Perhaps then her friends would have surrounded her in her final days. Perhaps Louise and her mother would have had a more meaningful time together, spared the undignified and excruciating dilemma over when and whether Louise would kill herself. Perhaps Louise could have really and truly died in peace.

4. *It suggests that it should be easier to help people die.* Louise's assisted suicide took place in the underground, amid the shadows of people who lied and broke the law in order to facilitate her so-

called death with dignity. The attitude of the article is implicitly critical of the fact that this subterfuge was necessary. The subliminal message, often voiced out loud by assisted suicide advocates, goes something like this: unreasonable people who refuse to allow others to control their own destiny are insensitive, thoughtless and cruel. They force dying people to endure unnecessary suffering. Such judgmental attitudes caused Louise's friends to abandon her when all she wanted to do was control the time and place of her own death. Her caring doctor was prevented from actively participating in her patient's final "treatment" because euthanasia by lethal injection is forbidden. Mero, a compassionate clergyman, was forced to risk imprisonment in his mission of providing care and comfort to the suffering.

The Other Side of the Story

The bitter irony is that the members of the little group surrounding Louise, with their pro-euthanasia agenda, were the ones who were thoughtless, insensitive and cruel, for they took from Louise, in Dr. Hendin's words, "her own death."[53]

• *Louise was unable to give informed consent to her suicide because she was denied information about hospice care.* According to what is revealed in the story, both the doctor and Mero allowed Louise to believe the either/or scenario: that she would have to die in a "facility" or kill herself at home. Apparently, neither discussed the option of hospice care with Louise or described the palliative care that could have reduced her discomfort. Thus, it appears that Louise was presented with a false premise from which to choose how to proceed.

• *The medical assistant pushed Louise into going forward with the assisted suicide.* The assistant who suddenly embraced Louise as a friend is suspect. Was she part of a pro-euthanasia group? Did she have an agenda? We are not told. Was not Belkin even a little curious about this? Regardless of her motives, the assistant is a powerful actor throughout the drama, urging Louise on to self-destruction.

• *Ralph Mero's "compassion" was available to Louise only if she carried out her designated role.* This is the most insidious part of the story. It is important to remember how emotionally vulnerable most terminally ill people are as the end of life approaches. Louise was certainly no exception. In her crisis, the "compassionate" Ralph Mero appears—a minister, no less—and tells Louise, "I'll be with you and I'll support you." From that point on it is quite clear that Louise has become dependent on the moral judgment and emotional support of Mero, to the extent that she even wanted to rely on him for medical advice as to how far her decline had progressed.

Through the early part of the process, Mero held Louise's hand. He patiently and gently went over the guidelines for the assisted suicide. He presented himself as a source of strength, a nonjudgmental rock to lean on in this difficult and emotional time. But when Louise hesitated and refused to be pressured into suicide, what did this altruistic man of compassion do? Did he hold her hand and discuss alternatives to killing, such as hospice care? Did he pray with Louise so that together they could seek God's guidance? He is a minister, after all. Did he assure her that whatever her choice might be, he was her friend and would be there to the end? No. He withdrew:

> Over the next few days, Mero checked in with Louise and her mother by telephone, but kept the conversation short. "I was measuring my phone calls," he says. He wanted to remain in the background and allow Louise to control the timing and pace. Her growing dependence on him was making him uncomfortable, and he needed to keep it clear in her mind, and his, that she was the driver and he was just along for the ride.[54]

In fact, when Louise seemed to be choosing a course other than the one he envisioned for her, he made it clear by his absence that she was on her own if she elected to die a natural death.

Imagine how painful it must have been for Louise when her minister, the man she was leaning on for strength and guidance, was suddenly holding her at arm's length, especially after being so intensely a part of her life over the previous weeks. The message from Mero was harsh and powerful: kill yourself and I am your man; stick it out to the end and I am out of here.

• *The reporter also pushed Louise toward killing herself.* As if all of that weren't disturbing enough, what are we to make of the reporter, Lisa Belkin, and her participation in these sad events?

Recall when the doctor informs Mero and Belkin that Louise is likely to slip quickly and become mentally incompetent, and therefore unable to kill herself or receive Mero's assistance: Belkin immediately flies to Seattle, unaware that Louise has not been told of this prognosis. During an interview on this occasion, Louise tells Belkin that she wants to wait a week or so before killing herself. Belkin is appalled:

> I was surprised, confused and extremely uncomfortable.... Without thinking, I blurted out a question: "Your doctor feels that if you don't act by this weekend, you may not be able to..."
>
> My words were met with a wrenching silence. Louise blanched, her pale skin turned even paler. I was horrified with myself....
>
> "She didn't...she never...I didn't know that," Louise said, sharply looking at her mother.
>
> "That's what she told me," her mother offered gently.
>
> Louise became silent....
>
> "It's O.K. to be afraid," her mother said.
>
> "I'm not afraid. I just feel as if everyone is ganging up on me, pressuring me," Louise said. "I just want some time."[55]

Indeed, Louise *was* being pressured, even by the reporter who at this point crossed the line from observer and chronicler to participant.

• *There is no compassionate voice of opposition.* "No Simple Suicide" presents a one-sided version of assisted suicide. Except for one brief passage, people who resist legalizing euthanasia are not heard from, nor are the many reasons given why opponents of the death culture are so devoted in their resistance. Notice also that the one quotation selected for use in the article by Belkin, presumably from a longer interview, describes opponents to euthanasia as "harsh," reinforces the false stereotype that opposition is based primarily on religion and does not express any concern for Louise's well-being.

Such short shrift was not given to proponents of assisted suicide. At one point in the article, Mero describes his work for Compassion in Dying as an experiment to "show, demonstrate, prove, that when people make a claim for humane treatment, it can be provided in a way that does not jeopardize vulnerable people or pose a threat to the social fabric."[56] Leaving aside the perversion of the word "treatment" in that sentence, we can assume that Mero hoped that by inviting Belkin to observe his work, he could get readers to accept his vision of a world where the ill can be routinely euthanized.

But as this analysis of "No Simple Suicide"—an article typical of this genre—demonstrates, what actually happened to Louise was just the opposite of the impression that the story sought to convey. Instead of receiving compassion from those she trusted, a sick and vulnerable woman *was pushed* by them into suicide in order to further their agendas. In Dr. Hendin's words, Louise's "death was virtually clocked by their [Mero's, the doctor's, her mother's, the medical assistant's, Belkin's] anxiety that she might want to live. Mero and the doctor influence the feelings of the mother and the friend so that the issue is not their warm leave-taking...but whether they can get her to die according to the time requirements of Mero, the doctor, the reporter, and the disease.... Individually and collectively, those involved in [Louise's assisted suicide] engender a terror in Louise with which she must struggle alone, while they reassure each other that they are gratifying her last wishes."[57] (Ralph Mero was unavailable for comment about my criticisms.)[58]

ANOTHER TRAGIC SCENARIO, SIMILAR to the one in which Louise found herself, unfolded in Australia in 2002. For a time, Nancy Crick believed she had terminal cancer. Prodded by euthanasia advocates who wished to use her assisted suicide as a bludgeon against laws prohibiting such an action in that country, Crick created a Web site to publicize her planned self-destruction.

Crick's case and her decision to allow her suicide to be used as a political wedge led to planned suicide becoming a political and media sensation. Euthanasia advocates vocally urged her on, assuring Nancy and the country that her self-destruction would be a win for self-determination and modernity. Some media outlets requested to be present to videotape her death. Instead of supporting her life, most of the public clamor pressed Crick toward suicide.

(When Crick temporarily wavered, opting for palliative care, the disappointment of euthanasia advocates was obvious. One of them grouched that one of Nancy's few remaining pleasures was smoking and she wouldn't be able to smoke in a hospital. Crick even received notes from assisted suicide advocates criticizing her for wavering in her desire to self-destruct!)[59]

When Crick finally decided to take her poison, twenty-one "friends" and family joined her, adding further social pressure to the decision to die and making it difficult for her to change her mind. They even *applauded* when she swallowed the poison.[60]

Crick's death elated euthanasia advocates, especially her doctor, Dr. Philip Nitschke. He was labeled with the moniker "Dr. Death" in Australia after his participation in assisted suicides (when the act was briefly legal in the Northern Territory) and because of his advocacy for buying a ship to commit mass euthanasia in international waters. For months he had orchestrated the publicity surrounding Crick's promised assisted suicide, but in the end he did not even have the courage to be with her when she died. Yet despite his absence, Nitschke claimed triumphantly that with Crick's death, "mass civil disobedience" had begun in the euthanasia movement.[61]

But then something happened that the euthanasia campaigners had not anticipated as they planned a public relations campaign around the Crick death. Crick's autopsy disclosed that she was *not dying of cancer*. In fact, she wasn't dying at all. Rather, a twisted intestine had caused her health difficulties. Her pain apparently resulted from a hernia and bowel adhesions, conditions that might have been corrected by surgery.[62]

After Crick died, the media reported that she actually knew beforehand that she was not dying of cancer. Moreover, so did the primary booster of her suicide, Dr. Philip Nitschke! He and Crick had been told weeks before her suicide that Crick did not have terminal cancer. Proving that those in the right-to-die movement believe that their advocacy of assisted suicide means never having to say they're sorry, Nitschke brushed aside the report. Claiming to be "annoyed" that people were making an issue of Crick's non-cancer, Nitschke admitted that deceiving the media about her condition beforehand was "a mistake," but he called the matter "irrelevant" because Crick had thought that "death was preferable" to living with her ailment.[63]

Still, there was little doubt that the news of Crick's non-cancer was a blow to the euthanasia cause. Dr. David Van Gend, a spokesman for TRUST, an Australian anti-euthanasia organization, reacting to the macabre circuslike atmosphere that euthanasia advocates and the media had made of a desperate woman's suicidal state, said, "An atmosphere of pressure and expectation was put on this lady from which she could not retreat without extreme loss of face," a circumstance that he criticized as "akin to the psychological and emotional entanglement of a cult. She was a vulnerable lady."[64]

Dr. Hendin's analysis about the travesty of "No Simple Suicide" and Dr. Van Geld's observation about the appalling events leading to Crick's death are exactly right. What happened to Louise and to Nancy Crick—and will happen to others if the euthanasia movement continues to metastasize—is not merely a "threat to the social fabric." It is, in fact, a rending.

TWO

CREATING A CASTE OF
DISPOSABLE PEOPLE

MORE THAN TWENTY YEARS AGO, I WAS an attorney working for a firm that represented a sixteen-year-old girl whom I will call Sally. Several years earlier, Sally had had surgery to correct a progressive case of scoliosis, a back problem commonly known as curvature of the spine. At the time of her operation, Sally was a bright, happy, alert twelve-year-old with long blond hair. Her mother said she had a ready laugh, and photographs showed a smile to knock your socks off.

As Sally was wheeled out of her room on a gurney for her surgery, she turned to wave to her parents, a half-fearful smile on her face. CLICK/FLASH: her parents snapped a picture. This would be the last smiling picture that would ever be taken of Sally.

Less than an hour later, Sally's heart stopped, owing to the negligence of her anesthesiologist. CPR was successful within a minute. Inexplicably, surgery continued. Then Sally had a second cardiac arrest. This time her heart was still for twelve minutes before resuscitation succeeded in saving her life.

Sally's brain, starved of oxygen, was severely injured. She was now a quadriplegic and had a profound cognitive disability. She could not feed herself, speak, or, some said, interact meaningfully with others. The hospital doctors did what they could for her; then Sally was transferred to a state hospital where she lived in what used to be called pejoratively "the basket ward."

This was as difficult and tragic a case as I had ever seen in my legal career. A young girl's life was ruined, her family destroyed by grief and self-recriminations, which contributed mightily to her parents' subsequent divorce. Four years after her injury, Sally's father rarely spoke her name, and her mother had put her own life on hold so that she could devote herself almost entirely to her disabled daughter's care. The point of the lawsuit was to obtain enough money from the negligent doctor's malpractice insurance company to ensure that Sally would be cared for properly for the rest of her life.

Early on I decided that it was my professional duty to visit with my client, even though she would not know who I was or why I was there. But month after month I found excuse after excuse to put it off. I was busy, after all. Many clients required my attention. Besides, I worked hard. I deserved that fishing trip.

These were all rationalizations, of course. I was not so busy and in demand that I couldn't spare a few hours for the drive to the hospital and back. And even if the hectic pace of an active civil litigation practice kept me tied to my desk or in courtrooms, there were always the weekends. Finally I faced the hard fact: the real reason I hadn't visited Sally was that I was afraid.

It isn't easy seeing the Sallys of this world. They remind us too much of our own mortality, of life's caprice, of the possibility that we or a loved one could, like Sally, lose the ability to control our body, the ability to communicate, perhaps even to perceive. Is it any wonder, then, that many of us ignore such people and, when confronted with the reality of the severely disabled (and sometimes even the not-so-severely disabled), wish they would just go away?

As time passed and the case moved closer to trial, my shame at my cowardice finally overcame my fear. One day the unexpected settlement of a case opened up a block of free time. I found myself phoning Sally's mother to arrange the visit. Twenty-four hours later I pulled into the parking lot next to the state hospital building in which Sally now resided.

I sighed nervously as I got out of the car. I did not want to do this! I still remember my heart pounding as I opened the door, walked to the elevator and pushed the up button. My hands were sweating.

The elevator door opened. I walked down a hall and entered Sally's ward. On my right was a long, narrow room filled with profoundly disabled people: dwarfs with heads enlarged by hydrocephaly; people of all ages apparently in comas; one uncon-scious or sleeping young woman, her face half-covered with small tumors while the other half was as clear as the skin of a magazine cover girl. A nurse later told me that she had one of the rarest condi-tions known to medical science.

Then, quietly, almost imperceptibly, my fear evaporated and was replaced by feelings of comfort, then warmth, and then, much to my amazement, joy. Here was a very human place. Curtains were hung and bright colors were painted throughout. There were plants around. Window shades were open to admit sunlight. The place smelled clean, fresh—not antiseptic. The nurses were deeply caring toward, indeed, loving of their patients. The mood in the ward was relaxed and gentle. I realized this was a home in the truest sense.

Then the nurses wheeled Sally to me. I would not have recog-nized her. She was lying in a bed, her eyes open but seemingly unaware and unable to focus on her surroundings. The pretty, opti-mistic face I knew from her presurgery photographs was gone, obliterated and distorted by her antiseizure medication. Many of her teeth were now missing. Her hair was short and stringy.

Yet none of that mattered. Sally was profoundly disabled, but that did not prevent her humanity from shining brightly through the veneer of difference.

I held her hand and began to sing to her. For some reason, I chose the late Dean Martin's theme song: "Everybody loves some-body sometime. Everybody loves someone somehow." As I sang, Sally's eyes focused and she looked up at me. She smiled and lifted her head. The nurses gathered around. Sally began to "sing" too, although it sounded more like a moan because she could not form words. Still, there was no doubting the happiness in her eyes and the smile on her face. Tears were in all our eyes (except Sally's) as we all joined in singing together. It was a precious moment that will remain with me for the rest of my life.

I came away from that experience a better man, unalterably convinced of two things: Sally had bad taste in music, and she was fully and completely a human being, worthy of the same love, care and respect as all of us. (Sally's case ultimately was settled for a very large sum, enough to assure her the best of medical care for the rest of her life.)

A Changed World

Before the euthanasia consciousness seeped into America's cultural bloodstream, society expected the Sallys among us to receive proper and humane care. The equality-of-human-life ethic demanded it. They, like all human beings, were equally endowed with the inalienable human right to life.

The actual practice of caring for disabled people did not always come up to the ideal, of course. Some of our most vulnerable citizens were subjected to horrible conditions and truly terrible abuse. That did not mean, however, that the equality-of-human-life ethic itself was compromised. Quite the opposite. It was the belief that each of us has inherent equal worth that caused us to demand reform and improved care whenever such gross misconduct was exposed.

Times change, and not always for the better. People like Sally are for the most part viewed quite differently today. "In a short time, we have gone from the attitude that all of our patients are human who deserve care—no matter what their level of functioning—to believing that some people aren't people anymore," says Sharon S. Orr, a registered nurse who has spent a career caring for profoundly brain-damaged people.[1] She would know. One of her charges was a young woman named Nancy Cruzan, who was the subject of a United States Supreme Court decision that made legal history.

As we move ever deeper into the twenty-first century, the once broad consensus in favor of the equality-of-human-life ethic has been substantially undermined. Not that we don't decry physical and mental abuse of the physically and mentally disabled. Of course we do. But a growing number of people no longer believe that cognitively disabled people possess the same intrinsic human worth or the same right to live as those of us who are able-bodied, "productive," and generally pleasing to look at. Indeed, to a disturbing degree, many in the legal and medical and bioethics communities, in academia, within religious institutions and among the general public view these helpless people as pointless and useless burdens to themselves, their families and society. Some have always believed this; what has changed is that such beliefs have become respectable and mainstream.

When a value as fundamental as the equality-of-human-life ethic is weakened, it changes our attitudes toward each other, our behavior, our concept of what constitutes a humane and compassionate society. We no longer speak much of people such as Sally and Nancy Cruzan as possessing an inherent right to live. Instead, we proclaim their inalienable "right to die."

HOW IS IT THAT IN THE EARLY 1980s, when I met Sally, no one even contemplated taking away her food and fluids? Yet only fifteen or so years later, some polls show that most Americans believed that it was right for Terri Schiavo to be dehydrated to death even though she was not terminally ill and did not need high-tech medical life support to survive.

In order to understand the radical changes that transformed medical ethics during the last twenty years, we must discuss two related but distinct concepts: The first is the absolute right of all patients, no matter what their condition, to receive humane care. The other is the right of patients or their surrogate decision makers to refuse or discontinue unwanted medical treatment.

Humane care consists of basic nonmedical services that each human being is absolutely entitled to receive in a medical setting: warmth, shelter, cleanliness and such. No matter how ill a patient, no matter the level of his or her disability, humane care can never be withdrawn ethically—even if the patient would prefer so. For example, if a patient wanted to die by hypothermia, being left uncovered in front of an open window during a blizzard, medical personnel would have to refuse the request.

Medical treatment consists of action taken by doctors or other healthcare professionals whose purpose is to provide a medical benefit to the patient. Obvious examples of medical treatment are surgery, prescribed medications, diagnostic tests and the like. Unlike the case with humane care, *the patient must consent to receive medical treatment* and may at any time refuse or discontinue it. This right exists even if the refusal of treatment will likely result in death. Thus, a cancer patient is entitled to refuse chemotherapy and the heart-disease patient can refuse bypass surgery.

It was not too many years ago that food and fluids were considered humane care. That is no longer true, at least for food and water supplied through a feeding tube. Such care has been redefined as medical treatment, creating a vehicle to intentionally end the lives of cognitively disabled people while retaining the pretense of ethical medical practice.

This did not just happen. It resulted from a deliberate campaign. As bioethicists and others among the medical intelligentsia began to worry about the cost of caring for dependent people and the growing number of our elderly, and as personal autonomy increasingly became a driving force in medical ethics, some looked for a way to hasten the deaths of the most marginal people without seeming to be actually killing the patient and thereby arousing hostility and opposition among the public.

Removing food and fluids provided by tube was seen as the answer. After all, it was rationalized, use of a feeding tube (whether in the stomach or through the nasal passage) requires a minor medical procedure. Moreover, the nutrition supplied by tube is not steak and potatoes but a liquid formula prepared under medical auspices so as to ease digestion. The term "artificial nutrition" was coined, making it appear that what was being withheld or withdrawn was not food and water but medicine, that is, medical treatment. From such small beginnings—changes in definitions and terminology—have come profound consequences. The "food and fluid" cases have rippled through traditional medical ethics and public morality, undermining one of the primary purposes for which our government has been instituted: the protection of the lives of all its citizens.

Dehydration Nation

The theologian and philosopher Richard John Neuhaus has written: "Thousands of ethicists and bioethicists, as they are called, professionally guide the unthinkable on its passage through the debatable on its way to becoming the justifiable until it is finally established as the unexceptional."[2] Neuhaus's point is that the loosening of ethical guidelines generally occurs first among self-described healthcare "bioethicists," theorists, philosophers, physicians, academics and others, long before entering the realm of public attention. These ivory-tower types argue behind the scenes in the medical literature, within professional organizations, in universities and at conventions about the alleged need to "reform" existing standards of morality, ethics, healthcare protocols and public policy. The debates, which receive little if any media attention, rage intramurally for a few years and eventually culminate in a rough consensus that gives both "liberals" and "conservatives" something of what they want: an agreement that policies should change, tempered by "guidelines" to prevent abuse.[3]

The next step is usually a series of legal test cases in which the judges generally lean on the testimony of expert witnesses—often the very doctors and bioethicists pushing the new agenda—who assure the judge that the healthcare profession has worked it all through and reached an ethical consensus. Most judges decide the case along the lines of this so-called consensus. After all, the judge will reason, I am trained in law, not medicine. If doctors and professional ethicists think it is right, who am I, a mere judge, to determine otherwise? The judge's own prejudices and fears about disability or dying may also play a part in the decision.

The court's imprimatur in turn legitimizes a new morality among the public, who often look to the law to tell them what is right and what is wrong. The media pick up the baton, running sympathetic stories that play on the emotions of the moment rather than the likely consequences. Soon, opinion polls reflect the public's increasing acceptance of policies they would have disdained only a few years previously, which stimulates politicians to frame those policies as statutory law or at least deters them from leading any opposition. In the end, as Neuhaus wrote, what once was unthinkable policy becomes the starting point for the slide down the next portion of the slippery slope.

This general pattern can be seen at work in the dehydration cases. The fundamental moral consensus that required the cognitively disabled to receive humane care, including nutrition and fluids for the duration of their natural lives, was attacked in this manner and eventually broken in the 1980s.[4] In March 1986, the first concrete step was taken to legitimize the intentional dehydration of unconscious, nonterminally ill patients. The American Medical Association Council on Ethical and Judicial Affairs, responsible for deliberating upon and issuing ethics advisories for the AMA, issued

the following opinion: Although a physician "should never intentionally cause death," it was ethical to terminate life-support
treatment, even if:

> death is not imminent but a patient's coma is beyond doubt irre-
> versible and there are adequate safeguards to confirm the accuracy of
> the diagnosis and with the concurrence of those who have responsi-
> bility for the care of the patient.... Life-prolonging medical treatment
> includes medication and artificially or technologically supplied respi-
> ration, nutrition and hydration.[5]

There it was. For the first time, food and fluids provided by a feeding tube were "officially" deemed a medical treatment that could be
withdrawn ethically, the same as turning off a respirator or stopping
kidney dialysis.

The opinion, written in passive prose, appears very narrowly
drawn. Only those who "beyond doubt" were permanently unconscious were supposed to be eligible for terminating the "treatment."
And protective guidelines were supposed to protect against abuses.
In actuality, a Pandora's box had been opened wide.

Once "consensus" was reached to allow intentional dehydration, at least in some situations, the issue was ripe for adjudication.
Lawsuits were soon filed requesting legal sanction for making disabled patients die by dehydration. The case of Nancy Cruzan had
the greatest impact. Indeed, not only did the Cruzan case open the
door to removing food and fluids from cognitively disabled patients,
but it also became intertwined with the debate on assisted suicide.

On January 11, 1983, Nancy lost control of her car on an icy
road in Missouri and crashed. She was thrown from her car and
landed facedown in a water-filled ditch. Nancy's heart stopped, but
paramedics revived her.

Nancy's injuries included profound cognitive disability. In
books about her case, she is usually described as unconscious from
the time of the accident, but that does not appear to be true.[6] For a
period of time after the accident, Nancy was able to chew and swallow food and drink fluids. Indeed, she was first put on a feeding
tube to make her long-term care easier. There was also evidence that
she could hear and see; she smiled at amusing stories and sometimes cried when visitors left.[7]

While the actual level of her abilities was (and still is) in some dispute, no one contends that Nancy required intensive-care hospitalization or skilled nursing care. She was not on a respirator, nor did she receive dialysis. She was not terminally ill. All she required to maintain her life was humane care: nutrition, fluids, warmth, cleaning, and turning to prevent bedsores or pneumonia.

If Nancy was unconscious, as claimed by her parents and other proponents of cutting off her food and fluids, then she was in no pain. The same cannot be said of her mother and father. Who can doubt that seeing a loved child so profoundly disabled over many years was an agonizing experience for the Cruzans? Perhaps the depth of their pain was the reason they began consulting with the Society for the Right to Die about ways to bring an end to Nancy's life.

The year after the AMA ethics council's opinion was published, in May 1987, the Cruzans filed a lawsuit seeking to force hospital employees where Nancy was living to remove their daughter's food and fluids. Hospital administrators and especially the nurses who cared for Nancy, who saw her as a living, breathing human being deserving of respect and proper care, resisted. They were unable, however, to persuade Judge Charles E. Teel of the Jasper County Circuit Court to let Nancy live. He ordered the hospital to do as the Cruzans requested.

The Missouri Department of Health appealed the decision. On November 16, 1988, the Missouri Supreme Court reversed the trial court, finding: "This is not a case in which we are asked to let someone die.... This is a case in which we are asked to allow the medical profession *to make Nancy die* by starvation and dehydration" (emphasis added).[8]

It was on to the United States Supreme Court. The Court's decision in *Cruzan v. Director, Missouri Department of Health* dealt primarily with the evidentiary standard established in Missouri law, which was that life support could be withdrawn from an incompetent patient only if there was "clear and convincing evidence" that the person would have wanted the treatment terminated. The Court upheld this requirement as constitutional, ruling that such a strict standard was properly in keeping with the state's obligation to protect the lives of its citizens. Since no clear and convincing evidence had been offered in the trial that removing food and fluids was what

Nancy would have wanted—as opposed to what her parents desired for her—Missouri could thus require that Nancy's life support continue.[9] (Unfortunately, the Court also accepted by implication that tube-supplied food and fluids is a form of medical treatment that can be withdrawn like any other form of treatment. Pro-euthanasia advocates often claim that this aspect recognized a new "right to die." It did not. It involved the right to refuse medical treatment, a different matter entirely.)

What at first appeared to be a resounding victory for those who believed in protecting the lives of cognitively disabled persons soon turned sour. The Cruzans went back to the original trial court. This time, two of Nancy's former coworkers came forward to describe a conversation that, they testified, had occurred many years before, while the participants were engaged in their work activities. The details were sketchy, as in the Schiavo case later on, but the gist of the testimony was that Nancy had indicated she would not want to live in a coma. Nancy's exact words could not be described, nor whether she had made the statement or simply agreed to a statement made by another. But that was all judge Teel (who had originally determined that Nancy could be dehydrated) required to rule that the Cruzans had provided clear and convincing evidence that Nancy would want her treatment ceased.

There was no appeal. By this time, the Missouri Department of Health had abandoned the case, deciding to allow Nancy's parents to have their way. Those who opposed the ruling—and who did not believe that the testimony came anywhere near to "clear and convincing"—were not parties to the case and thus were powerless to intervene. Nancy's food and fluids were withdrawn on December 14, 1990. She died twelve days later. The cause of death listed on her death certificate: dehydration.

Since Nancy Cruzan's death, the starving and dehydration of cognitively disabled patients has become routine in hospitals and nursing homes all around the country. Moreover, such killings have definitely not been limited to people who, in the words of the AMA ethics council opinion, are "beyond doubt" permanently unconscious. When the parents of Christine Busalacchi, a twenty-year-old auto accident victim, sought permission to end their daughter's life, doctors described her condition as a persistent vegetative state

(PVS). In PVS the patient has sleep and wake cycles but lacks reflex response and does not interact with his or her environment. The patient's eyes may be open, but he or she is believed to be unaware. This is distinct from a coma, where the patient's eyes are closed. Christine's father, Pete Busalacchi, believed that his daughter was "One hundred percent gone."[10] Dr. Ronald Cranford, testifying in favor of dehydrating Christine, dehumanized her by saying, "She's got a shell of a body, lying there with a brain stem."[11]

Yet nurses and medical personnel who had close interaction with Christine told a different story. Their descriptions do not come close to the PVS label. Some testified they had heard her grunt to indicate her choice of soap opera on television. They told of her smiling and interacting with favorite nurses. Nurse Sharon Orr recalls, "Christine was awake and alert. She would push buttons to call us. She would eat a bite and push a button, saying another bite please. We fed her with a spoon."[12] A videotape of Christine released to the media showed that she could indeed eat food by mouth, press a switch to ask for food, and obey simple requests. Thus, while there is no doubt Christine was profoundly disabled, it is highly unlikely that she was permanently unconscious.[13]

But Dr. Cranford discounted the observations of Christine's nurses, claiming that they were too emotionally involved to see the truth about her condition. This conforms to a pattern common in these cases, whereby judges in food and fluid cases often discount nurses' opinions and observations, even though they have the closest relations with patients. By contrast, testifying doctors, whose word has greater sway, may only have spent a few minutes examining the person.

Compelling evidence of her consciousness was not enough to save Christine's life. Nancy Cruzan had broken the ice. A new health-policy paradigm was taking control. It was not the presence or absence of consciousness that mattered. What counted was the view that death was the answer to profound cognitive disability. Since dehydration was considered appropriate for the unconscious, why not also the conscious who required a feeding tube? Christine soon followed Nancy into death by means of intentional dehydration.

The slide down the slippery slope from dehydrating the unconscious (assuming for the sake of argument that Cruzan was unconscious) to dehydrating the conscious but cognitively disabled (Busalacchi and other conscious cognitively disabled people who have met a similar fate) belies the argument that policies permitting the killing of patients can be strictly controlled. The carefully shaded moral distinctions in which the health care intelligentsia of bioethicists and policymakers take so much pride are of little actual consequence in the real world of cost-controlled medical practice, in busy hospital settings, and among families suffering the emotional trauma and bearing the financial costs of caring for a severely brain-damaged relative. Once killing is seen as an appropriate answer in a few cases, the ground quickly gives way, and it becomes the answer in many cases.

The deadly logic of its earlier decision to permit the withdrawal of tube feeding from unconscious people soon led the AMA to expand the list of those whose lives could be ended by dehydration. In 1994, a brief eight years after its first ethics opinion reclassifying tube feeding as medical instead of humane treatment, the AMA Council on Ethics and Judicial Affairs made a crucial revision. Where once the patient had to be "beyond doubt" permanently unconscious to permit withdrawing food and fluids, now "even if the patient is not terminally ill or permanently unconscious, it is not unethical to discontinue all means of life-sustaining medical treatment [including food and fluids] in accordance with a proper substituted judgment or best interests analysis."[14]

This shows how the slippery slope works. Once the killing of one group (in this example, the unconscious) is permitted, those killed in actual practice also include another group (in this example, the conscious, cognitively disabled). When it became clear that the original guidelines were not being adhered to, the guidelines were simply expanded rather than enforced more rigorously. This, in turn, formally legitimized practices that a few years before had been deemed completely unacceptable. For example, now that the practice of dehydrating conscious, cognitively disabled people is permitted in almost every state—so long as no family members object—the next step down the slope is already advancing: forced removal of feeding tubes from unconscious patients whose families want their lives sustained. This new bioethics agenda, known as "futile care theory," will be discussed in detail in Chapter 6.

Is Dehydration Painful?

Proponents of dehydration contend that deaths by dehydration are peaceful. An accurate discussion of this sensitive issue requires the making of proper and nuanced distinctions about the consequences of removing nourishment from incapacitated patients. This generally becomes an issue in one of the following two diametrically differing circumstances:

1. Depriving food and water from profoundly cognitively disabled persons who are not otherwise dying, a process that causes death by dehydration over a period of ten to fourteen days. As I will illustrate below, this may potentially cause great suffering.
2. Not forcing food and water upon patients who have stopped eating and drinking as part of the natural dying process. This typically occurs, for example, at the end stages of cancer when patients often refuse nourishment because the disease has distorted their senses of hunger and thirst. In these situations, being deprived of unwanted food and water when the body is already shutting down does not cause a painful death.

But the patients we are discussing here were not terminally ill. Indeed, those who are conscious can feel hunger and thirst.

St. Louis neurologist, Dr. William Burke, who opposes withholding food and water from cognitively disabled patients, claims that death by dehydration is painful:

> A conscious person would feel it [dehydration] just as you or I would. They will go into seizures. Their skin cracks, their tongue cracks, their lips crack. They may have nosebleeds because of the drying of the mucus membranes, and heaving and vomiting might ensue because of the drying out of the stomach lining. They feel the pangs of hunger and thirst. Imagine going one day without a glass of water! Death by dehydration takes ten to fourteen days. It is an extremely agonizing death.[15]

Dr. Ronald Cranford, the neurologist who testified in most of the news-making dehydration cases—always in favor of death—testified in a lawsuit in California involving the intended dehydration of a conscious but profoundly cognitively disabled patient named Robert Wendland (see below). During cross-examination, Dr. Cranford was asked whether patients could feel the pain of being dehydrated to death. Admitting that the eyes, lips and tongue of a person being dehydrated "get extremely dry," and acknowledging that "anything that is dry for a long period of time may crack," and "anything that may crack may bleed," Cranford testified that in his experience it is rare for dehydrating patients to go into seizures. That being duly noted, even Cranford's description of dehydration demonstrates the awfulness of the process, which he testified usually takes between ten and fourteen days but in some cases up to twenty-one days:

> After seven to nine days [from commencing dehydration] they begin to lose all fluids in the body, a lot of fluids in the body. And their blood pressure starts to go down.
>
> When their blood pressure goes down, their heart rate [goes] up.... Their respiration may increase and then the patient experiences what's called a mammalian's diver's reflex where the blood is shunted to the central part of the body from the periphery of the body. So, that usually two to three days prior to death, sometimes four days, the hands and the feet become extremely cold. They become mottled. That is you look at the hands and they have a bluish appearance.
>
> And the mouth dries a great deal, and the eyes dry a great deal and other parts of the body become mottled. And that is because the blood is now so low in the system it's shunted to the heart and other visceral organs and away from the periphery of the body....[16]

Of course, most of the people who are dehydrated are so incapacitated they cannot tell us what they experience as they slowly die. But we do know of one person who experienced deprivation of food and most liquids while in a profoundly disabled state—but who lived to tell us her harrowing tale.

In 1995, thirty-three-year-old Kate Adamson was felled by a brainstem stroke, which left her entirely paralyzed and unable to communicate with the world. She later recovered and wrote *Kate's Journey: Triumph over Adversity*.[17] Adamson is now a writer and lecturer, speaking, as she puts it, "on behalf of the rights of the disabled and weak to life, and life with dignity."[18]

Adamson has been very vocal in opposing the dehydration of people with cognitive disabilities—partly because of the pain she is convinced such deaths cause. And she would know: During her early care, doctors misdiagnosed Adamson as having a brain tumor and unlikely to regain consciousness. But she wasn't unconscious. Her condition was actually the "locked-in state," in which the patient appears totally unaware and unresponsive—and may be so diagnosed—but is actually fully conscious, though unable to communicate.

Believing that Adamson would never recover, doctors urged her husband, Steven, to leave her condition untreated so that she would "go gently into that good night."[19] He refused. Then, during the course of her care, Adamson needed to have a feeding tube inserted in order to provide adequate nutrition. Because her level of consciousness was misperceived and she was believed mistakenly to be totally unaware, she received inadequate anesthesia and thus felt the pain of her surgery. As painful as this was, Adamson now says that being deprived of all nourishment and most liquids for eight days during a subsequent treatment for a serious intestinal malady was even worse.

I became aware of Adamson during the height of the intense public controversy over the dehydration of Terri Schiavo. Adamson appeared on *The O'Reilly Factor*, on the Fox News Network, where host Bill O'Reilly asked her whether being denied food and water was painful:

> *O'Reilly:* When they took the feeding tube out, what went through your mind?
>
> *Adamson:* When the feeding tube was turned off for eight days, I thought I was going insane. I was screaming out in my mind, "Don't you know I need to eat?" And even up until that point, I had been having a bagful of Ensure as my nourishment that was going through the feeding tube. At that point, it sounded pretty good. I just wanted something. The fact that I had nothing, the hunger pains overrode every thought I had.
>
> *O'Reilly:* So you were feeling pain when they removed your tube?
>
> *Adamson:* Yes. Oh, absolutely. Absolutely. To say that—especially when Michael [Schiavo] on national TV mentioned last week that it's a pretty painless thing to have the feeding tube removed—it is the exact opposite. It was sheer torture, Bill.[20]

In preparation for an article I wrote on the issue of whether dehydration is necessarily humane, I contacted Adamson for more details about the pain she experienced while misdiagnosed as unconscious and having no food and little fluids. She described being deprived of food and water as "far worse" than experiencing the pain of abdominal surgery with inadequate anesthesia:

> The agony of going without food was a constant pain that lasted not several hours like my operation did, but several days. You have to endure the physical pain and on top of that you have to endure the emotional pain. Your whole body cries out, "Feed me. I am alive and a person, don't let me die, for God's sake! Somebody feed me."

What about the thirst? I asked:

> I craved anything to drink. Anything. I obsessively visualized drinking from a huge bottle of orange Gatorade. And I hate orange Gatorade. I did receive lemon flavored mouth swabs to alleviate dryness but they did nothing to slack my desperate thirst.[21]

Apologists for dehydrating cognitively disabled patients might respond that Adamson was not actually cognitively impaired, while patients who are not conscious don't feel anything. Yet persistent unconsciousness is often mistakenly diagnosed. Moreover, it is undisputed that *conscious* cognitively disabled patients are dehydrated in nursing homes and hospitals throughout the country. Dr. Cranford, for example, openly admits that he removes feeding tubes from conscious patients.[22] Thus, many other people may also have experienced the agony described by Adamson and worse, given that dehydrating to death generally takes about a week longer than the deprivation she experienced.

At this point, defenders of removing feeding tubes from people with profound cognitive disabilities might claim that whatever painful sensations dehydration may cause, these patients receive palliating drugs to ensure that their deaths are peaceful. But note: Adamson either did not receive such medications, or if she did, they didn't work. Moreover, because these disabled people usually can't communicate, it is impossible to know precisely what they experience. Thus, when the lawyer Janie Hickock Siess asked Dr. Cranford what level of morphine would have to be given to the conscious Robert Wendland to prevent him from suffering from the symptoms of dehydration, he testified that the dose would be "arbitrary" because "you don't know how much he's suffering, you don't know how much aware he is…. You're guessing at the dose."[23] At the trial, Cranford stated that he would probably put Wendland back into a coma (that is, back into the unconscious state from which he had emerged sixteen months post-injury) to ensure that he did not feel agony![24] Thus, even according to dehydration advocate Cranford, the prospect of agony in conscious people who are dehydrated to death is too real to ignore.

Causing suffering via dehydration is only the beginning of our worries about these food-and-fluids cases. The attitude that it is better to die than to become cognitively disabled has so pervaded the culture of health care that some doctors are beginning to worry about a rush to write off newly unconscious patients and consign them to death by cutting off life support before they have a chance to recover. According to Dr. Vincent Fortanasce, a board-certified neurologist and psychiatrist, too many doctors are making diagnoses of permanent unconsciousness prematurely—after only a few days or a week—when it takes at least three to six months to make a firm diagnosis.[25] "Eighty to ninety percent of the cases I see have been improperly diagnosed," Fortanasce says, "often by doctors who are not qualified to make the determination. Unfortunately, that's the real practice in medicine today."

Dr. Fortanasce recounts one example of this rush to write off unconscious patients from his own practice. A sixty-year-old patient collapsed and was diagnosed as PVS by his internist, who strongly urged the family to discontinue all life support, including nutrition. The family was reluctant and so they sought a second opinion from Dr. Fortanasce. "I came in, took the appropriate tests. The patient was not PVS. He had experienced a severe brain seizure. I prescribed continued life support and medication. A week later, the patient walked out of the hospital in full possession of his faculties. Had the family listened to the internist, the man would be dead today."[26]

The frequency of such cases is unknown: so far, no studies have been done. In most cases the withdrawal of food and fluids is done with the consent of the families, so no notice is taken. Unless someone objects to the dehydration or the premature withholding of life support, the patients die and no one is the wiser.

Litigating Life and Death

The legality of dehydrating the cognitively disabled has not yet been set completely in concrete, although not for lack of trying. Many relatives of the unconscious and cognitively disabled still refuse to permit their loved ones to be killed. A few courageous judges, such as Alabama's Pamela Willis Beschab, still hold the legal line against these killings. When relatives of Correan Salter, a stroke patient, wanted a court ruling permitting her dehydration, judge Beschab refused, writing, "Once the state accepts a policy that some lives are not worthy to be lived and some people would be better off dead, it takes the first step on a long and slippery slope from which there can be no turning back."[27] Unfortunately, most judges and family members are swept along by the prevailing cultural tide.

The following cases illustrate the acute and never-ending danger to the weakest and most helpless among us.

Michael Martin
"A-F-R-A-I-D": Michael Martin, a brain-damaged forty-one-year-old man, spelled out the word on the alphabet board.

"Are you afraid of somebody?" asked the speech pathologist at the Michigan hospital where Michael was being cared for.

Michael shook his head no.

"Are you afraid *for* somebody?"

Michael nodded his head yes.

The speech pathologist asked if he was afraid for the nurses, aides, or his roommate, David.

No.

"Are you afraid for yourself?"

Yes.[28]

Martin, a profoundly disabled man, didn't know it, but he too was about to be the center of a bitter dispute over whether he should live or die by dehydration. Martin's case deeply and bitterly divided a family. On one side was Mary Martin, his wife, who wanted Mike's life ended. Fighting to save him were Leeta Martin and Pat Major, Mike Martin's mother and sister.

"Do you like it here?" the pathologist continued.

Yes.

"Do you feel you get good care here?"

Yes.

"Are you afraid someone will take you from this facility?"

Yes.

The therapist then told Michael that he would be with them for "quite a while."

According to the chart notes, Michael then gave a big smile.[29] That hope was unduly optimistic. The judge of the Allegan County Probate Court, George A. Grieg, would soon issue a ruling allowing Mary Martin to order Michael's feeding tube removed in order that he die by dehydration.

What made the Michael Martin case significant was the relatively high level of Martin's functioning. When the court battle raged over him, he was not only conscious but also interactive, having learned in April 1992 how to use a communication augmentation system in which he pointed to letters so as to communicate. Through the system, he was able to say, "My name is Mike." According to the therapist's report, when asked to spell a word, "Mike spelled out the word [water]. When asked to find the character to clear this page, Mike was able to do it independently. Mike also indicated to us in response to a yes/no question, that the scanning device was too slow for him and he wanted it to be a little faster. When directed to the feelings page, Mike responded to the question of how he was feeling by indicating happy."[30] Unfortunately, Mike's feelings at this time would count for nothing in the coming legal drama over his potential killing.

In October 1992, as part of the court case then ongoing, Dr. Robert K. Krietsch, a board-certified physician specializing in physical medicine and rehabilitation, evaluated Michael Martin. Dr. Krietsch reported:

> When I first entered the room his radio was on and he agreed to allow it to be turned off When asked if he is able to see television and follow some shows, he indicates with an affirmative and also again, with a 'yes' head nod when asked if he likes certain types of shows. He brightened up with a large grin when asked if he liked cartoons.... When shown his poster with pictures of country western music stars, he again became quite animated with his expression, using a large grin, and was very cooperative in identifying by head nod and

attempted to point with his right hand on questioning who were the different stars that I pointed to…. He was 100% accurate on identifying all of these.

In open court, Judge Grieg recalled a visit he had with Martin where he had seen for himself that Martin was conscious and interactive:

> "I introduced who I was, that we were having a hearing on whether or not he still needed a guardian. What did he think? Did he think he still needed a guardian? He shook his head yes. I mean it was a definite movement. It came at an appropriate time—at the end of the question." Judge Grieg related how Martin would nod yes and no when asked various questions about former coworkers and family members. He described how he then asked Martin to show volitional movements: "I asked him, 'Can you move your hand?…. Is it your left one?' He shook his head no. I said, 'Is it your right one?' He said yes. I said, 'Can you move it for me,' and he raises it up and down."[31]

Michael Martin became disabled on January 16, 1987, when a train hit the car in which he and his entire family were driving, killing the Martins' daughter, Melanie, age seven. (Mary and the other two Martin children suffered injuries but fully recovered.) Michael Martin was unconscious for the first several months following the accident. Then he began to improve. By 1990, his treating neurologist, Dr. Walter Zetusky, measured his IQ between 63 and 67.[32]

Almost since the accident, Mary had believed that it was best for her husband to die. In August 1988, as Mike was slowly improving, she refused to permit antibiotics to be used to treat him for pneumonia. That, and her refusal to share information about his condition with Pat Major, his sister, and Leeta Martin, his mother, caused the two to seek Mary's ouster as Mike's guardian. That dispute ended with an informal settlement, but from that point forward, as in the Schiavo case, there were two opposing factions in the family.

Two years later, Mike developed a bowel obstruction. Mary had him transferred to Butterworth Hospital in Grand Rapids, Michigan. Unbeknownst to the rest of Mike's family, Mary asked hospital personnel to remove his feeding tube. That led to a meeting of the hospital ethics committee, which issued a statement favoring the dehydration; it stated in part: "While Mr. Martin is not in a persistent vegetative state, members of the Ethics Committee felt that the persistence of his condition and the level of his functioning were equivalent to a persistent vegetative state for purposes of considering the removal of nutritional support."[33]

In defense of the hospital committee, Mike's abilities were significantly reduced from what they had been only a few weeks before. Perhaps that was because he was ill or because he was in an unfamiliar place. (Experts who work with the cognitively disabled report that they may become depressed in a new environment, leading to an apparent lowering of abilities.) Regardless of the cause, the committee was working with incomplete information. It made no effort to contact Mike's neurologist, Dr. Zetusky, or staff members of the New Medico Neurological Center (where Mike was cared for before coming to Butterworth), who knew Mike very well and could have told the committee that prior to his transfer he had interacted meaningfully with his environment and obtained enjoyment in life.[34] Nor were Pat Major and Leeta Martin permitted to give the committee their opinions. Thus, whether through willful ignorance, negligence or a simple lack of facts, the committee issued a recommendation about Mike Martin's life and death without knowing the complete story.

Happily for Mike, a legal review of Mary's request had also been performed, and it would materially affect Mike's fate. Nervous about the previous legal scrap between Mary and her in-laws, the lawyers, in order to avoid litigation, recommended that the hospital should dehydrate Mike only if a court order permitted it to do so. That forced Mary to seek a judge's permission to end Mike's life, giving Pat Major and Leeta Martin the opportunity to stand up for his right to live.

The case would take years. The first round went to Pat and Leeta when Judge Grieg ruled that Mike could not be dehydrated because he had not prepared a written advance medical directive indicating that this would be his desire.

Round two was Mary's. The Michigan Court of Appeals reversed Judge Grieg's decision, deciding that oral statements could constitute "clear and convincing evidence" (the standard of proof

required in Michigan) of Mike's stated desires regarding his care if
he were ever incapacitated. More worrisome was a ruling that
pushed Michigan law down the slippery slope: The undisputed fact
that Mike was conscious was not necessarily a bar to his dehydration. Rather, his medical condition and capabilities would be only
one factor among many considered.[35]

Mary won the next two rounds also. Judge Grieg ignored plen-
tiful evidence that Mike was currently happy and not in pain, and
that he wanted to live. As if Mike were now a nonentity, the only
thing that mattered in the decision was how Mike felt *before* he was
injured. Relying on testimony by Mary concerning a private conversation she claimed to have had in which he allegedly said he would
not want to live if he were incapacitated, Judge Grieg ruled that
Mary could stop Mike's food and fluids. He did not take into
account the admitted fact that Mary would lose a substantial
amount of the settlement from the railroad if she divorced Mike but
not if he died, nor Mary's admitted romantic involvements after
Mike was injured. Despite these apparent conflicts of interest, Judge
Grieg wouldn't even appoint a neutral attorney to look out for
Michael's interests. The Michigan Court of Appeals agreed with
Judge Grieg, affirming the trial court's death ruling.

Mike's fate was ultimately decided in the Michigan Supreme
Court, which ruled on August 22, 1995, that Mary's uncorroborated
testimony was not sufficient to constitute clear and convincing evidence. Mary tried to take the case to the United States Supreme
Court but was turned down.

What if there *had* been clear and convincing evidence that
before his injury, Mike had expressed a desire to die if disabled?
Indeed, what if he had signed a medical directive that his food
should be withheld? Shouldn't the strong evidence that he was not
in pain and that he enjoyed his life count for something? Shouldn't
the benefit of the doubt be given to life rather than death? And
shouldn't the fact that Mike was awake, aware and interactive by
definition preclude dehydration?

Apparently not. Although the Michigan Supreme Court's ruling saved Mike's life, it is ominous that it did not prohibit ending the
lives of *all* conscious but cognitively disabled people who rely on
feeding tubes, although it certainly set a stringent level of proof

required before such killings can take place. Indeed, Dr. Ronald Cranford groused that the court's decision "shows how the clear and convincing evidence standard of proof can be manipulated to deny a person's liberty interest," which, he opined, should "frighten the people of Michigan."[36] In other words, according to Dr. Cranford it is wrong to give the benefit of the doubt to life.

Robert Wendland

"Wife requesting transfer [of Robert] to discontinue tube feeding for euthanasia," the concerned nurse wrote in the notes that became a part of Robert Wendland's medical records. "Caloric needs have increased...[due to] his hard work in therapies. The shock of this decision and committee approval! Is very difficult for obvious reason of his progression."[37]

In 1993, Robert Wendland, then forty-two, came home from an all-night drunk and was confronted by his wife, Rose, and his brother, Mike. An angry argument ensued. Rose told him that if he continued drinking and driving he would end up dead, kill someone else or spend the rest of his life in a hospital, and that the family would all have to suffer for it.[38]

Robert dismissed her concerns, replying that if such a thing happened, if he could not live as a full man and support his family, he would rather be dead. These words would later be used as evidence in a bitter and angry litigation between Rose and Robert's mother, Florence Wendland, a case that would reach the California Supreme Court, make national headlines, be covered on network television news programs such as *Today* and *Good Morning America*, and be the subject of numerous articles in some of the nation's foremost bioethics, legal and medical journals.

One week after the argument, Robert was catastrophically injured in a terrible auto accident. He was unconscious, a condition from which doctors predicted he would never emerge. But then in January 1995, Robert began to stir. At first the changes were almost imperceptible: a grimace here, a hand movement there. Soon, however, there was no doubt that Robert was now conscious.

According to court testimony by his nurses and therapists, confirmed by the medical records, after he awakened, Robert's condition dramatically improved throughout the spring of 1995. He learned to maneuver a motorized wheelchair on command and avoid obstacles, and at least once he even wheeled himself out of the hospital. Just a few months after waking up, he was able to respond to requests such as "Hand me the ball" 80 to 100 percent of the time. As proved by a videotape taken of one of Robert's therapy sessions, he was able to retrieve and return colored pegs from a tray when asked to do so by a therapist, evidence of sophisticated neurological function.[39] He was able to support up to 110 pounds on one of his legs, which meant his muscle tone was returning.[40] Although unable to communicate meaningfully, he showed emotional responses to his environment. For example, his mother testified that when asked, "Do you want to kiss my hand, Robert?" he would sometimes take her hand to his lips and kiss it. When asked if he wanted her to kiss his hand, he would sometimes "hold his hand up to my lips and allow me to kiss it."[41]

By every measure, Robert's cognition level and physical abilities were far above those of "Sally." Yet whereas only some ten years before she had benefited from kind and loving care in a health-care world where no one seriously would have proposed taking action to end her life, Robert's doctors and his wife wanted to take away his tube-supplied food and fluids in order that he dehydrate to death.

In a better world, Rose's request would have been rejected out of hand by Robert's doctors and the Lodi Memorial Hospital Ethics Committee. But rather than give all benefit of the doubt to life, committee members seem to have done just the opposite. As far as is known, no one argued for saving Robert's life. The nurses and therapists, who spent the most time with Robert—many of whom were extremely upset by Rose's decision—were never asked their opinions. Indeed, Robert's mother (who had visited her son almost daily since his accident) and his sisters—all of whom would have argued against his dehydration—were not even told that it was being contemplated. (Robert's brother, Mike, who supported Rose, was aware of her decision.)

There were probably no disabled people on the committee who might have better defended Robert's right to life. (The exact makeup of the committee has been kept a closely guarded secret.) Moreover, the county ombudsman, whose specific job was to advocate on Robert's behalf, supported Rose's decision without taking the time to learn that Robert could maneuver a wheelchair.[42] The ombudsman testified in court that her primary concern was to determine whether Rose's decision was made in haste. Once she believed that it was not, the ombudsman had no problem with the dehydration.[43]

Robert would have died then and there but for an anonymous nurse who risked being fired by blowing the whistle to one of Robert's sisters. Robert's mother, Florence Wendland, and one of his sisters, Rebekah Vinson, decided to sue to save his life. They asked attorneys Janie Hickock Siess and John McKinley of Stockton, California, to represent them. When Siess learned the facts of the case, she was stunned. "I knew from my studies in law school about the *Cruzan* case that unconscious people could have their food and fluids terminated, but I had no idea that anyone would ever consider dehydrating a conscious human being. But here it was. The plans to end Robert's life had already been made. He was to be discharged from the hospital, picked up by an ambulance, brought to a skilled nursing facility, where he would be starved to death. I couldn't believe it. I thought, this can't be legal. What sane person would want to do this?"[44]

Siess and McKinley quickly obtained an injunction prohibiting the dehydration, setting the stage for a bitter six-year court battle between Rose on one side and her mother-in-law and sister-in-law on the other. The issue at stake: should the law permit Robert's feeding tube to be removed in order that he die by dehydration?

It is important to emphasize that Robert was not terminally ill. His doctor admitted on the witness stand that there was no medical reason to withhold food and fluids.[45] His life was threatened with termination solely because it was not viewed as worth living, a view Rose claimed Robert would have shared before he was injured, and thus, she contended, his death would protect his personal autonomy. Yet, whatever Robert's previous feelings about profound disability, post-injury he cooperated with his therapy, at least implying that he wanted to live. Moreover, he was sometimes able to answer yes and no questions by pushing a button. ("Is your name Michael?" No. "Is your name Robert?" Yes.) When asked whether he wanted to die, intriguingly, he did not answer.[46]

The Robert Wendland case, as Yogi Berra would have said, turned out to be déjà vu all over again. As in Michael Martin's case, a mother and sister faced off against a wife over whether a conscious, cognitively disabled man could be dehydrated to death. And as occurred in Michigan, the state supreme court would make the final decision.

The case proved to be a white-knuckle roller-coaster ride. Robert's mother, Florence, won the first round when her attorney prevailed upon the trial judge to rule that those seeking Robert's dehydration had not presented clear and convincing evidence that he would have wanted to die under his circumstances or that dehydration would be in his best interests. That approach was reversed by the California Court of Appeal, which substantially upheld Rose's view that statutory law in California merely required her to prove her "good faith" by clear and convincing evidence. (Alarmingly, the court also ruled that "there should be no presumption for continued existence" in California law.) [47]

One of the most disturbing aspects of the entire Wendland saga was the concerted effort to dehumanize and depersonalize Robert in order to make his dehydration easier for the courts to swallow. Thus, instead of celebrating Robert's progress from coma to interactivity as wonderful medical victories for someone who only months before had been unconscious, expert bioethicist witnesses denigrated his interactivity as mere "trained responses" rather than truly human behavior.[48] One went so far as to contend that Robert "is unable to think at all in the manner we conceive humans do."[49] Similarly, Robert's own court appointed appellate attorney argued that Robert "can respond to stimuli somewhat in the manner that an animal might."[50] Most disturbingly, illustrating how such dehumanizing and denigrating values can become embedded into law, the three-judge panel of the California Court of Appeal actively embraced Robert's dehumanization in their discussion explaining why they wished to reverse the trial judge's ruling.

The case reached its dramatic denouement when the California Supreme Court overruled the court of appeal and reinstated the trial judge's approach, noting, among other issues, that similarly fundamental decisions involving incompetent persons require very high standards of proof. (For example, a California conservator must prove beyond a reasonable doubt that a decision to sterilize a developmentally disabled conservatee is in the latter's best interests. As

Florence's lawyer argued compellingly, to "provide greater legal protections against sterilization than death is to turn the overarching purposes of constitutional safeguards upside down.")[51]

Unfortunately, Robert died of pneumonia several weeks before his mother and sister's great court victory. Tellingly, the person at his bedside as he died was not his wife, Rose Wendland, but his mother, Florence.

Terri Schiavo

In the decade after Nancy Cruzan died, Michael Martin, Robert Wendland and other food-and-fluids cases broke into the news, received varying levels of media attention, and soon were forgotten in the never-ending information barrage that is the hallmark of the modern world. But then suddenly, unexpectedly, seemingly out of nowhere, the desperate cause of one helpless, cognitively devastated young woman named Terri Schiavo sparked an intense cultural conflagration that increased widespread popular distrust for the courts and political branches of government; forced a state legislature, a popular governor, both houses of Congress and the President of the United States into tight political corners; attracted the concerned attention of a dying Pope John Paul II; and ignited bitter kitchen table debates all around the world.

Why Terri? In a sense, her case came as a surprise and yet was not exactly unexpected. The fight over assisted suicide and related life-and-death issues are like the irresistible force meeting the immovable object. Knowing that both value systems could not long occupy the same space, activists on both sides of these emotional issues expect to participate in a long series of epochal political clashes that will inevitably determine which value system—quality or equality of life—predominates in society. Indeed, not since Jack Kevorkian's heyday in the late 1990s had these crucial issues received as much sustained media attention and public debate as they did when attention focused on Terri Schiavo.

Yet no one quite expected the collision to occur when it happened or to be about a food-and-fluids case involving a woman supposedly in a PVS. But as they often do, events spontaneously developed and quickly reached critical mass, and then came the conflagration—not because "professional" activists drove it to the fore, but rather because of the grassroots political advocacy of hundreds of thousands, perhaps millions, of average people who saw profound injustice in Terri's pending dehydration.

Most people learned about Terri because of the Internet. Knowing that cases such as these are often won and lost in the sphere of public relations, Terri's parents, Robert and Mary Schindler, hit upon a brilliant stroke: They created a Web site, www.terrisfight.org, dedicated to organizing public opinion to save Terri's life. The site issued press releases, carried news of the case, linked copies of court documents, presented Terri's personal history and, most important of all, allowed millions of viewers access to powerful videos of Terri Schiavo apparently reacting to the world around her.

In one such scene, Terri is asked by a doctor to open her eyes. For a moment; nothing. Then Terri's eyes flutter and she opens them. She is apparently so earnest and eager to please—and this really touched my heart when I first saw it—that she opens her eyes so wide her forehead wrinkles.

In another scene, Mary Schindler, Terri's mother, comes into the room. She talks happily to her daughter: "Hi! Hi, it's Mommy. How are you?" As Mary adjusts Terri on the bed, it sure appears like she recognizes her mother and she smiles happily.

In a third scene, Terri appears to respond happily when music is turned on. And so it goes.

These videos made all the difference. Rather than being an abstract "vegetable" (a truly loathsome word to describe any human being), Terri came to be seen by many as a real person, obviously alive and fully human. Michael Schiavo's supporters and proponents of Terri's dehydration within the bioethics community stomped, fussed and insisted that the appearance of interactivity in the videos was actually reflexes and mirages, that Terri was PVS. But, rightly or wrongly, many viewers saw these complaints as being akin to the cheating husband who tells his wife after catching him *in flagrante delicto*, "Are you going to believe me or your lying eyes?" The videos told a different story than that of a supposedly vegetative woman whose brain was liquid, making it impossible for her to interact. And for her supporters, the real Terri came out of the shadows, a subhuman no more.

Most readers will be generally familiar with the overview of

Terri's Schiavo's case. She collapsed from unknown causes on the night of February 25, 1990. Her husband, Michael Schiavo, told police that he heard a thud, found her unconscious on the bathroom floor, and called the paramedics. Terri's life was saved, but her brain was catastrophically injured, resulting in permanent and profound cognitive impairment. She was eventually diagnosed as being in a persistent vegetative state—a matter of later dispute. Terri was not tethered to "machines." She did not need a respirator or kidney dialysis. The only form of "life support" she required was a feeding tube.

After Terri collapsed, Michael lived with his in-laws until May 1992, and the three worked closely together to provide Terri with optimal care and rehabilitation. For example, they took Terri to California for an experimental treatment involving the implantation of electrodes in her brain. But when the insurance money ran out, attempts at rehabilitation apparently ceased, and there were no further efforts in rehabilitative therapy from 1993 on.[52]

In February 1993, Michael and the Schindler family had an angry falling-out and became permanently estranged. The Schindlers first tried to wrest guardianship from Michael later that year because he refused to permit Terri to be treated for an infection. They would clash in court again in 1998, when Michael sought court permission to withdraw her tube feeding.

Between 1998 and Terri's death in March 2005, Schiavo and the Schindlers battled over her fate in all levels of Florida's judiciary, eventually in federal courts, and even more intensely in the court of public opinion—a struggle that eventually resulted in Florida and the United States government passing laws tailored to save her life. Notwithstanding these efforts, the courts remained unanimous and adamant in upholding Pinellas County Circuit Court judge George W. Greer's order, siding with Michael, that Terri Schiavo must die. With all legal options exhausted, the world watched—and her supporters agonized—as Terri slowly dehydrated to death over nearly fourteen days, passing away at age forty-one on March 31, 2005.

THE INTENSE PERSONAL, CULTURAL, LEGAL and political struggle over Terri Schiavo's life and death deserves far more attention than I can possibly devote to it here. Nor, in the limited space available, can I possibly unpack the many factual disputes that developed over more than a decade of intra-family acrimony and years of bitter litigation. But having observed the case closely for several years, having acted occasionally as an unpaid, informal adviser to the Schindlers, and having participated, sometimes heatedly, in the intense public debate over Terri's fate, I offer the following incomplete observations about why Terri's dehydration was such a profound injustice:

A Victim of Casual Conversations: Most people date the beginning of the Terri Schiavo case to the night she collapsed. But the root of the controversy goes back even further, all the way back, in fact, to sometime during the second term of President Ronald Reagan and a few casual conversations Terri purportedly had with her husband and his family—interactions she might not even have remembered on the day she fell ill.

According to Michael Schiavo, Terri told him on a few occasions during their marriage that if she were ever in a situation of being artificially maintained, she would want life support removed.[53] Michael's brother Scott backed him up, testifying that she told him she wouldn't "want to be kept alive on a machine."[54] (As noted above, Terri wasn't on a machine. But Judge Greer interpreted this statement to include a feeding tube.) Michael's sister-in-law, Joan Schiavo, testified that after watching a movie, Terri had stated she would not want "tubes"; that Terri approved of pulling the life support from the dying baby of a mutual friend; and that Terri said that if she ever wrote a "will," she would indicate that she didn't want "tubes."[55] (Others told a different story. For example, one of Terri's friends testified that Terri opposed removing life support from Karen Ann Quinlan, but this was disregarded by Judge Greer when he issued his first death order.)[56]

Little did Terri know that these and a few other purported statements, uttered in very casual circumstances—and possibly not intended to include feeding tubes since they occurred before the Cruzan Supreme Court case was decided, bringing the issue of dehydration to public light—would become the justification for withdrawing all food and water from her. Indeed, relying solely on these purported statements, Judge Greer ruled that Michael Schiavo had established "by clear and convincing evidence"—the highest evidentiary standard in civil law—that Terri would rather dehydrate to death than receive food and water supplied by a feeding tube.[57]

This aspect of Terri's case deserves far more attention that it has received. Many of us may have made similar casual statements in response to the death or disability of a relative or the emotions generated by a movie. But shouldn't much more be required to justify the intentional ending of a human life? At the very least, shouldn't we demand a well thought-out, informed and preferably written statement that not only indicates what is desired but also shows that reasonable alternatives have been fully considered?

For example, if Terri did say she didn't want tubes, did she even contemplate that this statement would be interpreted to include a feeding tube? Did she consider that the removal of her tube could mean enduring a dying process that might result in seizures, heaving, nose bleeds, cracked lips, parched tongue, and the extremities becoming cold and mottled? Did it occur to her that this type of death would devastate her parents and siblings? If she did, would that have made a difference to her?

And what did the statement "I don't want tubes"—assuming that she made it—mean, anyway? Perhaps Terri was thinking about the stark atmosphere of a neonatal intensive care unit in which babies are kept alive by battalions of beeping and buzzing medical machines. Or, if she was thinking of Karen Ann Quinlan's circumstance, she might have conceived of herself spending years on a respirator, which was the treatment in controversy in that matter. But Terri wasn't on a respirator. The only life support she needed was food and water. But these basics of life are precisely what a court would prohibit her receiving—*even by mouth*, despite the fact that proving food and water by mouth is not a medical treatment.[58]

Michael Schiavo Told Different Stories about Terri to Different Courts: Michael Schiavo's testimony about his wife's purported statements constituted the primary evidence that Terri would not want to live. But Schiavo's testimony is suspect because he told two different and conflicting stories to two different courts from which he sought two dramatically different types of court orders.

The first time he presented evidence about Terri's life expectancies, he was seeking a $16 million jury verdict for medical malpractice that, he claimed, had a part in causing Terri's injury. During the trial, Schiavo presented evidence that:

- Terri could be expected to live a normal life span. (This is important because the longer a person incapacitated by malpractice lives, the higher the jury award may be. In this action, Michael never told the jury that Terri wouldn't want to live and didn't want tubes. Nor was the jury informed that Michael would, within months of their verdict, begin refusing to provide Terri antibiotics and other medical treatment.)

- He would become a nurse and spend the rest of his life devoting himself to Terri's care.

- Money awarded to Terri in the malpractice case would be used for proper medical testing, rehabilitation, and the best of care. Indeed, the jury was presented with a proposed plan for further rehabilitation.[59]

The jury awarded $1.3 million. (Michael had earlier settled with a doctor for an additional $250,000.) Approximately $300,000 of the jury award went to Michael for loss of consortium, about $750,000 was awarded to Terri to pay for her ongoing care, and the rest went to lawyers' fees and costs. Michael was subsequently named guardian of Terri's person, and a bank became the guardian of her estate.

As soon as the money was in the bank—money Michael would inherit if Terri died since she didn't have a will—his decisions about Terri's care took a deadly 180 degree turn. Schiavo decreed that Terri was to receive no further rehabilitation. In the summer of 1993, when Terri developed a urinary tract infection, he refused to permit her to be administered antibiotics.[60]

A little more than five years later, when Schiavo wanted the court's permission to remove the feeding tube, he swore that she would not want to be maintained. Why didn't this clear inconsistency impact Judge Greer's belief in Michael's credibility? As hard as it is to understand now, this clear contradiction between what Michael told the malpractice jury and what he said later on wasn't brought up by the Schindlers' attorney in the trial—and all later attempts by subsequent lawyers to use this issue as one of the reasons to have a new trial were denied.

Conflicts of Interest: Michael Schiavo had profound personal and financial conflicts of interest that should have precluded him from serving as Terri Schiavo's guardian and requesting her death by dehydration. First, the financial: When Michael requested permission to cease Terri's nutritional support, she still had an estate valued at more than $700,000. Indeed, according to Richard L. Pearse Jr., the guardian *ad litem* initially appointed to represent Terri's interests, as of April 4, 1998, Terri's trust fund held $713,828.85. "Thus," wrote Pearse, "Mr. Schiavo will realize a substantial and fairly immediate financial gain if his application for withdrawal of life support [tube-supplied food and water] is granted."[61] At the time, Schiavo's brother and sister-in-law had not yet publicly supported his claim that Terri would want to die. To Pearse, Schiavo's testimony alone was insufficient to justify the removal of tube feeding, because, he opined, his "credibility is necessarily adversely affected by the obvious financial benefit to him of being the ward's sole heir at law in the event of her death while still married to him."[62] (Subsequent to the filing of the report, and perhaps in response to it, Schiavo's brother and sister-in-law came forward to claim that Terri had made similar statements in their presence.)

Of perhaps even greater concern was the acute personal conflict of interest between Schiavo's duty as a guardian for Terri, and the new life he had created for himself in the years after her collapse. Pearse described this matter tersely as Michael "getting on with his life."[63]

In 1996, Michael Schiavo moved in with the woman with whom he had fallen in love. In the years that followed, the couple had two children. Few would have held this against him—if he had turned Terri's care over to her parents. Instead, Schiavo insisted that he retained all the rights of a husband—including the right to inheritance and retention of marital property—as he simultaneously enjoyed connubial bliss and sweet domesticity with his new family.

In most situations, Schiavo's cohabiting with another woman and siring two children by her would constitute a clear abandonment of his marriage. At the very least, his "complicated" domestic situation gave rise to the appearance of divided personal loyalties.

This fact could have materially affected the public's perceptions about who had the high moral ground in the struggle over

Terri's care. Yet most media accounts of the Schiavo controversy inexplicably omitted this crucial fact from their reportage. Most reports merely identified Schiavo as Terri's "husband"—thereby leaving the distinct impression that he had been as loyal to Terri all those many years as he promised the malpractice jury he would be, and adding heft in the public's mind to the claim that he was only fulfilling a promise to Terri that he would never let her be maintained by artificial means.

For instance, while *Newsweek*'s extensive report laudably mentioned both sides of many of the controversies in the case—indeed, more than most other stories—it omitted the relevant facts of Michael's personal life.[64] Similarly, in the *New York Times*' many early articles, opinion columns and editorials, Michael's extracurricular activities were completely ignored. Its October 23 editorial merely stated:

> Michael Schiavo, her husband and legal guardian, went to court seeking to cut off the feeding tube that was keeping her alive. He testified that Ms. Schiavo, who did not have a living will, would not have wanted the feeding to continue.[65]

Imagine how different the readers' impression of the case would have been if the editorial had included the total context, stating: "Michael Schiavo, who remains legally married to Ms. Schiavo but has lived for years with and sired two children by his fiancée, went to court seeking to cut off the feeding tube."

Richard Pearse, Terri's initial guardian *ad litem*, perceived these conflicts of interest as crucial evidence in determining how to decide Terri's fate properly, writing in his report to the court in December 1998, "Given the inherent problems already mentioned, together with the fact that the ward has been maintained on the life support measures sought to be withdrawn for the past 8 years, it is the recommendation of the guardian *ad litem* that the petition for [tube] removal be denied."[66] But Pearse was soon kicked off the case based on allegations of bias asserted by Michael Schiavo's lawyers, and no new *ad litem* was ever appointed in the state guardianship case to represent Terri's interests.

Once Pearse was out of the picture, the conflict-of-interest issue lost all traction. As we've seen, the media mostly brushed these matters aside in their reporting, while the courts cared not a whit about potential adverse influences that would, under similar circumstances, almost surely have resulted in a court order preventing Schiavo from managing Terri's property. (Indeed, Michael was never permitted to be the guardian of Terri's estate.) But for Terri's supporters, the widespread disregard of these facts constituted a bitter injustice and a clear reason to transfer Terri's care from the husband, who so clearly had moved on with his life, to her parents and siblings, who wanted nothing more than to love her unconditionally, care for her and provide for her needs for as long as she lived.

The Rule of Terri's Case: "If following a legal procedure will likely result in Terri dying, it will be adhered to," Bob and Mary Schindler's attorney Patricia Anderson told me early in 2004. "But if a procedure could make that outcome more difficult to attain, it will not be followed."[67] Anderson called this judicial giving of the benefit of every doubt to Terri's death, rather than her life, "the Rule of Terri's Case."

Anderson's complaint was well founded. For example, under Florida law, Terri should have had a court-appointed guardian *ad litem* to represent her interests exclusively throughout the court proceedings. But as we have already seen, after Richard Pearse was dismissed, Terri was never again provided the services of a guardian *ad litem* during the court case that determined her fate.

Similarly, when in October 2003 the state of Florida passed "Terri's Law," permitting Florida's governor to suspend the planned removal of a feeding tube in certain cases, it also required the appointment of a guardian *ad litem*.[68] But after the *ad litem*, Jay Wolfson, urged that she be allowed a swallow test, David A. Demers, chief judge of the Sixth Judicial Circuit, who had appointed Wolfson, refused to renew his authority.[69] This, despite Governor Jeb Bush specifically informing Demers that he needed further information from Wolfson to properly carry out the governor's responsibilities under Terri's Law.[70] (This law was subsequently declared unconstitutional by the Florida Supreme Court as a violation of the separation-of-powers doctrine.)[71]

Then there was the evidence that came to light after the initial trial in the case that could have resulted in a materially different outcome had the Schindlers been granted a new trial, either in state court or in federal court after Congress passed a law granting federal jurisdiction and requesting a *de novo* review of the case—a request summarily refused by the federal courts at all levels. Among the evidence that was never permitted to be fully litigated and that could have affected the "clear and convincing" evidence finding that Terri would want to be denied tube-supplied food and water:

- The different stories Michael Schiavo told different courts about Terri's likely life span and her desires for care if incapacitated, as recounted earlier.

- The affidavits of three nurses who cared for Terri in the mid-1990s, signed under penalty of perjury, which called Michael Schiavo's good faith toward Terri into significant question. One of these affidavits was especially damning. According to Carla Sauer Iyer, for example, Terri had potential for rehabilitation, potential she would note on the chart but which "would always be deleted by the next time I saw the chart." Moreover, she testified, "Throughout my time at Palm Gardens [nursing home], Michael Schiavo was focused on Terri's death. Michael would say, 'When is she going to die?' 'Hasn't she died yet?' and "When is that bitch gonna die?'.... Other statements which I recall him making include, 'Can't you do anything to accelerate her death—won't she ever die?' When she wouldn't die, Michael would be furious."[72]

- While most physicians diagnosed Terri as being PVS, and the two guardians *ad litem* who briefly represented Terri agreed, there was credible evidence presented after the original trial that she was responsive and perhaps capable of being improved through rehabilitation.[73] This was not a matter of a judge having to decide which side of a case had the most credibility. Terri was there for the rehabilitating. But despite repeated requests by Terri's family, Judge Greer would have none of it. Rather than permit attempts at rehabilitation that would at least have demonstrated once and for all whether Terri was beyond all improvement, Judge Greer ordered that no attempts to improve Terri's condition be made.[74]

The law is supposed to protect people like Terri Schiavo. Instead, in hearing after hearing, the courts, following the Rule of Terri's Case, seemed to work overtime to skirt these protections. Yes, many hearings were held over several years. But never, once the original trial was held, did any state or federal court permit the sum and substance of the Schiavo case to be reexamined in open court—even despite a federal law passed in a strong bipartisan vote requesting the federal courts to do so.[75] Indeed, rather than conduct an independent *de novo* review of the facts of the case as provided by the federal law, U.S. District Court judge James D. Whitemore instead defied the spirit of the federal law by declaring that "the state court judge applied the heightened clear and convincing evidence in determining her intentions."[76]

Perhaps the most clear-cut example of this phenomenon is the repeated waiving by Judge Greer of Michael Schiavo's statutorily mandated duty as Terri's legal guardian to file an annual "guardianship plan." Florida law explicitly states:

> Each guardian of the person *must* file with the court an annual guardianship plan which updates information about the condition of the ward. The annual plan *must* specify the current needs of the ward and how those needs are proposed to be met *in the coming year.* [My emphasis.][77]

The plan must describe the "plan for provision of medical, mental health, and rehabilitative services in the coming year." If a guardian fails in this duty:

> The court *shall* order the guardian to file the report within 15 days after the service of the order upon her or him or show cause why she or he should not be compelled to do so.[78]

Moreover:

> The court *must* review the initial and *annual* guardianship report to determine that the report: (a) meets the needs of the ward.... [My emphasis.]

And:

> The approved report constitutes authority for the guardian to act in the forthcoming year. The *powers* of the guardian *are limited by the terms of the report.* [My emphasis.][79]

In other words, Judge Greer was duty-bound to review Michael's care plan for Terri each year *prospectively*, not retrospectively, which makes sense since its purpose is to ensure that the plan is appropriate to the ward's *future needs*. Moreover, the approved guardianship plan *constituted Michael's authority to act as Terri's guardian,* and his actions would have been limited by the contents of the plan in each year. Thus, it would appear that if the statutes were followed, Michael would have had no legal authority to direct Terri's care in the absence of an approved plan.

Yet despite these very clear statutory mandates, Judge Greer *six times* granted Michael's requests for "time extensions" for the July 2001–June 2002 plan, to the point that it had not been filed by January 2004—nearly three years past due. Greer also just now, in 2005, approved a time extension for Schiavo to file his guardianship report for the period between July 2002 and June 2003. By granting these repeated extensions Judge Greer sent a clear message to Michael Schiavo: I am not going to require you to comply with the mandates of Florida law.

In 2004, I asked Schindler lawyer Pat Anderson why, in her opinion, hard-and-fast rules that govern other guardianships did not apply to Terri. She chuckled bitterly, "It's the Rule of Terri's Case. Both the guardian and the judge treat Terri as though she were already dead and in no need of these statutory protections."[80]

Conclusion

As we have seen, there is a clear pattern in these food-and-fluids cases: The higher the patient's perceived awareness—as in Wendland and Martin—the greater the likelihood that the disabled patient's life can be saved. Conversely, those who, like Terri, exhibit more limited capacities are increasingly seen—or at least treated— merely as inconvenient "biologically tenacious" lumps of flesh.[81]

By this standard, no matter how hard her family fought, no matter how long it took, Terri's diagnosis of PVS doomed her. Her quality of life simply did not measure up in a society that no longer perceives human life to have intrinsic value simply and merely because it is human. To those with a certain mindset, this meant she was no longer *fully* human, no longer a person, no longer one of "us." In the end, perhaps Terri Schiavo had to die because those with the power to decide simply believed that she was better off dead.

THREE

EVERYTHING OLD IS NEW AGAIN

F OR MORE THAN TWO THOUSAND YEARS, mercy killing has been culturally disdained and illegal in the West and most of the rest of the world. Some euthanasia advocates claim that these life-affirming policies were instituted as part of some vast conspiracy by church leaders to impose religious hegemony on society and to promote suffering as a form of sacrament. While it is true that pragmatic concerns, humanitarian values and religious tradition intertwined to create the particular cornerstone of Western civilization that I earlier labeled the equality-of-human-life ethic, this moral principle is not in and of itself a religious belief. Indeed, the ethical precepts of modern medicine that prohibit killing date back well before the dawn of Christianity to the writings of Hippocrates, a Greek physician who lived in the fifth century B.C., who gave his name to the famous Hippocratic Oath, and whose ethical prescription was for doctors to "First, do no harm."

That is not to say, of course, that the killing of the weak and ill has never been carried out. Some ancient Greek societies, Hippocrates notwithstanding, so disdained children born with birth defects that they found a convenient way around their legal proscription against killing by exposing these unfortunate infants on hillsides. So did the Romans. It is also true, as euthanasia advocates are fond of pointing out, that some hunter-gatherer societies traditionally expected the old and disabled to remain by the side of the trail when they couldn't keep up. Some of these cultures also routinely killed babies born with birth defects.

Unlike the reasoning behind today's advocacy to legalize euthanasia and assisted suicide, the purpose behind these acts of killing generally involved a perception of absolute necessity: a stark choice between maintaining the life of the individual and the continued existence of the society or tribe. These death practices—targeting the weak and "abnormal"—generally waned or ceased altogether as life became less harsh.

In the contemporary West, we judge cultures as "advanced" or "civilized" in part by the manner in which they care for their weakest and most vulnerable members.[1] Cultures that disrespect their dying, elderly and disabled, or that do not provide for them in a caring and compassionate manner, generally are seen as backward, if not downright oppressive. Traditionally we have measured our own progress toward a genuinely humane and enlightened society against these same standards.

This appears to be changing. An ethical tug-of-war has emerged between those who continue to hold to the equality-of-human-life ethic and those who wish to replace it with a different, less egalitarian principle, sometimes described (euphemistically, in my opinion) as the "quality-of-life" ethic. It was described as early as 1970 in a prescient editorial in *California Medicine,* published by the California Medical Association, whose members were familiar with the debates then ongoing among the medical intelligentsia. The editors saw radical change in the offing:

> The traditional Western ethic has always placed great emphasis on the intrinsic worth and equal value of every human life regardless of its stage or condition…. This traditional ethic is…being eroded at its core and may eventually be abandoned…. [H]ard choices will have to be made…that will of necessity violate and ultimately destroy the traditional Western ethic with all that portends. It will become necessary and acceptable to place relative rather than absolute values on such things as human lives…. One may anticipate…death selection and death control whether by the individual or by society.[2]

In 1970, the ideas of death control or death selection were utterly beyond the pale for most people. Agonizing memories were still too fresh. After the destruction under the Third Reich (the mother of all death cultures) and the lessons of the Holocaust, the equality-of-human-life ethic was at its zenith and the watchword was "Never again!"

But now, a mere thirty-five years later, many perceive the traditional Western "sanctity of life" ethic as religious imposition. On one hand, we claim to feel compassion for people with developmental disabilities and pass laws for their public accommodation. On the other hand, some of us barely object if such people are killed, and a few even applaud. Thus, even as the Special Olympics celebrates the achievements of people with cognitive difficulties, and the Americans with Disabilities Act promotes equality for those among us with physical impairments, our society countenances the death by intentional neglect of infants born with Down syndrome and spina bifida, and blithely accepts the premise that suicide by the disabled is "rational."[3]

We don't come to this crossroads without a road map. Others in this century have trod this same path—with disastrous results—most particularly the supporters of eugenics in the United States, England and, most notoriously, Germany. Knowing this, we can have the courage to learn from our calamitous past and choose a better, more humane approach to overcoming today's difficult bioethical challenges.

It is a delicate matter to bring up the horrors of eugenics and the Holocaust when intellectually engaging today's public policy disputes. Contemporary apologists for euthanasia/assisted suicide protest that those earlier proponents of the death culture were different people living in a different time, many driven by intense bigotry and, in Germany at least, a fierce racial ideology and social Darwinism that fueled the madness. And it is true: Today's euthanasia advocates are not racist or anti-Semitic. Nor do they seek to create a master race. Indeed, they are far more likely to wear the mantle of compassion than of bigotry, and to identify with libertarianism rather than with notions of totalitarianism embraced by the National Socialists.

These very real differences in motivation should not, however, lull us into becoming receptive to the policies they advocate. Wicked ideas are hardest to detect in their own time, even when they are variations on a theme that has previously been tried with catastrophic results. For although there are many substantive differences between the values that drove the earlier eugenics-based death cultures and the ones emerging in our day, a careful analysis of the *actions* being advocated—rather than just the words used to promote those actions—leads to the uncomfortable inference that the differences are not as profound as many would like to believe.

Germany Abandons the Equality-of-Human-Life Ethic

Between 1939 and 1945, the activity that is called euthanasia made the transition from being a theoretical idea that had been current for more than forty years to being actually carried out. During those years, many German physicians participated willingly and enthusiastically in a program specifically established to kill off their most chronic patients. Euthanasia, in turn, led directly to the death camps of Auschwitz, Treblinka and Dachau as, in the words of the psychiatrist and Holocaust historian Robert Jay Lifton, "the medicalization of killing" became "a crucial…terrible step [toward] systemic genocide."[4] During these six years, doctors and nurses intentionally killed more than two hundred thousand helpless people: the cognitively or physically disabled, people with mental disease, infants born with birth defects, the senile elderly, even severely wounded German soldiers. German euthanasia practices were the first movement of the symphony of slaughter that took the lives of millions of Jews, Gypsies, homosexuals, Communists, labor union members, Jehovah's Witnesses, Catholics and other "undesirables" whose deaths we memorialize in the term *Holocaust.*

The medical professionals who killed their own patients did not act under duress, coercion or menace, or out of fear for their own lives. They were not drafted into performing euthanasia; they eagerly volunteered. "Those responsible believed in the necessity of what they were doing," writes Michael Burleigh of the London School of Economics.[5] In fact, German doctors who participated in euthanasia viewed the killing of certain patients as a final treatment—an act that compassionately served the interests of the patients as well as their families and the Reich as a whole.

Many people mistakenly believe that German crimes against humanity were all Hitler's idea, purely a product of Nazi ideology. In actuality, doctors who later participated in mass killing had, in

Lifton's term, developed a "'euthanasia' consciousness," a value system in which some lives are viewed as unworthy of protection.[6] This unethical approach to the practice of medicine was already well developed in Germany by the time Hitler came to power in 1933. Indeed, the German medical, legal and academic intelligentsia had aggressively promoted euthanasia as a proper and ethical public policy since the late nineteenth century, when Hitler was a child.

The first notable advocate of euthanasia in Germany was Adolf Jost, who publicized his ideas in *The Right to Death*, published in 1895. Jost considered the state to be a "social organism," a view later adopted by many Germans, Hitler included, and he argued that the life and death of each individual must ultimately belong to the collective. According to Lifton, Jost's thesis was: "The state must own death—must kill—in order to keep the social organism alive and healthy."[7]

In 1913, euthanasia was popularized and legitimized in Germany through the publication of an open letter ("Euthanasie") written by Roland Gerkan, a man dying of lung disease. His text reads like that of a contemporary euthanasia advocate: "Why, instead of permitting us to die gently, today, do you demand that we embark upon the long martyr's road, whose final goal is certainly the same death which you deny us today?"[8] Gerkan even penned a model law legalizing euthanasia for anyone with an incurable illness, suggesting—just as modern euthanasia advocates do—that "protective guidelines" be enacted to protect against abuse, including the requirement that the person who wanted to be killed petition judicial authorities for permission, that the case be reviewed by two qualified physicians to determine the likely outcome of the disease, and that legal protection against liability be assured for "whosoever painlessly kills the patient as a result of the latter's express and unambiguous request."[9] The law would apply not just to the dying but also to the elderly and the "crippled."[10]

Gerkan's thesis provoked much debate among German physicians, academics, lawyers, ethicists and church leaders. But the issue, then seen mainly as an intellectual exercise, was soon overshadowed by a more pressing matter for the German people: World War I.

The nation suffered terribly during the war, not only from the killing of its soldiers in battle but also from the privations caused by shortages of food and other resources at home. During the war, lack of resources led to a harsh utilitarianism. Some Germans were considered expendable. Mental patients, for example, were deemed not worth feeding, which led to their intentional mass starvation.[11]

At the end of the war, the country was reeling. Bitter in defeat, economically ruined, politically torn by factional fighting that would ultimately lead to the Nazi takeover, the country desperately searched for national meaning and a way to bind its wounds. Such was the social mood when, in 1920, two venerable German professors published a book on the subject of euthanasia: *Permitting the Destruction of Life Not Worthy of Life.*[12] The book consisted of two separate essays, one by each co-author: Karl Binding, an intellectual star and one of Germany's premier legal experts, and the physician Alfred Hoche, then considered one of Germany's most prominent medical humanitarians.

The importance of the publication of *Permitting the Destruction of Life Not Worthy of Life,* a full frontal attack on the equality-of-human-life ethic and described by Lifton as "the crucial work," is difficult to overstate.[13] The high-profile respectability of its authors and their explicit endorsement of legalizing the killing of weak and vulnerable Germans deeply influenced the value system of the general public and the ethics of the medical and legal communities. As a consequence, Hoche and Binding's book became a cornerstone of the intellectual foundation upon which the coming euthanasia practices would be built.

Reading *Permitting the Destruction of Life Not Worthy of Life* is a chilling experience, not only because of its crass embrace of killing the defenseless but also because of the ways in which it mirrors many of the concepts propounded by today's euthanasia advocates. Binding and Hoche believed that there were people living in Germany whose lives were so degraded and undignified that they constituted "life not worthy of life." Who were these "useless eaters," as they later came to be known?

1. *Terminally ill or mortally wounded individuals* were those who "have been irretrievably lost as a result of illness or injury, who fully understand their situation, possess and have somehow expressed an urgent wish for release."[14] This view is virtually identical to euthanasia policies being urged upon us today.

2. *"Incurable idiots,"* whose lives the authors saw as *"pointless"* and *"valueless,"* were considered to be killable because they were an economic and emotional "burden on society and their families." Hoche put it this way: "I have discovered that the average yearly (per head) cost for maintaining idiots has till now been thirteen hundred marks.... If we assume an average life expectancy of fifty years for individual cases, it is easy to estimate what *incredible capital* is withdrawn from the nation's wealth for food, clothing, and heating—for an unproductive purpose" (emphasis in original).[15] Today's advocates do not denigrate the mentally retarded as "idiots," nor do most go as far as Hoche and Binding did in calling for their death. However, the economic cost of caring for those labeled as having a low quality of life is frequently noted by euthanasia advocates.

3. The *"unconscious,* if they ever again were roused from their comatose state, would waken to nameless suffering" and should be spared this.[16] The United States and other Western nations already ascribe to this criterion.

As euthanasia proponents always do, Binding and Hoche called for protective guidelines to govern the killing practice, including the need to make an application to an oversight board, the investigation by at least two physicians, a finding that the patients are "beyond help," with a report of the final act of killing to be given to the board.[17] Those who participated as killers, whether medical personnel, family members or others, would, as in today's legislative proposals, be free from legal liability or criminal culpability for their lethal acts. These ideas later came to haunt Hoche, who would turn against the German euthanasia program—even though much of its rationale derived from his own writings—after one of his relatives became a victim.[18]

AT THE SAME TIME THAT HOCHE and Binding were urging euthanasia upon Germany, another pernicious social revolution caught on in Germany as well as in the United States and Britain: the eugenics movement. Eugenicists claimed the right to determine which human traits were better than others and to establish a hierarchy of "hereditary worth." They intended to promote the desirable traits through selective "breeding," using the new science of genetics. Humans with traits considered worth keeping were encouraged to procreate. Those with undesirable characteristics were discouraged and even forcefully prevented from having children. Eugenics profoundly violated the equality-of-human-life ethic and resulted in terrible oppression wherever it found official acceptance.[19]

In Germany, eugenics theory created a growing obsession with purifying and strengthening the "Nordic race." Many Germans fervently believed that unless "inferior" Germans were kept from breeding, the *Volk* would weaken and eventually cease to exist. Moreover, Adolf Jost's idea that the state, rather than the individual, was the paramount decision maker also became widely accepted, popularizing the notion of forced sterilizations of those who were deemed "useless breeders." Hitler was quite clear in *Mein Kampf* that he supported eugenics, seeing it as a method to "fight for one's own health." The alternative, according to Hitler, would be a national disaster, an end to what he called "the right to live in the world of struggle."[20]

When the Nazis took power in 1933, they quickly enacted laws authorizing involuntary sterilization. (Actually, they were years behind the United States, where some states began to pass eugenics laws in 1908.) To be kept from "breeding" were the mentally retarded, the blind and the deaf, and "cripples" such as those with a clubfoot or a cleft palate. Relatives of such people were even urged to sterilize themselves voluntarily so as to prevent the "defect" from being passed on to the next generation. It is estimated that in the end, up to 350,000 Germans were sterilized in the years 1933–1945.[21]

IN THE YEARS FOLLOWING THE APPEARANCE of *Permitting the Destruction of Life Not Worthy of Life,* there was much debate about the so-called right to die that had been so forcefully propounded by Binding and Hoche. It soon became clear that the populace was in general agreement with the authors. For example, a 1925 survey among parents of children with mental disabilities disclosed that 74 percent of them would agree to the painless killing of their own children.[22] One can only imagine the attitudes of nonparents.

Well aware that the German public supported euthanasia, the new Nazi government proposed legalizing the practice in 1933. A front-page *New York Times* article described the proposal as making it possible for physicians to end the tortures of incurable patients. Protective guidelines were to be included in the law, including the necessity that the patient "expressly and earnestly" request to die, or if the patient was unable to do so personally, that relatives make the request, "acting from motives that do not contravene morals."[23]

This legislation never became law because of an outcry from the churches. But that did not stop the Nazi government from campaigning to increase public support for the killing of "useless eaters." Toward this end, many propaganda films were produced depicting mentally retarded people as lower than beasts, a tactic also—not coincidentally—employed against Jews. But it was not only the cognitively impaired "idiots" who were at the receiving end of pro-euthanasia advocacy in Germany throughout the Nazi period. Various media also pushed the idea that physically disabled people also had lives not worth living, and moreover, that their deaths would be best for themselves, their families and the state.

The 1939 German motion picture *I Accuse* (*Ich Klage An*) is a classic of this genre. *I Accuse* is particularly relevant to today's bioethical arguments, particularly voluntary euthanasia and assisted suicide. Wildly popular among German audiences (more than fifteen million paid to see it), the film called for legalizing voluntary euthanasia and functioned as an apologia for murdering disabled infants.[24] According to Richard Sobsey, professor of psychology at the University of Alberta and director of the university's Development Disabilities Center, *I Accuse* cleverly promoted killing as an acceptable answer to medical difficulties by intensely personalizing the issue of suffering caused by serious illness, while at the same time depersonalizing killing as it related to disabled infants in order to make their murder easier to accept.

The movie is pure melodrama. The primary character of *I Accuse* is a woman pianist who grows progressively disabled due to multiple sclerosis. Unable to play her beloved piano, deeply worried about becoming a burden to her physician husband, she begs for euthanasia. "The audience was supposed to relate to her deeply and [accept facilitating] her desire to die as correct and compassionate,"

Sobsey says.[25] Thus, *I Accuse* promoted euthanasia as beneficial, compassionate and supportive of autonomous decision making in the same manner as do contemporary euthanasia activists.

As the wife and husband struggle with her MS, a subplot develops around the third main character, a university professor, who lectures students on how in nature only the "fit" survive. He illustrates his teaching with graphic documentary scenes of asylums from Nazi film archives, which depict the patients as grotesque and inhuman. It is in this context that the parents of a disabled infant beg the doctor to kill their child as an act of mercy.

"The movie never shows the baby," Sobsey notes. "This was a way of depersonalizing the infant and making his or her ultimate killing less shocking."[26]

The baby is killed off camera, and this is presented as a difficult but necessary act to protect the overall health of the *Volk*. The wife commits suicide with her husband's help, a scene played, to the sound of a mournful piano, for all the pathos it is worth. The husband is arrested, but also lauded, along with his wife, for selflessness, wisdom and courage in deciding that she should die. To reassure audiences that abuses will not occur with voluntary euthanasia, one character in the movie remarks, "The most important precondition is always that the patient wants it."[27]

The movie ends with the husband's impassioned accusation to the judges against the law that forbids euthanasia (the real accusation in *I Accuse*):

> No! Now, I accuse! I accuse the law which hinders doctors and judges in their task of helping people. I confess...I have delivered my wife from her sufferings, following her wishes. My life and the lives of all people who will suffer the same fate as my wife depends on your verdict. Now, pass your verdict.[28]

With the German people thoroughly propagandized, the stage was almost set for the horror that was to follow. But just as Frankenstein's monster needed a bolt of lightning to come alive, one last development was required for euthanasia to become a reality in Germany: the perversion of traditional medical ethics.

For millennia, physicians have owed their sole professional allegiance to their patients. That changed dramatically in Germany.

Many doctors and nurses came to accept the idea that they owed a duty to the state—as well as to their patients—in their delivery of medical services. As a consequence, some doctors and nurses soon became among the most dangerous people in Germany.

As the Thirties came to a close, Germany had reached a dangerous point: Many physicians and most Germans believed that there was such a thing as individuals "not worthy of life," and that it was proper to terminate the lives of such "useless eaters." Forced sterilizations were commonplace and popularly accepted as a proper method to strengthen the state. Doctors had accepted a dual loyalty, believing they owed a professional duty to the state in their practice of medicine as well as to their individual patients. The ground was now thoroughly prepared for mass murder.

Euthanasia Comes to Germany

For Hitler, the German euthanasia program was the culmination of his long-held desire to legitimize euthanasia in Germany. He had pulled back from the initial proposal at the beginning of his years as dictator for fear of opposition from the churches during a time when he was consolidating his still tenuous grasp on political power. According to Robert Jay Lifton, Hitler had decided that "the best time to eliminate the incurably ill" would be at the outbreak of his long-planned European war, a time when the general belief in the intrinsic value of human life could be expected to be lessened.[29] But as we have seen, many Germans were well ahead of their Führer. Indeed, by 1938, more than a year before the outbreak of actual hostilities, the German government had received an outpouring of requests from the relatives of severely disabled infants and young children seeking permission to end their lives. Requests for euthanasia of the dying and disabled also were sent, some written by patients themselves and others by people who wanted euthanasia for relatives.

At this time, Hitler was looking for a good case with which to begin active euthanasia in Germany. In late 1938, the opportunity arrived via a letter from the father of "Baby Knauer," an infant born blind with a leg and part of an arm missing. The boy's distraught parents, accepting the general value system of their time, were deeply ashamed to have brought a useless eater into the world. And, seeing the killing of their son as the solution to their problems, they wrote Hitler requesting permission to have their child "put to sleep."

Hitler was quite interested in the case and sent one of his personal physicians, Karl Rudolph Brandt, to investigate. Brandt's instructions from the Führer were to verify the facts of the baby's condition and, if found to be as described, to assure the child's doctors and his parents that no one would face punishment or liability if he was killed. Brandt was then to witness the euthanasia and report back to Hitler. The doctors in the case who met with Brandt agreed that there was "no justification for keeping the child alive," and Baby Knauer soon became one of the first victims of the Holocaust.[30]

By this time, Hitler, Brandt and other Nazi social engineers had developed a detailed plan for implementation of a euthanasia program, and Hitler decided that the long-awaited moment had come. Unlike the German sterilization laws, no statute was ever enacted to legalize euthanasia. Rather, Hitler signed a decree permitting medicalized killing of disabled infants and appointed Brandt and a Nazi party member, Philip Bouhler, to head the program. Sympathetic physicians and nurses from around the country—many not even Nazi party members—cooperated in the barbaric scheme.

Disabled children were the first to suffer medicalized killing. Formal "protective guidelines" were created along the lines originally proposed by Karl Binding and Alfred Hoche, including the creation of a panel of "expert referees," which judged who was eligible for killing and who was not. (The panel reviewed a questionnaire filled out by the child's doctor, not the child's actual medical records.) At first it took a unanimous verdict of all panel referees to allow a patient to be killed. Ironically, among the selected referees was Ernst Wentzler, the inventor of an incubator for prematurely born children, who unfortunately was also a devotee of Binding and Hoche. Wentzler was so committed to euthanasia that even in 1963 he recalled his work in sorting through the euthanasia requests as having been "a small contribution to human progress."[31]

Beginning in early 1939, babies born with birth defects or with congenital diseases fell victim to the euthanasia program. Their doctors would admit these unfortunate infants to medical clinics, where they would then be euthanized. Most of these children were voluntarily turned over to medical authorities by their own parents; some (but certainly not all) knew, or at least suspected, that their disabled children were being sent to their deaths.

The practice quickly became systematized. Regulations made it mandatory for midwives and doctors to notify authorities whenever a baby was born with birth defects. These cases would be reviewed by euthanasia referees to determine if the children were eligible for euthanasia. Those deemed unworthy of life were killed either by intentional starvation or by an overdose of a drug, most typically a sedative called Luminal.

Once the principle was established that some human beings could be killed because they were disabled, it did not take long to add others to the list of expendables. These next victims were severely mentally ill and retarded adults, a category soon expanded to include the criminally insane and people with medical conditions such as epilepsy, polio, schizophrenia, senile diseases, paralysis and Huntington's disease. This was known as the T4 program.* As with the children's euthanasia order, the matter was officially a secret.

The adult victims were usually killed at designated medical clinics and hospitals, which had been turned into eradication centers in a dress rehearsal for the brutality being planned against Jews and others at death camps. Indeed, just as occurred in the later genocide, the T4 program became highly bureaucratized as government workers "coldly and calculatingly organized the murder of thousands of people" and kept meticulous records of what they were doing.[32] For example, secretaries "shared their offices with jars of foul-smelling gold-filled teeth, listening to dictation which enumerated 'bridge with three teeth,' 'a single tooth,' and so on."[33] Ironically, because euthanasia was considered a healing medical treatment, disabled Jews, as official undesirables, were not included in the program. Eventually, this "discrimination" was ended. But for disabled Jews, there were to be no protective guidelines, since, by definition they were thought to embody "dangerous genes" in an individual medical sense and "racial poison" in a collective ethnic sense.[34] Disabled

---

*T4 was a code name based on the address of the German Chancellery, Tiergarten 4.

adults were generally killed with carbon monoxide (the same method chosen by Jack Kevorkian for ending the lives of some of his victims in the United States fifty years later).

Modern euthanasia proponents, understandably wanting to distance their cause from these horrors, assert that German euthanasia is irrelevant to today's proposals because the German program was conducted in total secrecy. In fact, so many people were involved in the killing bureaucracy that it was not long before many Germans began to understand what was happening. As Hitler's henchman Heinrich Himmler put it in 1941, "This is a secret that is no longer a secret."[35]

To their credit, many Germans were appalled by the killing. Some even found the courage to resist. According to the late disability rights activist Hugh Gallagher, "There were actually public demonstrations against the euthanasia program, which were anathema to the Nazis. Even some party members were appalled but they convinced themselves that the 'Führer must not know [about the program].'"[36] One of the most powerful voices in opposition to euthanasia was the Catholic archbishop Clemens August von Galen, who courageously preached against the euthanasia program from the pulpit on August 3, 1941, stating in words that are still relevant today:

> If you establish and apply the principle that you can "kill" unproductive human beings, then woe betide us all when we become old and frail! If one is allowed to kill unproductive people, then woe betide the invalids who have used up, sacrificed and lost their health and strength in the productive process.... Poor people, sick people, unproductive people, so what? Have they somehow forfeited the right to live? Do you, do I have the right to live only as long as we are productive?... Nobody would be safe anymore. Who could trust his physician? It is inconceivable what depraved conduct, what suspicion would enter family life if this terrible doctrine is tolerated, adopted, carried out.[37]

Not wishing to arouse domestic discontent by arresting the popular clergyman—von Galen had threatened to meet the Gestapo in full regalia if they came for him—Hitler did nothing. Still, the Führer vowed revenge at the end of the war, promising to "balance the accounts" with Archbishop von Galen, so that "no 't' remains uncrossed, no 'i' left undotted."[38]

In response to the opposition that his euthanasia policy generated in some quarters, in August 1941 Hitler ordered Brandt to suspend the T4 program. (He never rescinded the infanticide program.) But that was not the end of it. Participating doctors did not need an order from Hitler to kill their "patients." They had become true believers, convinced they were performing a valuable medical service for their "patients" and their country. The protective guidelines were cast aside as the meaningless documents they had always been. From then until a few weeks *after* the end of the war, some doctors went on a killing rampage, known today as "wild euthanasia." Doctors during the later war years killed any patient they pleased, often without medical examination, usually by starvation or lethal injection.

It is important to reiterate that throughout the years in which euthanasia was performed in Germany, whether part of the officially sanctioned government program or otherwise, the government did not force one doctor to kill a patient. Nor were any doctors ever punished for refusing to euthanize a patient. It was the participating doctors themselves who had become the zealots.

Then, it was finally over. After the Nuremberg Trials, the Allies hanged Brandt and a few other physicians for crimes against humanity. But most doctors and nurses who had been involved in mass killing went unpunished, many continuing in their fields of practice. One physician who appears to have participated in the euthanasia Holocaust, Dr. Hans Joachim Sewerling, was even elected president of the World Medical Association in the 1980s. When the American Medical Association discovered his background and protested, Sewerling resigned, blaming a "Jewish conspiracy" for his troubles. However, he remained in good standing with the German Medical Association, which made him an honorary member of its board of trustees.[39]

Early Euthanasia Activism in the United States

During the 1920s and 1930s the United States faced the same social forces and erosion of values that influenced Germany. Indeed, on the brink of World War II—and even for a short time into the war— euthanasia was steadily gaining respectability and acceptance among the American people.

The roots of the pre–World War II American euthanasia movement sprang from the infamous eugenics movement. While not leading to mass killing as it did in Germany, American eugenics advocacy led to oppression via the legally sanctioned forced sterilization of more than sixty thousand people. Indeed, eugenics had so thoroughly polluted the moral thinking of America—especially among the elites—that the legal go-ahead to forced eugenic sterilization came from the United States Supreme Court in its notorious 1927 opinion, *Buck v. Bell*.[40]

The life story of Carrie Buck is as sad as her case was unjust. Carrie, the daughter of a prostitute, became pregnant out of wedlock at age eighteen, apparently after being raped by a relative of her foster father. The ashamed foster family had her involuntarily institutionalized in an asylum. Rather than protect their patient, Carrie's doctors, believing they had a duty to protect society against the "unfit," decided to sterilize her as a way to carry forward their eugenic theories.

Carrie Buck sued, and the test case eventually reached the Supreme Court. In a ruling that vividly demonstrates how judges' own prejudices can sometimes overcome facts and logic, Chief Justice Oliver Wendell Holmes issued the majority opinion. "Three generations of imbeciles is enough!" he declared.

> We have seen more than once that the public welfare may call upon the best citizens for their lives. It would be strange if it could not call upon those who already sap the strength of the State for these lesser sacrifices [sterilization], often not felt by those concerned, in order to prevent our being swamped by their incompetence. It is better for all the world…[if] society can prevent those who are manifestly unfit from continuing their kind.[41]

And so the real reason Carrie Buck was sterilized, along with tens of thousands of other Americans, was not because she was genetically "defective" but because she was poor and powerless and seen as an undesirable. Later in her life, she was released from the asylum, married twice, sang in a church choir and took care of elderly people until her death in 1983.[42] But involuntary sterilization laws remained on the books in a few states into the 1960s.

In his splendid history of the American eugenics movement, *War Against the Weak*, Edwin Black notes bluntly that "Murder was always an option." The proposed method of death was called the "lethal chamber," a device intended to induce a painless death for "people deemed unworthy of life."[43]

A Merciful End, Professor Ian Dowbiggin's thoroughly researched history of the euthanasia movement in the United States, shows that the general acceptance and practice of eugenics led directly to a campaign for the legalization of euthanasia. By the 1930s, several American euthanasia advocacy organizations had been formed. One of the movement's foremost leaders of this era, Charles Potter, energetically called for legalizing both voluntary euthanasia and mercy killing for a wide category of supposedly deficient people. As Dowbiggin explains, Potter argued that euthanasia "was a worthy reform not just because it served humane, individual objectives and empowered people," but also because it "served social purposes." Echoing the values promoted in *Permitting the Destruction of Life Unworthy of Life*, Potter estimated in 1935 that the savings New York alone would achieve by killing "imbeciles and idiot infants and monsters" instead of caring for them would approximate $30 million annually.[44]

Along similar lines, Dr. Foster Kennedy, the president of the Euthanasia Society and a professor of neurology at Cornell, opined in a speech, "If the law sought to restrict euthanasia to those who could speak out for it, and thus overlooked those creatures who cannot speak, then I say as Dickens did, 'The law is a ass.'"[45] Kennedy later said that "defective children" up to the age of five should be permitted to be killed upon the request of parents or guardians "if after careful board examination" it was determined that these children had no "future or hope."[46]

The American public responded favorably to arguments for voluntary euthanasia, which then as now were couched in terms of the "right to die," a term that was first used in Binding and Hoche's *Permitting the Destruction of Life Not Worthy of Life*. Indeed, a 1939 public opinion poll of New York State doctors surveyed by the

Euthanasia Society, published in the *New York Times*, found that 80 percent of respondents favored voluntary euthanasia for adults.[47] The high number was probably unreliable, the poll having been taken by an advocacy group. Still, an independent survey done the same year showed that belief in voluntary euthanasia was becoming mainstream, with "roughly 40 percent of all Americans polled said they supported legalizing government-supervised mercy killing of the terminally ill." The time certainly seemed "ripe" for attempting to legalize euthanasia in the United States.[48]

Whatever chance euthanasia had to become accepted public policy in the United States at that time was obliterated with the country's shock and horror over the Holocaust. After the war, euthanasia theory fell into near total disrepute and the movement grew quiescent. It did not, however, die, as the events of the last fifteen years clearly demonstrate. Indeed, many of today's euthanasia advocacy groups trace their roots back to euthanasia organizations formed in the 1930s.

Heeding the Warnings of History

The bioethicist Arthur Caplan has written, "Those who see analogies [to the Nazi period] must be specific about what they believe is similar between now and then. Blanket invocations such as... 'euthanasia, if legalized, will lead to Nazi Germany,' are to be avoided unless they can truly be supported in the scope of the claim being made."[49] He is absolutely right. Just because the Nazis said or believed something, or adopted certain public policies, doesn't mean, ipso facto, that the belief or policy is inherently evil or immoral. For example, Hitler created the German autobahn; this does not mean that President Dwight Eisenhower was wrong when he facilitated the creation of the interstate highway system.

What relevance, if any, do the euthanasia horrors of Nazi Germany bear to euthanasia proposals in our own time? Some experts on that era see little relevance. Robert Jay Lifton, for one, has written, "One can speak of the Nazi state as a 'biocracy.' The model here is a theocracy, a system of rule by priests of a sacred order under the claim of divine prerogative."[50]

There is no doubt that today's euthanasia advocates are not

driven by the ideological madness that sees biology as destiny and the cleansing of the gene pool as a divine imperative. But Michael J. Franzblau, M.D., a clinical professor of dermatology at University of California San Francisco Medical Center, and a committed Nazi hunter, whose work was primarily responsible for exposing Dr. Sewerling's euthanasia past, does see "a direct connection." Franzblau says,

> If we codified euthanasia and assisted suicide, we would unalterably alter the relationship between physicians and patients. It is frightening to consider that many of the arguments made today by euthanasia advocates echo almost precisely the arguments originally made by Binding and Hoche, and after them, Hitler and the Nazis as they implemented the euthanasia program. There are certain lines that should not be crossed. Permitting doctors to become killing agents is one of them.[51]

It is indeed intriguing how closely many of the concepts advocated in *Permitting the Destruction of Life Not Worthy of Life* resemble in word and rationale many of the pro-euthanasia sentiments expressed in our current debate. Examples of this can be found by comparing Binding and Hoche's text with the 1996 majority opinion of the U.S. Court of Appeals for the Ninth Circuit when it ruled, in *Compassion in Dying v. The State of Washington*, that Washington State's law banning assisted suicide is unconstitutional. Binding asserts that the "freedom to end [one's] own life...is the primary human right."[52] Similarly, Judge Stephen Reinhardt, writing on behalf of seven other jurists, opined, "There is a Constitutionally protected liberty interest in determining the time and manner of one's own death."[53]

> *Binding:* "We are dealing with a legally permissible act of healing, which is most beneficial for patients in severe pain, and with the elimination of suffering.... This is not a matter of killing them."[54]
>
> *Reinhardt:* "We have serious doubts that the terms 'Suicide' and 'assisted suicide' are appropriate legal descriptions of the specific conduct at issue here."[55]
>
> *Binding:* "The permission of the suffering patient is not legally required."[56]
>
> *Reinhardt:* "We should make it clear that a decision [to end a patient's

life] of a duly appointed surrogate decision maker is for all legal purposes the decision of the patient himself."[57]

Binding: "It is also completely unrestricted legally for a third party to help it along and encourage a decision to do it."[58]

Reinhardt: "We recognize that in some instances, the patient may be unable to self-administer the drugs and that administration by a physician, or a person acting under his direction or control, may be the only way the patient may receive them."[59]

Binding: "The motto or rallying cry for this movement has been the expression 'the right to die.'"[60]

Reinhardt: "The terms 'right to die'…and 'hastening one's death' more accurately describe the liberty interest at issue here."[61]

Hoche: "I consider it less important to work out all of the details than to admit that implementing this program obviously presupposes that all conceivable safeguards along these lines must be provided."[62]

Reinhardt: "While there is always room for error in any human endeavor, we believe that sufficient protections can and will be developed by the various states."[63]

Hoche: "The idea of gaining relief from our national burden by permitting the destruction of life…will (from the start and for a very long time) encounter lively, strident, and passionately stated opposition."[64]

Reinhardt: "Those who believe strongly that death must come without physician assistance…are not free…to force their views, their religious convictions, or their philosophies on all other members of a democratic society."[65]

Happily, the United States Supreme Court reversed the Ninth Circuit decision in 1997 (see Chapter 5). But that a large majority of U.S. Circuit Court of Appeals judges could so closely mimic the values and attitudes expressed by Binding and Hoche—views that helped lead directly to the Holocaust—is cause for alarm.

Many in the disability rights community are quite troubled by the similarities between current euthanasia thought and the intellectual foundations of the German experience. Carol Gill, director of the Chicago Center for Disability Research, also disabled by polio, notes that "disability has supplanted death in people's minds as the worst thing that can happen."[66] Similarly, Diane Coleman, the founder of the disability rights organization Not Dead Yet, says,

"Our priorities are all mixed up. When we demand services that would help us [the disabled] to live in liberty we are resisted at almost every turn. But if we ask to die, lawyers, doctors, bioethicists and everyone else come out of the woodwork and are more than happy to help."[67]

These fears and prejudices about and against the disabled are shared by many physicians and sometimes affect their approaches to treatment. Gill notes that when "doctors don't believe the lives of disabled patients are tenable," they feel that ending the life of the patient by nontreatment (or, presumably, euthanasia) "is doing the patient and the family a favor."[68] In such medical attitudes there surely are disturbing echoes from Germany's past.

Behavior is generally preceded by attitude. We tend to act out what we believe. That is why comprehending how the German euthanasia program could proceed—the widespread acceptance of apportioning relative worth to different categories of human lives, the lessening of the doctor's responsibility to the individual patient, and so on—is so important. These phenomena send messages that should resound through the decades: Making a virtue out of killing will have unpredictable consequences; deforming the traditional physician-patient relationship will be at the patient's peril; degrading the inherent perceived value of some humans leads directly to their oppression. The fact that we are flirting with some of the same ideas and value systems that led to horror in Germany is definitely cause for concern.

Take the equality-of-human-life ethic. Here, startling similarities can be found between attitudes in those awful times in Germany and contemporary attitudes. To say, as modem euthanasia advocates do, that the lives of some people should be protected by the law while the lives of others should not be presumes that some human lives are inherently more valuable than others. This creates a subjective approach to the right to live, rather than the objective view inherent in the equality-of-human-life ethic.

Absent a strong adherence to the objective standard, decisions about life and death and access to appropriate medical care become power-based. That is what happened in Germany during the Holocaust. Another example of a subjective approach to the right to live, albeit on a much smaller scale, is Oregon's health-care rationing for

Medicaid recipients. Under this plan, a list of more than seven hundred treatments was created and each treatment was given its own number. Every year, a cutoff number is determined, reflecting the amount of money available to fund Medicaid operations. Payment will be made for all appropriate treatments below the cutoff number; any treatment assigned a higher number will not be covered.

As first proposed, the Oregon plan placed healing treatment for end-stage AIDS patients very low on the list of treatment priorities, all but ensuring that Medicaid AIDS patients who wanted curative treatment at that stage in their disease would not receive it. AIDS activists were appropriately outraged, seeing this as a devaluation of the lives of people with AIDS. They were determined not to let Oregon abandon members of their community, no matter what the patients' prognosis. Through effective political advocacy, the activists successfully amended the plan so that AIDS patients who want healing treatment can obtain it, regardless of the stage of their disease.

If it is true that the politically powerful are better off in a quality-of-life-based system, the converse is true for people who are less organized and less powerful. In Oregon, although late-stage AIDS patients on Medicaid need not fear being cut off from treatment, categories of patients with little or no organized power—very low birth-weight babies and late-stage cancer patients, to name two—are on the nonpayment side of the cutoff.

We must not come to perceive killing as a virtue, as did the Germans of generations past. We have already decided that a whole class of patients, those assessed as PVS, can be killed by dehydration without consequence, and this has led directly to concerted efforts to expand the designation of those eligible for this "beneficence" to the conscious but cognitively disabled.

Those who sorted through the brutality of the Holocaust in the years following the war earnestly wanted to learn how it could have happened and to ensure that it never happened again. One man deeply involved in researching these issues with the Nuremberg Tribunal was Dr. Leo Alexander, who served with the U.S. Office of Chief Counsel for War Crimes. Dr. Alexander wrote a penetrating and important analysis about the foundation of the Holocaust in the

July 14, 1949, issue of the *New England Journal of Medicine*, whose relevance is unblunted today:

> Whatever proportions these crimes finally assumed, it became evident to all who investigated them that they had started from small beginnings. The beginnings at first were merely a subtle shift in emphasis in the basic attitudes of the physicians. It started with the acceptance of the attitude, basic to the euthanasia movement, that there is such a thing as a life not worthy to be lived. This attitude in its early stages concerned itself merely with the severely and chronically sick. Gradually the sphere of those to be included in this category was enlarged to encompass the socially unproductive, the ideologically unwanted, the racially unwanted and finally all non-Germans.[69]

Looking at the state of the 1949 culture of American medicine, Dr. Alexander then warned:

> In an increasingly utilitarian society these patients [with chronic diseases] are being looked down upon with increasing definiteness as unwanted ballast. A certain amount of rather open contempt for the people who cannot be rehabilitated with present knowledge has developed. This is probably due to a good deal of unconscious hostility, because these people for whom there seem to be no effective remedies, have become a threat to newly acquired delusions of omnipotence…. At this point, Americans should remember that the enormity of the euthanasia movement is present in their own midst.[70]

FOUR

DUTCH TREAT

URING WORLD WAR II, THE GERMANS occupied the Netherlands for nearly five years. It was one of the most heroic times in that nation's notable history. The Dutch resisted the Nazis at every turn, some citizens risking their own lives to protect Jews and otherwise refusing to bend to the will of their cruel occupiers.

Dutch medical professionals were major participants in the resistance. The German commander of the occupation, Arthur Seyss-Inquart, now known derisively as "the Butcher of Holland," wanted to remake Dutch medical ethics in the German image. Toward that end he issued several orders, one of which required Dutch physicians to perform their professional services as "a public task," one that he defined as assisting as a "helper...in the maintenance, improvement and re-establishment of [the patient's] vitality, physical efficiency and health."[1] But Dutch physicians unanimously rejected the order. Some went so far as to take down their shingles rather than violate their sacred duties to heal and protect their patients and to maintain a healthy separation between private obligation to each patient and public duty to the state.

Seyss-Inquart was furious. First, he tried to coerce the doctors into compliance with his order by stripping them of their licenses to practice. The doctors paid no heed; they stopped signing birth and death certificates but never stopped treating their patients. Seyss-Inquart then took lethal action. One hundred doctors were arrested at random and shipped to concentration camps in the East, from whence few returned. Still, Dutch doctors did not budge. They were literally willing to die before they would betray any of their patients.

Eventually it was the Germans who blinked in this ethical struggle, deciding not to take more drastic action against the doctors of a hostile, occupied nation. As a consequence, Dutch medical ethics were not subverted and euthanasia never entered medical practice in the Netherlands during World War II.

The Butcher of Holland was hanged after Nuremberg, in part because of his treatment of the Dutch medical community. Yet, in a painful irony, some of the very policies that Seyss-Inquart could not force upon heroic Dutch doctors during World War II have been willingly embraced by their modem counterparts—and not in microscopic proportions. Today, a majority of Dutch doctors openly accept euthanasia and assisted suicide as appropriate medical procedures.

Dr. I. van der Sluis, a Dutch opponent of his nation's euthanasia policies, told me exactly when and how such a radical change in values and ethics occurred. "There was never propaganda in favor of euthanasia in my country before 1960," van der Sluis recalled. "Then came the cultural revolution of the late 1960s and early 1970s, which hit the Netherlands very hard. Traditional ethics collapsed in almost every area, including in the medical community. It got to the point that if you didn't accept the 'new ideas' you were a suspect person."[2]

A visit to Amsterdam reveals the truth of van der Sluis's woeful observations. On the one hand, the city is the epitome of beautiful European charm, crisscrossed by canals, filled with magnificent architecture, giving all the appearance of Old World dignity and propriety. Amsterdam, like other Dutch cities, is a model of energy conservation. People generally walk, bicycle or take public transportation to get where they wish to go. Indeed, it sometimes seems that more people in the streets are on bicycles than in cars. The trolley system is efficient and affordable. Most notably, almost all of the people are open and friendly.

On the other hand, Amsterdam, once a community of proper merchants, is a city where decadence has become commonplace. In postcard racks in front of tourist-oriented stores are cards vividly depicting the Pope defecating, along with other equally tasteless offerings. In the main downtown shopping district, where families stroll in the evenings, restaurants are situated next to open-air slot-machine casinos, which are next to clothing stores whose neighbors are pornography emporiums with storefront window displays of sexual toys and explicit, full-color, gynecologically oriented photographs. Then there's the famous, or infamous, red-light district, where prostitutes sit in the windows. "Coffee shops" abound, with names like The Grasshopper and Mellow Yellow, where marijuana and hashish are legally sold and their pungent scents hang in the breeze, even in the early morning, when patrons can be seen slumped in their chairs inside.

The look of Amsterdam comes from the Dutch belief that they can manage vice by licensing it. The same attitude has carried over into their attitude toward death and disability. Because some doctors believed that euthanasia was appropriate, it was quasi-legalized in 1973 by a court decision. The idea was to create a compromise between proponents and opponents of legalization, whereby euthanasia would technically remain illegal but would be permitted in those few cases in which, supposedly, no other method could be found to alleviate a patient's agony. So long as Dutch doctors followed the guidelines set by the court, and later by statute, there would be no legal troubles. The idea was for euthanasia to be available as a rarely used safety valve to prevent needless suffering.

As we shall see, however, it hasn't even come close to working out that way. Instead of the medical establishment's managing and controlling death, the reverse seems to have occurred: The death imperative is controlling the practice and ethics of Dutch medicine. In the last thirty years Dutch doctors have expanded euthanasia practice exponentially, going from killing the terminally ill who ask for it, to killing the chronically ill who ask for it, to killing the depressed who have no physical illness who ask for it, to killing newborn babies in their cribs because they have birth defects, even though they cannot possibly ask for it. Dutch doctors also engage almost routinely in nonvoluntary euthanasia without significant legal consequence—even though such homicides are regarded as murder under Dutch law. And despite this abysmal record, the country formally legalized euthanasia in 2002, eradicating the last vestige of restraint in the system—the unlikely prospect of prosecution.

The Dutch System of Euthanasia

By the early 1970s, the Netherlands, deeply influenced by the cultural upheavals of the Sixties, cast aside traditional values and ethical norms. In this milieu, as occurred to a somewhat lesser degree in the United States, the prevailing value system was turned on its head in many cultural areas such as drug use, sexual morality and family issues.

Unlike in the United States, however, the euthanasia movement in the Netherlands quickly established a strong beachhead, finding respectability and broad public acceptance, at least in theory. Euthanasia became a popular topic of discussion and analysis among Dutch physicians and laypeople, with many coming to accept it as an appropriate response to the few cases at or near the end of life where suffering can supposedly not be alleviated.

These new attitudes profoundly affected Dutch law, beginning with a 1973 case in which Geetruida Postma, a Dutch physician, was charged with murder after she terminated the life of her seriously ill mother by giving her a lethal injection.[3] Postma appears to have intentionally used her mother's death to legitimize euthanasia among the populace and in law. Indeed, it is unlikely that the matter would have come to the attention of the authorities had she not insisted that her actions be made known.[4]

During the trial, an unrepentant Postma testified that she acted out of compassion, stating that her mother was partly paralyzed, could hardly speak, had pneumonia and was deaf. She further asserted that she killed her mother at the elder woman's request.

The highly visible case soon became a *cause célèbre*, much discussed and debated throughout the country, a rallying point for legalizing euthanasia, and the catalyst for the establishment of Holland's first voluntary euthanasia organization, the Voluntary Euthanasia Society. Postma's case generated such support that during the proceedings, doctors in her province signed an open letter to the Netherlands minister of justice stating that euthanasia was commonly practiced among physicians.[5]

The court found Dr. Postma guilty of murder. However, the court also accepted the premise that most Dutch doctors supported euthanasia in some cases. That being so, the court reasoned, the law should follow the medical consensus rather than the democratically enacted statute. Thus, in a departure from the usual Dutch practice that requires changes in law to be made exclusively by members of Parliament, the court decided instead to issue a legal precedent permitting euthanasia in some cases.

Dr. Postma received only a one-week suspended sentence and a year's probation. To justify its action, the Dutch court relied heavily on expert testimony by the district's own medical inspector (illustrating the nonadversarial nature of the trial), who set forth certain conditions under which the average physician allegedly thought euthanasia should be considered acceptable. These conditions established the first boundaries for euthanasia practice in the Netherlands. Among these were the requirements that the patient be considered incurable, implying that the patient must suffer from a physical illness; that the patient's suffering be subjectively unbearable; that the request for termination of life be in writing; and that there should be adequate consultation with other physicians before euthanasia was carried out.[6] Inclusion of these conditions in the court's decision, which was not appealed, became the basis for subsequent public and government acceptance of euthanasia in the Netherlands.

With the Postma decision, the Dutch stepped boldly onto a steep slippery slope. Other court decisions soon followed, each widening the boundaries of acceptable medicalized killing and further liberalizing the conditions under which euthanasia would not be punished. Thus, even though killing by doctors remained technically illegal, it soon became entrenched in Dutch medical practice.

In 1993, the Dutch Parliament legally formalized the informal system of euthanasia permissiveness that had been crafted by the courts. The "guidelines" were formalized by statute to which doctors were required to adhere if they were to avoid punishment for euthanizing or assisting the suicides of patients.[7] These guidelines included the following:

- The request must be made entirely of the patient's own free will and not under pressure from others.
- The patient must have a lasting longing for death.
- The request must be made repeatedly over a period of time.
- The patient must be experiencing unbearable suffering.

- The patient must be given alternatives to euthanasia and time to consider these alternatives.
- There must be no reasonable alternatives for the relief of suffering other than euthanasia.
- Doctors must consult with at least one colleague who has faced the question of euthanasia previously.
- The patient's death cannot inflict unnecessary suffering on others.
- Only a doctor can euthanize a patient.
- The euthanasia must be reported to the coroner, with a case history and a statement that the guidelines have been followed.[8]

In actual practice these guidelines offered scant protection for the weak, vulnerable and despairing, nor, as we shall see, did they inhibit doctors from euthanizing patients who fell outside the guidelines' parameters.

At this point it is important to recall that when euthanasia was first accepted in the Netherlands, it was supposed to be a rare event, to be resorted to only in the most unusual cases of "intolerable suffering." The guidelines were designed specifically to keep euthanasia occurrences few and far between by establishing demanding conditions that had to be met, at the risk of criminal prosecution. Over time, however, doctors began to interpret the conditions loosely and even to ignore them. In the few circumstances where the law took notice, it accommodated expanded euthanasia through continual loosening of the meaning of the guidelines.

This is the typical pattern of the euthanasia movement. Killing by doctors is always presented to the public as a "rare" occurrence, an option used only when nothing else can be done. Proponents soothingly assure a doubtful public, as the New York euthanasia advocate Dr. Timothy Quill puts it, that euthanasia will be restricted to "the patient of last resort, [to be] taken only when hospice care stops providing comfort and dignity," when "all alternatives have been exhausted."[9] Unfortunately, when put into actual practice, as the Dutch experience clearly demonstrates, it quickly ceases to be rare or resorted to only when all else fails. Instead, in the words of Dr. K. F. Gunning, perhaps the most notable Dutch opponent of euthanasia, "Once you accept killing as a solution for a single problem, you will find tomorrow hundreds of problems for which killing can be seen as a solution."[10]

In the twenty-plus years since euthanasia was redefined in the Netherlands as a legitimate tool of medical practice instead of a serious crime, cultural biases have changed. No longer constrained by conscience or culture, thanks to a redefinition of euthanasia as medical treatment instead of killing, Dutch doctors now terminate categories of people whose assisted deaths would have once provoked outrage, and do so in numbers that were not anticipated when the practice was first promoted in 1973. "Since my country came to accept euthanasia, there has been a steady increase in the categories of people who can be killed," says Dr. Gunning. "The numbers of cases in which doctors consciously cause their patients' death in my country is frightening."[11] Rather than being rare, statistics show that euthanasia is now almost a matter of medical routine.

The Remmelink Report

In 1990, responding to the heated debate about Dutch euthanasia and the many anecdotes being told internationally about involuntary killings of patients by doctors, the Dutch government decided to determine how euthanasia was actually being carried out and appointed an investigative committee. Called the Committee to Investigate the Medical Practice Concerning Euthanasia, it was commonly known as the Remmelink Commission, after the committee's chairman, Professor J. Remmelink, then the attorney general of the Dutch Supreme Court.

The Remmelink Commission conducted three studies. In the first, a retrospective study, more than four hundred physicians were interviewed about their opinions on the practice of euthanasia. Then for six months the same physicians were asked to record and report their actions in cases with a fatal outcome. Finally, a representative sampling of deaths was taken from the register at the Central Statistics Office, and the physicians who had been involved in the care of the deceased were asked to provide information about the cases. In all three instances, the doctors' anonymity was guaranteed.

The commission's two-volume report, known as the Remmelink Report, was issued in 1991.[12] It was intended to reassure the public that euthanasia was rare and that the existing guidelines were effective in controlling the practice. This was done, in part, by severely restricting the definition of "euthanasia" to the deliberate termination of another's life at his or her request, usually accomplished by a lethal injection of a sedative and a curare-like poison. Cases that did not explicitly fit this category were not called euthanasia. A doctor's lethally injecting a patient without request, which as we shall see is not an uncommon occurrence in the Netherlands, was called not involuntary or nonvoluntary euthanasia but rather "termination of life without patient's explicit request." (Some Dutch doctors call the act "life-terminating treatment," proving that the Dutch are not above resorting to euphemisms.) Other acts of intentional killing, such as purposefully overdosing a patient with pain-control medication for the purposes of killing him, also fell outside the Remmelink Report's working definition of euthanasia.

Although it dubiously narrowed the definition of euthanasia, to its credit the Remmelink Report did include the complete statistical data upon which its conclusions were based. Independent analysis of this rich source of information had a profoundly negative impact on the world's view of Dutch euthanasia. According to the Remmelink Report, about 130,000 people die each year in the Netherlands.[13] Of these, approximately 43,300, or about one-third, die suddenly—from catastrophic heart attacks, stroke, accidents and the like—thus precluding medical decision making about end-of-life care.[14] That leaves approximately 90,000 people whose deaths involve end-of-life medical decision making each year.

With that in mind, here are the figures about euthanasia-related deaths in 1990, derived from the Remmelink Report's published statistical data:

- 2,300 patients were euthanized (killed) by their doctors upon request and 400 people died through physician-assisted suicide, for a total of 2,700 doctor-induced deaths.[15] That is approximately 3 percent of all deaths involving end-of-life medical care. The equivalent percentage in the United States would be approximately 41,500 deaths.
- 1,040 died from involuntary euthanasia, lethal injections given without request or consent—three deaths every single day.[16] These deaths constitute slightly more than 1 percent of all cases involving end-of-life medical care. (The same percentage in the United States would be approximately 16,000 involuntary killings per year.)

- Of these involuntary euthanasia cases, 14 percent, or 145, were fully competent to make their own medical decisions but were killed without request or consent anyway.[17] (The same percentage in the United States would be more than 2,000 who would be killed.) Moreover, 72 percent of the people killed without their consent had never given any indication that they would want their lives terminated.[18]

- 8,100 patients died from an intentional overdose of morphine or other pain-control medications.[19] In other words, death was not a side effect of treatment to relieve pain, which can sometimes occur, but was the *intended result* of the overdose. Of these, 61 percent (4,941 patients) were intentionally overdosed without request or consent. The equivalent percentage in the United States would amount to approximately 78,000 deaths.

These figures are startling. Of the approximately 90,000 Dutch people whose deaths involved end-of-life medical decision making in 1990, 11,140 were intentionally killed (euthanized) or assisted in suicide—or 11.1 percent of all Dutch deaths involving medical decision making! This is approximately 8.5 percent of Dutch deaths from all causes. Of these killings, *more than half were involuntary* (1,040 involuntary lethal injections and 4,941 involuntary intentional overdoses). Applying these percentages to U.S. population figures, the equivalent would be 170,000 deaths each year caused by euthanasia or assisted suicide, with about 85,000 of these involuntary, more than the current number of U.S. suicides and homicides combined.[20]

It should also be kept in mind that the Remmelink statistics probably underestimate the actual number of deaths caused by euthanasia and assisted suicide. A study conducted by the Free University at Amsterdam revealed that two-thirds of Dutch general practitioners have certified a patient's death as resulting from natural causes when in fact it was euthanasia or assisted suicide.[21] Another Dutch study arrived at a similar conclusion, finding that only 28 percent of doctors were honest about their euthanasia killings when filling out death certificates.[22] Moreover, a study conducted by the Medicolegal Group of Limburg University in Maastricht found that 41.1 percent of doctors who participated in the survey admitted to having engaged in involuntary euthanasia.

A more recent Dutch study, written up in the *New England Journal of Medicine* in November 1996, found that only 41 percent of all euthanasia deaths were reported to the authorities. This same study revealed that 23 percent of physicians interviewed had killed patients without having received an explicit request. Also mentioned is a new wrinkle not touched upon in the Remmelink Report: At least half of Dutch physicians take the initiative by *suggesting* euthanasia to their patients.[23] In a similar vein, a 2003 study published in the British medical journal *The Lancet* found that "the rate of euthanasia had significantly increased" between 1995 and 2001, while "the rate of ending life without a patient's explicit request" remained virtually unchanged.[24]

Guidelines That Do Not Protect

In 1999, a statistical analysis of Dutch euthanasia practices published in the *Journal of Medical Ethics* concluded that the Dutch promises of "effective regulation ring hollow" and that killing by doctors in the Netherlands "remains beyond effective control."[25] And for good reason: As University of Haifa professor Raphael Cohen-Almagoran, a self-described ideological believer in euthanasia, admitted in his 2004 book *Euthanasia in the Netherlands: The Policy and Practice of Mercy Killing*, Dutch euthanasia policy:

> does not work because all of the guidelines, without exception, are broken time and time again. It is not always the patient who makes the request for euthanasia or physician-assisted suicide. Often the doctor proposes euthanasia to the patient. Sometimes, the family initiates a request. The requirement that the request be voluntary is thus compromised. On occasion, the patient's request is not well considered.... [T]here have been cases in which no request was made and patients were put to death.... Once cannot expect a policy that would work 100 percent of the time, but given the many frequent breaches of all the Guidelines, the Dutch should invest effort to find remedies and prevent abuse and lawlessness.[26]

Cohen-Almagor was so shaken by his findings that he no longer supports the legalization of euthanasia, although, being ideologically committed to "giving patients better control over life and death," he still supports assisted suicide.[27]

Beginning with the Remmelink Report and continuing thereafter with virtually every other study of Dutch euthanasia practices, report after report has demonstrated clearly that guidelines do not protect and do not restrict. And why should they? The Dutch government has clearly indicated it has no interest in forcing doctors to toe the line by rarely prosecuting doctors who violate euthanasia regulations, and in the rare case of a conviction, never imposing meaningful punishment. For example, a Dutch nurse was given a two-month suspended sentence for killing an AIDS patient, receiving the sanction not because she killed but because she was not a physician.[28] Meanwhile, when doctors kill people who have not asked to die, they generally receive no punishment of any kind. For example, the *British Medical Journal* reported on a general practitioner who killed his elderly comatose patient with a lethal injection, and was convicted of murder but received no penalty of any kind despite having violated virtually every protective guideline.[29] As a Dutch ethicist retorted when I brought these matters up in a February 2003 "Brainstorm" debate sponsored by the Fulbright Commission in Lisbon, "Yes, we have guidelines to tell doctors proper methods of practice, but of course, they should not be enforced."

But the issue goes much deeper than law enforcement authorities refusing to enforce the rules. What euthanasia really did to the Dutch was to alter profoundly the nation's conception of right and wrong. With the widespread acceptance of a euthanasia consciousness in the Netherlands, the guideline limitations became mere window dressing that made little actual difference at the bedside to doctors or, indeed, to much of the general public. Finding the proverbial exception to the rule became a standard practice, which in turn soon changed the exception into the rule. The official guidelines then expanded to meet the actual practice.

These cases have real faces. Dr. Gunning tells of one such tragic circumstance: "A friend of mine, an internist, was asked to see a lady with terminal lung cancer, who had a short time to live and was very short of breath. After the examination, he asked the patient to come to the hospital on Saturday for a few days so that be could alleviate her distress. She refused, being afraid of being euthanized there. My friend assured his patient that he would be on duty and that no such thing would happen. So the lady came. On Sunday night she was breathing normally and feeling much better. The doctor went home. When he came back on Monday afternoon, the patient was dead.

The doctor's colleague told him, 'What is the sense of having that woman here? It makes no difference whether she dies today or after two weeks. We need the bed for another case.'"[30] In other words, the woman was euthanized against her explicit wishes simply to accommodate the killing doctor's priorities.

The psychiatrist Dr. Herbert Hendin, medical director of the American Foundation for Suicide Prevention, is one of the world's foremost experts on Dutch euthanasia. Over the last several years, Hendin has held extensive discussions with Dutch doctors who euthanize patients and has reviewed the records of actual cases. Dr. Hendin believes that many doctors in the Netherlands feel justified in performing involuntary euthanasia because a system that permits them to kill "encourages some to feel entitled to make [euthanasia] decisions without consulting the patient."[31] As an example, Hendin recounts his interview with a pro-euthanasia doctor who justified killing a nun who had requested not to be killed on the basis of religious belief, because *he felt* she was in too much pain.[32]

It is not only the many involuntary killings that violate Dutch guidelines. Dr. Hendin describes his conversation with a Dutch doctor who has euthanized between fifty and one hundred patients. One of the cases in which he consulted was that of an elderly woman who wanted to die, not because she was ill but because she was haunted by memories of being a concentration camp survivor.[33] How could this case possibly meet the guidelines? The woman was not ill. The doctor in question was a family practitioner, not a psychiatrist, and there appears to have been no sustained attempt to alleviate the poor woman's anguish. Despite this, in an act that reeks of tragic irony, the doctor put her to death and is now afflicted himself by his memory of her.[34]

To prove the existence of cases that violate the official guidelines, it is not necessary to rely on anecdotal evidence. Such cases have even been documented in euthanasia-friendly documentaries originally produced in the Netherlands and later shown in the United States. One such documentary, broadcast over public television on the program *The Health Quarterly* in 1993, revealed how broadly the Dutch guidelines are interpreted—that is to say, how commonly they are ignored.[35]

One case documented in the film concerns a man named Henk

Dykema, who at the time of filming was asymptomatic HIV-positive. Dykema feared the afflictions that he expected to befall him and had been asking his doctor to kill him for more than a year. The film shows the doctor telling Henk that he might live for years at his current stage of infection, but the patient wants none of it. The doctor, a general practitioner, then discussed Henk's case with a colleague, also a general practitioner. Significantly, no psychiatrist was consulted or involved. Finally, the doctor agreed to provide a poisonous drug cocktail to Dykema, even though he was not suffering any significant physical symptoms.[36]

Dykema's assisted suicide was clearly not a last resort, as required by the Dutch guidelines. He and his doctor did not explore all other possible options, such as psychiatric treatment, which could well have alleviated his anxiety and depression. Nor was he told of the actions the doctor could have taken to relieve his suffering when he did become ill. The doctor didn't even wait until Henk had actual symptoms of AIDS. As Dr. Carlos Gomez, a specialist in hospice medicine at the University of Virginia and an expert on euthanasia issues, aptly put it, Dykema's physician was "responding to anticipation of suffering…which may or may not have been true. In a sense the physician was saying, 'You're absolutely right, your end is going to be a disaster.'"[37] Dr. Hendin, analyzing Dykema's case from a psychiatrist's perspective, commented, "the patient was clearly depressed. The doctor kept establishing that the man was persistent in his request, but did not address the terror that underlay it."[38] Now consider this: had the doctor called in suicide prevention experts to help Henk live instead of helping to kill him, Dykema might well have survived long enough to benefit from the protease inhibitors and other drugs that now extend the lives of HIV patients for many years.

The documentary shows another patient who was euthanized, a psychiatrist named Jan Stricht, who asked for euthanasia because he had blood clots on the brain. The malady was not terminal. Dr. Stricht, the viewer is told, might have lived "one year or twenty years."[39] Nor had the affliction caused significant physical pain. Rather, Dr. Stricht was emotionally upset at his greatly reduced physical capacities, caused primarily by significant difficulties in depth perception and other such motor deficiencies.

Dr. Stricht's own physician, a general practitioner, described the case as one of "mental suffering." The depressed man was feeling the effects of being dependent on others for the necessities of life: "I can depend on other people to do things, but the bad thing is they want to do it their way and not my way, so they don't help me.... I have to eat what they decide that I have to eat, which I don't want to eat at all.... Or, I want to drink, and they say, 'You drink too much. It's wrong to do.'"[40] Stricht's upset at his growing dependence was seen by the doctor as legitimate reason to provide euthanasia. Tellingly, the doctor took no effort to address and correct Stricht's legitimate complaints about the quality of his caregiving.

The documentary also shows Maria, a twenty-five-year-old woman with anorexia nervosa, asking for euthanasia. She is in remission but fears a recurrence of her malady, saying: "I've thought about dying day and night, and I know that if relief does not come, I will return to the old pattern, the pattern of self-punishment, hurting myself. I know it. I feel it, and therefore I hope the release will come soon and I die."[41] Maria's doctor agrees to euthanize her, stating, "It is not possible to have a good quality of life for her." This case was even too much for the authorities, who brought charges against the doctor. However, the euthanasia consciousness had so permeated the justice system that a judge ruled that Maria's killing was justified because her suffering had made her life unbearable.

Similar tragedies can be found in many published investigations of Dutch euthanasia. For example, the *Oregonian* reported on a woman with skin cancer who was euthanized. She was not in pain, nor was she in a terminal stage of her illness. Rather, she was upset by the scars on her face and demanded euthanasia from her doctor, or else—the threat being that she would "jump from the balcony." Her doctor, to his later expressed regret, accommodated her wish to die.[42]

Studies indicate that families, rather than patients, generally decide when the time has come for euthanasia. According to Dr. Hendin, doctors called in such cases "usually advocate euthanasia," because they "support the relatives' desire to be free from the burden of caring for the patient."[43] One such case occurred when a wife told her husband to choose euthanasia or a nursing home. Not wanting to be cared for by strangers, he chose death. The doctor killed him, despite knowing of the coercion.[44]

Dr. Gunning tells of another such case related to him by a close physician friend of his who supports euthanasia: A man was hospitalized with terminal cancer and was in great pain. His son came to his father's doctor and said that the family wanted to bury the old man before they went on holiday. The doctor agreed and overdosed the man with pain-control medication. The next day, much to his shock, the old man was sitting up, feeling great. The intended overdose had not killed him but had killed the pain.[45]

Dancing with Mr. D, a revealing book written a few years ago by a Dutch doctor, Bert Keizer, demonstrated how farcical the protective guidelines have become in the Netherlands. Keizer works in a nursing home, where he cares for—and sometimes kills—disabled, elderly and dying people. He looks upon euthanasia as a necessary and proper, albeit distasteful, part of his job. As depicted in the book, so do his colleagues, his patients and their families.

Keizer is brutally honest in revealing his own attitudes about his patients. He depicts the lives of frail and dying people as pointless, useless, ugly, grotesque. Those with whom Keizer interacts all seem to share these views, including his colleagues, family members of patients, and the patients themselves. This allows Keizer to kill patients without any consequence other than having a few bad dreams.

And kill his patients Keizer does, again and again. One man he euthanizes probably has lung cancer but the diagnosis is never certain. A relative tells Keizer that the man wants to be given a lethal injection, a request later confirmed by the patient. Keizer quickly agrees to kill the man. Demonstrating the utter uselessness of "protective guidelines," he never tells his patient about treatment options or how the pain and other symptoms of cancer can be palliated effectively. He never checks to see if the man has been pressured into wanting a hastened death or is depressed. Keizer doesn't even take the time to confirm the diagnosis with certainty. When a colleague asks, why rush, and points out that the man isn't suffering terribly, Keizer snaps, "Is it for us to answer this question? All I know is that he wants to die more or less upright and that he doesn't want to crawl to his grave the way a dog crawls howling to the sidewalk after he's been hit by a car."[46]

Keizer either doesn't know or doesn't care that with proper medical treatment, people with lung cancer do not have to die in such unmitigated agony. The next day, he lethally injects his patient, telling his colleagues as he walks to the man's room to do the deed, "If anyone so much as whispers cortisone [a palliative agent] or 'uncertain diagnosis,' I'll hit him."[47]

Another of Keizer's patients is disabled by Parkinson's disease. The patient requests to be killed, but before the act can be carried out, he receives a letter from his brother, who uses a religious argument to urge him to change his mind. The letter causes the man to hesitate, upsetting Keizer, who writes, "I don't know what to do with such a wavering death wish. It's getting on my nerves. Does he want to die or doesn't he? I do hope we won't have to go over the whole business again, right from the very start."[48] Keizer involves the nursing home chaplain to assure the man that euthanasia will not upset God. The man again thinks he wants to die. Keizer is quick with the lethal injection, happy the man has "good veins," and the man expires before his uncertainty can disturb his doctor's mood again.

The guidelines in the Netherlands clearly protect nobody. But when you think about it, that is not their purpose. Their real purpose is to allow the Dutch people to ignore reality and pretend that killing can be controlled. But if doctors aren't punished for violating the killing regulations, if physicians like Keizer can kill patients when a cancer diagnosis isn't even finalized, if a young anorexic woman can be assisted in suicide because she fears she will keep punishing herself, if a doctor kills a woman on the basis of what the doctor himself calls "a case of vanity," if the guidelines allow families to push the death agenda regardless of the desires of their ill relatives, whom can they protect?

The answer is very clear to anybody willing to look beyond the romantic myths of euthanasia to the way it actually works in the real world: nobody.

Death on Demand Comes to the Netherlands

The Dutch psychiatrist Boutdewijn Chabot has written, "If one accepts, as I do, that persistently suicidal patients are indeed terminal, then one must ask whether a persistently suicidal state can be diagnosed as an incurable disease. I believe in some cases, like that of my patient, it can."[49]

Hilly Bosscher was just such a deeply depressed and suicidal woman. She had lost her two sons, one to suicide in 1986 and the other to brain cancer in 1991. Her marriage, never very good and often abusive, took a turn for the worse after her first son's death and was dissolved in 1990. Bosscher had briefly received psychiatric treatment years earlier for the depression and suicidal thoughts she experienced after her son's suicide. On the day her second son died, she failed in an attempt to kill herself. She still wanted to die but hesitated at self-destruction for fear that she would be hospitalized if she tried and failed again. However, she moved the graves of her two sons to the same cemetery and purchased a burial plot for herself so that she could be buried between them.[50]

Bosscher began to attend meetings of the Dutch Euthanasia Society, where she met Dr. Chabot, who attended meetings to troll for patients. She told Chabot that she didn't want therapy "because it would loosen the bonds with her deceased sons."[51] Chabot took her as a patient anyway and met with her on four occasions between August 2 and September 7, 1991. Chabot did not attempt to treat her. Rather, he interviewed her to determine her prognosis. After these interviews and his consultations, despite the complete absence of any physical illness, he agreed to help Bosscher kill herself, which he did on September 28, 1991.

Chabot was charged with the crime of assisted suicide. His lawyer was Eugene Sutorius, a charming man with a quick smile and a sharp legal mind that any attorney would admire. Sutorius was no stranger to euthanasia cases, being a legal adviser to the Dutch Voluntary Euthanasia Society and the lawyer primarily responsible over many years for pushing the boundaries of euthanasia in the Dutch courts. Sutorius recalled for me his legal argument on behalf of Dr. Chabot:

> My...plea was [that] the doctor acted justifiably in [a situation of] a conflict of duties—one, the preponderant duty, which is preserving human life, and the second is fighting suffering or preventing it.... In this case, the duties could not be reconciled, one could not be fulfilled

without violating the other.... So, I said, he could not escape the [patient's] request, and the request would be reasonable and understandable, and it would be according to his prognosis inevitable that the suffering would just continue.... So I argued that a doctor may, under very strict circumstances, be justified in giving the priority to the other duty, the duty to relieve suffering. And that, they [the court] accepted.[52]

According to Sutorius the prosecutor vigorously presented the case, but even so there was never much question of Chabot's actually being meaningfully punished:

The public prosecution, as a body, sees that this is not criminality in the normal sense. That he [the prosecutor] is not fighting real criminals here; he is fighting doctors that encounter a problem.... So, even the prosecutor, while bringing the case, he's more interested in making sure that we have strict definitions and order than he is in punishing the professional. He's trying to create a precedent. It's either yes or no, but he wants to make sure that there's order in society and that these things are done decently.[53]

Both the prosecutor and Sutorius got what they were looking for in the Chabot case. The lower court refused to punish the psychiatrist in any way, a decision blessed by the Dutch Supreme Court, with the minor caveat that Chabot erred by not having a colleague independently examine the patient. The basis of the ruling was that the law cannot distinguish between suffering caused by physical illness and suffering caused by mental anguish—which, of course, is where the logic of euthanasia inevitably leads. Thus, Dutch guidelines now permit doctors in the Netherlands to kill their depressed patients on the basis of patient demand caused by depression, even if the patient refuses treatment that might overcome the suicidal fixation. In other words, in the Netherlands, people with a significant depression can obtain death virtually on demand.

Killing Babies

In the Netherlands, infants are killed because they have birth defects, and doctors justify the practice. One Dutch pediatrician explained, "Some patients, if you withhold or withdraw treatment, the child will not die immediately. It might take hours or days or weeks. And then, I think it's better to support the child to die, and to help the child to die, and that's actually what we are doing, of course, in very rare occasions."[54]

Thanks to another "prosecution" of a doctor who euthanized an infant, the courts have begun to open the door for euthanasia to legally enter the pediatric ward. Dr. Henk Prins killed a three-day-old girl who was born with spina bifida, hydrocephaly and leg deformities. The doctor—a gynecologist, not a pediatrician or a medical expert in such cases, although experts were consulted—was defended by Sutorius. Prins testified in the trial court that he killed the child, with her parents' permission, because of the infant's poor prognosis and because the baby screamed in pain when touched. Yet the child was in agony because she was neglected medically. The open wound in her back, the primary characteristic of spina bifida, had not been closed, nor had the fluid been drained from her head, even though these medical treatments, which are standard in spina bifida cases, would have substantially reduced her pain. The trial court refused to punish the doctor. Indeed, the judge praised Dr. Prins for "his integrity and courage and wished him well in any further legal proceedings he may face."[55]

A 1997 study published in *The Lancet* revealed how deeply pediatric euthanasia had metastasized into Dutch neonatal medical practice. According to the report, doctors killed approximately 8 percent of all infants who died in the Netherlands in 1995. Assuming this to be typical, this amounts to approximately 80 or 90 infanticides per year. Of these, one-third would have lived more than a month. At least 10 to 15 of these killings involve infants who do not depend on life-sustaining treatment to stay alive. The study found that 45 percent of neonatologists and 31 percent of pediatricians who responded to the questionnaire had killed infants.[56]

A follow-up study of end-of-life decisions made for infants, published in April 9, 2005, found that nothing had changed. In 2001, in 8 percent of cases, drugs were administered to infants "with the explicit intention to hasten death."[57]

In 2004, Groningen University Medical Center made international headlines when it admitted to permitting pediatric euthanasia and published the "Groningen Protocol," infanticide guidelines the hospital used when killing 15 to 20 disabled newborns each year."[58] The Protocol creates three categories of killable infants: those with "no chance of survival"; those who have "a poor prognosis and are dependent on intensive care"; and infants with "a hopeless prognosis," including those "not depending on intensive medical treatment but for whom a very poor quality of life...is predicted."[59] Par for the course, authorities refused to prosecute even though pediatric infanticide is murder under Dutch law.

Apologists for the infanticide applauded Dutch doctors for going public with the Protocol. "As things are," Eduard Verhagan, head of Groningen's children's clinic, told the Associated Press, "people are doing this secretly and that is wrong. In the Netherlands we want to expose everything to let everything be subject to vetting."[60]

Secrecy? What secrecy? It has been widely known for years that Dutch doctors kill disabled and dying babies—as demonstrated in *The Lancet* study of 1995 infanticides (published in 1997), cited above. Indeed, a 1990 report of the Royal Dutch Medical Association (KNMG), "Life-Terminating Actions with Incompetent Patients," set forth "requirements for careful medical practice" when ending the lives of handicapped newborns. The standard for permitting pediatric euthanasia was based on what Dutch doctors call an "unlivable life."[61] If this sounds familiar, it is: It differs little in its bigoted view of the value of disabled people from the attitudes expressed by Binding and Hoche in 1920 in *Permitting the Destruction of Life Not Worthy of Life*.

According to current Dutch medical ethics, the "livableness" of a life depends on a combination of factors, including the following:
- The expected measure of suffering (not only bodily but also emotional—the level of hopelessness)
- The expected potential for communication and human relationships
- Independence (ability to move, to care for oneself, to live independently)
- Self-realization (being able to hear, read, write, labor)
- The child's life expectancy.[61]

If the infant's "prospects" don't measure up to what the doctor and the parents believe is a life worth living, the child can be neglected to death or, if that doesn't work, killed.

The Dutch government-supported documentary that I described earlier included the stories of infanticides of infants who were not terminally ill.[62] Indeed, viewers of the program learned that three out of eight neonatal intensive care units in the Netherlands already had adopted specific policies—endorsed by the Dutch Pediatric Society—permitting infanticide by lethal injection.

The publication of the Groningen Protocol isn't designed to end the secret that is not a secret. It is intended to legitimize eugenic infanticide and move it, in the typical Dutch fashion, from a technical crime tolerated by the so very tolerant Dutch, to outright legality. In other words, the last tenuous vestige of protection left in the Netherlands against infanticide—that is, its technical illegality—is to be stripped away, even for disabled babies not dependent on life support for survival.

Some Dutch doctors and ethicists rationalize these policies by resorting to hard utilitarianism, asserting that the value of a life "depends on how valuable that life is for other people." Most rhetorical justifications of Dutch infanticide, however, are couched in more compassionate tones, stressing that the killing is in the best interests of the child. Thus, the State Committee on Euthanasia of the KNMG declared support for killing newborns—as well as minors, mentally retarded persons, and the demented elderly—if "one can suppose that were the patients to express their will, they would opt for euthanasia." It is doubtful that actual disabled people are often let into the decision making about whose lives are livable and whose lives are best ended. They might have a contrary point of view.

INFANTS ARE NOT THE ONLY CHILDREN who are eligible for euthanasia. Pediatric oncologists have provided a *hulp bij zelfoding* (self-help for ending life) program for adolescents since the 1980s, in which poisonous doses are prescribed for minors with terminal illness.[63] Moreover, children who want physician-assisted death may be able to receive it without the consent of their parents. A 1986 report issued by the Central Committee of the Royal Dutch Medical Association explained its position on euthanasia of older minors:

> The Central Committee is not in favour of including an exact limit in the law with respect to the "rights" of parents in the case of a minor making a request for euthanasia. Nor is the Central Committee in

favour of giving a right of veto to one or both parents in such cases. The Central Committee does hold the view, however, that the physician should always consult the parents about their child's request for euthanasia. But with a view to the child's own good, *this does not imply that parents have the power of decision.* It goes without saying that where a young child is concerned, the state of affairs will be different from those where an older child is concerned

We would like to advocate not to include a separate age limit in the law, as it may be impossible as well as unjust in our opinion to lay down an exact age limit in this matter. Sometimes, a 15-year-old child can have a mature judgment. At all times, it will be a matter of acting carefully in medical respect. [Emphasis added.][64]

As these words are written, Dutch euthanasia advocates are agitating to reduce the age of consent to euthanasia to twelve years.

Falling Off a Vertical Cliff

Where next for Dutch euthanasia? In 2001, despite the many problems—only some of which have been described in this chapter—the Netherlands formally legalized euthanasia. The guidelines that have proved so inadequate to their protective task remain. Only now, doctors don't even have to report their killing activities to a prosecutor, but only to a euthanasia-supporting medical board.

But even this broad license isn't enough for the death fundamentalists that drive the Dutch euthanasia agenda. For example, on the day after the new law took effect, Els Borst, the Dutch minister of health, suggested that elderly people who are "tired of life" and who do not otherwise qualify for euthanasia should be given access to a "suicide pill" to end their lives. Borst cited two ninety-five-year-olds she knows as a reason for the Department of Justice to permit the distribution of a suicide pill: "They were bored stiff, but alas, not bored to death."[65]

Any pretense of control and "limits" is evaporating before our very eyes. In 2000, a Dutch doctor was found to have acted properly when he euthanized a healthy eighty-six-year-old man who wanted to die because he was "living a pointless and empty existence." The man was depressed about his "physical decline" due to aging and the deaths of friends. In other words, the euthanasia was justified based on the social decline of the patient. Despite this, the doctor was acquitted of any crime, the court ruling that the man's "hopeless existence" justified the euthanasia.[66] In 2003, this was overturned by the Dutch Supreme Court, but the court also ruled that the violation was "so minor that any form of punishment would be inappropriate."[67]

Many Dutch physicians were furious at the Supreme Court's ruling, and in response, the Royal Dutch Medical Association sponsored a study of whether and how to permit euthanasia for patients without a specific physical or psychological diagnosis. There was never any real doubt that the authors would propose liberalizing the already radical euthanasia license. In January 2005, authors of the investigation urged that doctors be allowed to kill "patients who are suffering through living." Jos Dijkhuis, an emeritus professor of clinical psychology who led the inquiry, stated to the *British Medical Journal* that "a doctor's task is to reduce suffering," and therefore, "we can't exclude these cases [those that can't be classified as having an explicit physical or psychological cause] in advance. We must now look further to see if we can draw a line and if so, where."[68]

Which raises an obvious question: Why bother? Any "strict guidelines" that were crafted would not be strict and would not be enforced.

Drawing Conclusions

One of the pioneers of Dutch euthanasia, Dr. Pieter Admiraal, who has killed more than one hundred patients, told me, "Of our doctors, 84 percent will give euthanasia, while 16 percent will not. Of these 16 percent, most will send patients to another doctor for euthanasia. Only a few will not participate either directly or indirectly.... If you come to euthanasia like we did, you will come to the same result."[69]

I doubt that the Dutch physicians who died resisting Nazi pressure to begin killing their weakest and most vulnerable patients would admire Dr. Admiraal and his colleagues today. They would be horrified and appalled.

Unlike the Dutch, Americans do not come to the decision about whether to accept legalized euthanasia blindly. We have the Dutch experience to guide us. On the basis of their experience with euthanasia, what can we learn about the death culture? First, as Dr. Gunning put it, the Dutch have proved that once killing is accepted as a solution for one problem, tomorrow it will be seen as the solution for hundreds of problems. Once we accept the killing of terminally ill patients, as did the Dutch, we will invariably accept the killing of chronically ill patients, depressed patients, and ultimately even children.

Second, the substantive differences between the Dutch and the U.S. health care systems mean that the U.S. experience with the death culture would likely be far *worse* than that in the Netherlands. The Dutch have virtually universal health coverage. In the United States, on the other hand, tens of millions of Americans are without health insurance, which means they often receive inadequate health care. Moreover, for-profit health maintenance organizations are putting great financial pressure on the health-care system and are imposing a financial conflict of interest between patients and their own doctors by punishing physicians financially if they provide too much care. Although cost containment is an issue in the Netherlands, financial pressures to hasten death are much more muted there than they would likely be here.

Third, the Netherlands is a much more tolerant society than we are, generally more accepting of differences among people, such as those of race, gender and sexual orientation. These nonjudgmental attitudes filter into the Dutch medical practice. It is to be expected that the prevailing American prejudices would filter more strongly into our medical practice. An editorial in the *New England Journal of Medicine* cited a plethora of studies that uncovered significant race-based inequality in the delivery of health care in the United States, and opined that the disparities in the delivery of health care apparently caused by racism need to be focused upon with the "rigor and attention given to other health concerns of similar magnitude."[70] These and other factors make it likely that legalizing and especially "routinizing" euthanasia in the United States would be especially dangerous for marginalized populations.

A legitimate question then: If euthanasia is so bad, why do a majority of the Dutch people support their country's policy? I put this very question to W. C. M. Kijn, a retired professor of medical ethics who served as a member of a government-appointed committee in the Netherlands that investigated whether euthanasia should be formally legalized and wrote the minority report recommending against legalization. Professor Klijn told me: "We Dutch pride ourselves on our history. We see ourselves as having been good in the past; therefore, we believe that we will always be good. It is an arrogance of goodness. Thus, even though there are striking resemblances to our euthanasia practices and those the Nazis sought to impose upon us, we assure ourselves: We resisted the Nazis. We are sophisticated, humane. We can't be doing wrong! To admit we are wrong on euthanasia would be to say that we are not the compassionate, sophisticated, enlightened people we think we are. It is very hard in the Dutch character to do that."[71]

Professor Klijn also believes that the Dutch, much like the people of the United States, have an almost reflexive response to arguments based on "personal autonomy." Because this concept is so deeply ingrained in the Dutch and the American value systems, many people, upon hearing the magic word "choice," quickly make up their minds and don't have the time or inclination to dig deeper. They don't see the whole picture: the abuses, the destruction of family cohesiveness, or the paternalism inherent in euthanasia, because the decision as to whether one lives or dies often depends more on the doctor's values than on the patient's.

Dr. van der Sluis, a secularist opponent of his country's euthanasia policies, raises another point germane to the ongoing debate in the United States. Many Dutch accept euthanasia so as not to be perceived as overly religious. "The proponents of euthanasia have falsely, but successfully, cast the argument as one of religion versus rationality," Dr. van der Sluis told me. "They assert that only fundamentalist Christians oppose euthanasia, and since few Dutch are fundamentalist Christians, they tend to support euthanasia." [72] Dr. Pieter Admiraal verified this point when he told me, "The only way to deny euthanasia is based on religion. Most Dutch are nonbelievers, and thus they must support euthanasia."[73]

Dr. Herbert Hendin discovered another interesting reason why euthanasia may be accepted by the Dutch: The case studies, only some of which are recounted here, are not widely discussed in the Netherlands out of "loyalty to the system" and in order not to threaten the delicate consensus that has developed concerning the

practice. Dr. Hendin writes that several Dutch euthanasia proponents admitted that they are not candid in their discussions about
euthanasia "for political considerations." They don't want to "play
into the hands of the Christian Democrats," the minority opposition
party that opposes euthanasia.[74] Moreover, Dr. Hendin discovered
that the Dutch are exquisitely sensitive to being criticized, and that
"savage criticisms" of Dutch euthanasia policies by "physicians in
the rest of Europe" have "forced the Dutch into a defensive position."[75] He also noted, "Virtually all of those who have played a role
in advancing the cause of euthanasia [in the Netherlands] on
humanitarian grounds were concerned about the problems in implementation yet seemed disinclined to express their doubts publicly."[76]
Hendin confronted one such proponent who had published an article in favor of euthanasia that broadly contradicted his private
conversations with Hendin. The doctor justified his hypocrisy on the
basis of his not "wish[ing] to be critical of the system or perhaps to
be viewed as being so in a culture in which uncritical support for
Dutch euthanasia policies is politically correct."[77]

More than twenty years of legitimized euthanasia may also
have desensitized the Dutch to activities that they once would have
found abhorrent. One documentary televised on the Dutch television network showed the actual killing of a man with amyotrophic
lateral sclerosis (ALS), generally known in this country as Lou
Gehrig's disease, by his doctor. Even this documentary, intended to
promote the legitimacy of euthanasia, showed how the Dutch
euthanasia guidelines offer little actual protection. For example, the
doctor who provides the required second opinion tells the patient
bluntly, "You have an incurable disease which will soon end in
death, and unless there is some intervention you will experience terrible suffering. You will probably suffocate."[78]

In fact, according to Dame Cicely Saunders, the creator of the
English hospice movement, if people with ALS receive proper care,
they do not suffocate. She has helped more than three hundred such
patients die with dignity in hospice, so she should know. (I have
confirmed this assessment with several U.S. neurologists and hospice doctors.) Yet neither the patient's doctor nor the rubber-stamp
consultant bothered to tell the patient this news, which might have
caused him to change his mind about being killed. (An edited ver-

sion of this documentary was shown in the United States on December 8, 1994, on ABC's magazine show *Primetime Live*.)

Another example of the desensitization of a nation to indecency was a program aired on Dutch television that was partly financed by the Dutch Ministry of Health, called *A Matter of Life and Death*. The broadcast consisted of six segments; in each, two seriously disabled patients were pitted against each other. Both tell the audience about themselves and their respective illness and describe their current prognosis. The audience then votes on which of the two should receive life-prolonging treatment and which should not. The Dutch government defended the show as an effort to stimulate discussion about reducing health-care costs.[79]

Then there is the case of the little girl who fell into a lake and drowned. Normally, such a story would not be national news. But in this case, "Two hundred people stopped eating sandwiches, playing Frisbee, or walking the dog, and stood. Some moved to the bank and watched the girl drown. No one tried to help."[80] The little girl's death, captured on video, shook the Netherlands in much the same way that the Rodney King video did this country, as the Dutch, "in a rare moment of self-examination," wondered and worried about the decline of their culture.[81]

Of course, these anecdotes don't prove anything one way or the other about whether euthanasia has adversely affected the Dutch national character. It is interesting to note, however, that some Dutch no longer trust their doctors. The Dutch Patients Association, a patients' rights group with sixty thousand members, distributes a wallet card to protect members from being involuntarily euthanized. The card specifically states that it is "intended to prevent involuntary euthanasia in case of admission of the signer to the hospital" and instructs that "no treatment be administered with the intention to terminate life."[82]

Nonetheless, the Dutch euthanasia virus is catching. A 2000 report found that 10 percent of Belgian deaths appear to result from euthanasia.[83] With Belgian doctors clearly eager to follow the lead of their Dutch neighbor, Belgium formally legalized euthanasia in 2002. Notably, the first Belgian case, the killing of a man with multiple sclerosis, violated the guidelines; and just as occurs routinely in the Netherlands, the doctor involved faced no consequences. Now Bel-

gium is set to legalize euthanasia for children. Two Belgian legislators justify their plan to permit children to ask for their own mercy
killing on the basis that young people "have as much right to
choose" euthanasia as anyone else. Yet, these same children who are
supposedly mature enough to decide to die would be ineligible to
obtain a driver's license.[84]

And, in a striking example of how a belief in beneficent killing
leads quickly to the fall off a vertical moral cliff, Belgian doctors in
Flanders have been found to commit infanticide in about the same
numbers as their Dutch counterparts. Moreover, according to a
study published in *The Lancet*, nearly 70 percent "of the physicians
questioned…had either used lethal drugs for this purpose [to end
infants' lives] or could conceive of situations in which they would
use them."[85]

Meanwhile, the Swiss have blazed a different trail to hastened
death. Recognizing that killing is not really a medical act, the Swiss
permit laypeople to assist suicides so long as the motive is "altruistic." Doctors are not permitted to euthanize patients nor to assist
suicides in their professional capacities, although doctors can, like
any other Swiss citizen, assist a suicide so long as their participation
is not for "selfish" reasons.[86] Most assisted suicides are facilitated by
assisted suicide lay organizations, such as one called Dignitas. These
groups set their own standards for agreeing to help suicidal people—which may include the disabled and some who are mentally
ill—end their lives. One need not be a Swiss citizen to gain access to
these death services; this has led to the recent phenomenon of people traveling to Switzerland to gain help in dying, known as
"suicide tourism."[87]

FIVE

INVENTING THE RIGHT TO DIE

I N 1992, JACK KEVORKIAN SERIOUSLY PROPOSED in the *American Journal of Forensic Psychiatry* that a pilot program of death clinics be established in Michigan. The clinics, which he called "obitoria," would be staffed by physician-killers known as "obitiatrists," who would be permitted legally to terminate patients who request it, in a procedure Kevorkian then called "medicide"* but now labels "patholysis."[1] Kevorkian foresaw that the first "patients" to receive medicide would be the terminally and chronically ill. However, he looked forward to the eventual widening of obitiatry to include people he labeled "patients tortured by other than organic diseases."[2]

At the time, such an idea seemed fantastical, almost laughable, appropriate to science fiction movies such as *Soylent Green* rather than serious intellectual discourse. Not anymore. Euthanasia is no longer confined to debates in ethics classes or late-night musing among friends over drinks. Indeed, in the last fifteen years determined and never-ending political and legal actions undertaken by euthanasia advocates and their lawyers brought assisted suicide to

---

*Kevorkian used the term for being killed by a doctor. But medicide really means to kill a doctor. When the Oakland County medical examiner Dr. Ljubisa J. Dragovic pointed out the actual meaning of "medicide" to local reporters, Kevorkian took some ribbing among the press. Later, after Kevorkian helped kill Ali Khalili, a physician, Dragovic told me he received an anonymous phone call on his voice mail, saying, "Ha, ha, ha. The first medicide has been accomplished." Dr. Ljubisa J. Dragovic, interview with author, August 21, 1996.

legal reality in Oregon and could make it a national constitutional right. Opponents can no longer afford the luxury of assuming that "it can never happen here."

Initiatives and Propositions

It is quite shocking to realize that the modern euthanasia movement has been with us for less than twenty years. It was only in 1988 that the first attempt was made to qualify a euthanasia legalization initiative on California's ballot. And that effort failed miserably; proponents were unable to obtain enough signatures to qualify for the ballot.

Rather than being discouraged by their California failure, death fundamentalists redoubled their efforts. In 1991 they tried again, this time succeeding in qualifying a euthanasia legalization initiative in the state of Washington. Known as Initiative 119, the proposal would have permitted doctors to lethally inject patients under some circumstances. The early polls had the proposal far ahead, with some polls exceeding 70 percent approval. But that was before the anti-119 forces were able to present the reasons why legalizing euthanasia is a dangerous and unwise idea. In the end, support for euthanasia plummeted in Washington, and Initiative 119 lost by 54 percent to 46 percent.

Encouraged by the relatively narrow margin of their loss, however, euthanasia advocates got right back to work. Again California was targeted, and Proposition 161, a proposal that was almost identical to Initiative 119, successfully qualified for the November 1992 ballot.

The campaign over Proposition 161 was a virtual replay of the earlier Washington struggle. Once again, early polls showed public support in the 70 percentile range. But as usually is the case in debates over legalizing euthanasia, the more California voters learned about euthanasia and the more they considered the consequences that would flow from permitting doctors to kill, the less they liked Proposition 161. Following Washington's lead, California rejected legalized euthanasia by 54 to 46 percent. Next, it was on to Oregon, where a different political strategy would lead to a dramatic victory for the death culture.

In Oregon, euthanasia proponents received that deeply longed-for, foot-in-the-door breakthrough in 1994 with the passage of Measure 16—albeit with a bare 51 percent of the vote—and nothing has been the same since.

The campaign for Measure 16 illustrates the step-by-step political tactic that euthanasia advocates believe offers their best hope of establishing a broad euthanasia license: When necessary, take a half-step back in order to propel the euthanasia cause two steps forward. But never stop agitating. Never stop pushing. Never stop propagandizing. Wear down opponents.

Realizing that Initiative 119 and Proposition 161 had been too ambitious in seeking to authorize doctors to lethally inject patients as in the Netherlands, the authors of Measure 16 wrote the law in minimalist terms to make it appear less threatening and radical. Instead of lethal injections, doctors would "only" be permitted to write lethal prescriptions that the patient would self-administer.

Both sides in the debate over legalizing euthanasia entered the Measure 16 campaign with reason for optimism. Opponents, buoyed by the victories in Washington and California, believed that an appropriately hard-hitting campaign would convince the people of Oregon to reject physician-induced death. Proponents believed that their clever shift of responsibility for suicide from doctors to patients would make the proposal more defensible. Moreover, initial polls showed support for the initiative in the high 60 percent range.

The "Yes on 16" campaign led by Oregon Right to Die chose as its poster woman a nurse named Patty A. Rosen, head of the Bend, Oregon, chapter of the Hemlock Society. Rosen claimed in commercials to have helped her daughter, who was dying from bone cancer, to kill herself some years before. In the ads she labeled herself a "criminal" because she had obtained the pills for her pain-racked daughter to swallow, and asserted that she had done so because her daughter "couldn't bear to be touched." Her voice cracking with emotion, Rosen recounted, "As she slipped peacefully away, I climbed into her bed and I took her in my arms for the first time in months." It was a poignant, touching bit of advocacy that left few viewers unmoved and fewer still thinking about the vital issues of the campaign, such as the potential for abuses; societal consequences; the availability and underutilization of compassionate caregiving opportunities like effective pain control (effective even for bone cancer when properly applied); and whether doctor-induced death would really reduce human suffering.

Emotionalism and fear mongering about suffering and death were not the only tactics of Measure 16's proponents. There was also an unsubtle appeal to Oregon voters' reputed parochialism, mixed in with a strong dose of Catholic bashing.

The Catholic Church was very closely associated with the "No on 16" campaign, as it had been with the campaigns to defeat Initiative 119 and Proposition 161. Catholics provided significant funds to the "No on 16" campaign, and church representatives were often selected by the media to express anti–Measure 16 sentiments. Soon, as had occurred in the Netherlands more than twenty years before, a false premise became the controlling paradigm; that Measure 16 was a battle between rigid religionists and compassionate rationalists.

In furtherance of this strategy, the "Yes on 16" campaign created ads that stank of anti-Catholic bigotry. One ad asked, "Are we going to let one church make the rules for all of us?" A notable pro–Measure 16 radio commercial was more specific in its anti-Catholic appeal:

> Who do you politicians and religious leaders think you are, trying to control my life? It's none of your business, so back off and back off now. I'm voting yes on 16 because what we have are some politicians and religious leaders who are playing politics all getting together to control my life. Listen, if I'm terminally ill I don't want my family to be forced to drain their savings for unnecessary costly medical care while I suffer just because the politicians and religious leaders say that's the way it has to be. And don't buy the garbage the Catholic Church is putting out. The safeguards in 16 are as long as your arm. Multiple medical opinions, two oral requests, and a written request that can be canceled at any time, a fifteen-day waiting period, and another forty-eight-hour waiting period. You know, there are just some people who believe they have a divine right to control other people's lives, and they'd better back off because it's none of their business. Vote yes on 16.[3]

Another ad complained that Catholic money was financing the opposition:

Their opposition is theological. They believe suffering is redemptive and that preserving physical life is always valued higher than relief of suffering, no matter how humiliating and intolerable that physical life is. And they apply that standard not only to themselves but also to every Oregonian. They want to impose their unique theological perspective on the entire state.[4]

In contrast to the proponents' hardball, pull-out-all-the-stops advocacy, the opposition forces, under the umbrella of the Coalition for Compassionate Care (CCC), took more of a surprisingly wiffle-ball approach to the campaign. Critics later contended that this go-soft approach was a form of unilateral political disarmament leading directly to the measure's narrow passage. This lack of aggressiveness is perhaps best illustrated by a crucial lapse during the critical last week of the campaign. Information surfaced that Patty Rosen had been, to put it kindly, less than candid about the death of her daughter in her commercials in support of Measure 16. In these ads, Rosen stated that her daughter had died from taking an overdose of pills. But a tape recording and transcript of a Rosen speech made in California two years previously on behalf of Proposition 161 revealed that she claimed to have actually given her daughter an injection because she feared the pills were not going to work.

Here was an opportunity rarely found in campaigns of this sort: Measure 16 proponents assured voters that passage of the measure would benefit the dying, yet the poster woman for the campaign had stated earlier that she feared pills alone would not be sufficient to kill her dying daughter. If Patty Rosen's credibility could legitimately be questioned in the minds of voters (she admitted in a newspaper article that she had given her daughter an injection), then so could the veracity of all the arguments supporting Measure 16. But no attempt was made to exploit Rosen's credibility gap, even though the opposition campaign was well aware of her deception and still had money in the bank.

In the end, it was a tragic matter of "so close, yet so far." Support for Measure 16 plummeted, as had support for Initiative 119 and Proposition 161—but not quite far enough. A bare 51 percent of Oregon's voters gave a state's formal imprimatur to physician-assisted suicide, for the first time in history.

Behind the "Oregon Death with Dignity Act"

Measure 16, formally called the Oregon Death with Dignity Act, classifies a prescribed fatal overdose of drugs as a medical treatment. It authorizes any patient who has been "determined by the attending physician and consulting physician to be suffering from a terminal disease" to make a written request for "medication for the purpose of ending his or her life."[5]

The following "safeguards" have been written into the act. The attending physician shall:

- Make the initial determination of whether a patient has a terminal disease, is capable and has made the request voluntarily.
- Inform the patient of:
  a. His or her medical diagnosis.
  b. His or her prognosis.
  c. The potential risks associated with taking medication to be prescribed.
  d. The probable result of taking the medication to be prescribed.
  e. The feasible alternatives, including, but not limited to, comfort care, hospice care, and pain control.
- Refer the patient to a consulting physician for medical confirmation...and for a determination that the patient is capable and acting voluntarily.
- Refer the patient for counseling, if appropriate (counseling is required only if depression or another mental condition causes "impaired judgment").
- Request that the patient notify next of kin.
- Inform the patient that he or she has the opportunity to rescind the request at any time...and offer the patient an opportunity to rescind at the end of the fifteen-day waiting period.
- Verify, immediately prior to writing the prescription...that the patient is making an informed decision.
- Fulfill the medical record documentation requirements.
- Ensure that all appropriate steps are carried out in accordance with this Act.

The law also requires a waiting period of fifteen days between the initial request "and the writing of a prescription."[6]

These so-called safeguards are mostly smoke and mirrors

designed, like those in the Netherlands, to give the appearance that the patient is in control. Measure 16 proponents insisted during the campaign that the only people eligible for doctor-hastened death are people at or near the brink of death. This was not true. The law defines terminal illness as "an incurable and irreversible disease that…will, within reasonable medical judgment, produce death within six months." The measure thus assumes that doctors who diagnose a terminal condition can be accurate in predicting the expected time of death. But as an Oregon hospice doctor, Gary L. Lee, put it, "The 'six months to live' provision is bogus. Doctors usually can't predict the time of death in that fashion. I have had the experience where people were supposed to die, and didn't. I have seen cases where cancer suddenly cleared up for no apparent reason. You never know who is going to die. You just never know."[7]

In another telling lapse in the initiative's language, there is nothing in the definition of terminal illness requiring that the expected death will occur "despite appropriate medical treatment" or other such language, so as to weed out people who will be unlikely to die if they receive proper medical care. Nor is there any requirement, as in the Netherlands, that assisted suicide be the only option to alleviate suffering.

Worries about doctors killing patients are assuaged in Measure 16 with the blithe assurance that under the law, doctors can't do the deed; the patients have to kill themselves. Yet nowhere in the initiative is there a stated requirement for self-administration of a lethal dose or, indeed, a prohibition against a physician's administering a lethal dose. The law merely says that the law does not specifically authorize such action.*

---

*Worries that self-administered assisted suicide would eventually morph into physicians' lethally injecting those who cannot swallow prescribed poison were validated after Measure 16 went into effect. In 1999, ALS patient Patrick Matheny committed assisted suicide after obtaining a lethal prescription—which he received via Federal Express. (Erin Hoover Barnett, "Man with ALS Makes Up His Mind to Die," *Oregonian*, March 11, 1999.) According to media reports, Matheny's brother-in-law provided "help" to him after he had difficulties self-administering the poison. That is not supposed to happen under the protective guidelines. Law enforcement officials conducted a perfunctory investigation to see whether the self-administration provision of Oregon's assisted suicide law had been broken—but they were so lacking in curiosity that the brother-in-law who admitted helping Matheny wasn't even ques-

Proponents also assure that depressed people will not be helped to die under Measure 16 because doctors are supposed to refer those they believe to be depressed for "counseling." Yet the medical literature makes it clear that most doctors are not adept at identifying depression in their dying patients.[8] This means that many depressed people could easily slip through the Oregon suicide machinery without referral to a mental health professional.

But suppose a doctor believes that a suicidal patient is depressed and refers him or her to counseling. Even that "safeguard" is more mirage than substance, given Measure 16's definition of counseling:

> Counseling means a consultation between a state licensed psychiatrist or psychologist and a patient for the purpose of determining whether the patient is suffering from a psychiatric or psychological disorder, or depression causing impaired judgment.[9]

Nowhere does the law mandate a formal psychiatric evaluation to accurately diagnose depression. Even if depression is diagnosed, there is no requirement that it be treated. Moreover, since depressed patients are not prevented from killing themselves, so long as they do not have "impaired judgment"—at best a vague and undefined legal term—assisted suicides of depressed people are likely under Measure 16.

There's more. Incompetent patients might be allowed to receive a lethal dose of drugs under the act, since the doctor need only determine that the patient is "capable" before assisting in a suicide, not that the patient is "competent." This is a crucial distinction. Under the act, every person is capable who is not "incapable," defined as lacking "the ability to make and communicate health care decisions." Thus the ability to communicate decisions replaces the necessity of being competent to make decisions. Besides, depression is a mood disorder, not a thought disorder. Depressed people know they are not Napoleon or Cleopatra. They know that two plus two equals four.

---

tioned. Then David Schuman, an Oregon deputy attorney general, opined that the state constitution and the Americans with Disabilities Act would likely require the state to offer "reasonable accommodation" to "enable the disabled to avail themselves of the [Death With Dignity] Act's provisions." (Correspondence of Deputy Attorney General David Schuman to state Senator Neil Bryant, March 15, 1999.)

But because they are depressed, they are likely to make self-destructive decisions—which they can justify with apparent rationality but which they would not make were they free of depression.

Measure 16's consulting-physician protection is also a joke. To be a consulting physician, a doctor need only be "qualified by specialty or experience in making a professional diagnosis and prognosis of the patient's disease."[10] That's no different from requiring that the consulting doctor be licensed, since the fact of licensure, by definition, means that the doctor is "qualified to make a professional diagnosis." (This is why it is legal for ob/gyns, for example, to perform plastic surgery, often with regrettable results.) Thus, a Kevorkian-type doctor who possesses few skills and little up-to-date training could make a specialty out of rubber-stamp death consultations. And as for being an attending physician, any doctor obtains that status as soon as a patient or surrogate decision maker asks him or her to become the patient's primary physician. Thus, under Measure 16, a doctor with only a brief and superficial relationship with the patient can prescribe the deadly doses of drugs, and under the law, the doctor need not even be present when the lethal prescription is taken. (In 2004, doctors were present in only 6 out of 37 cases of assisted suicide.)[11]

With so much missing from Measure 16's guidelines, they can hardly be called strict. Nor, as we shall see, do they protect. What they do, like all euthanasia guidelines, is falsely assure.

The Oregon Court Cases

Lee v. Oregon
Shortly after Measure 16 passed, Hospice's Dr. Gary Lee and others, including a man dying of AIDS and a diabetic, filed suit against Oregon's Death with Dignity Act. The suit was based on the belief that "Oregon's new assisted suicide law rests on a judgment that the lives of terminally ill and disabled patients are less deserving of protection than others."[12] The plaintiffs contended that the law "violates the constitutional guarantees to terminally ill and disabled individuals of equal protection of the law and due process with regard to the right of an individual to life."

The lawsuit succeeded at the trial court level. U.S. District Court judge Michael Hogan ruled that Measure 16 was unconstitutional because it created a two-tiered system of justice. In his decision he wrote:

> Measure 16 singles out terminally ill persons who want to commit suicide and excludes them from protection of Oregon laws that apply to others. Residents of Oregon are entitled to protection from committing suicide if found to be a danger to themselves, and after evaluation by a psychiatrist or other state certified mental health specialist.... Under Measure 16, the very lives of terminally ill persons depend on their own rational assessment of the value of their existence, and yet, there is no requirement that they be evaluated by a mental health specialist.[13]

Judge Hogan noted that doctors must treat their patients with medical competence but Measure 16 established a lower standard of care for the terminally ill. Hogan also believed that the law left the terminally ill open to coercion, exploitation and victimization after the time the lethal prescription is filled by the patient:

> Measure 16 abandons the terminally ill person at the time the physician provides a lethal prescription. It fails to even acknowledge the most critical time, that of death. It provides a means to commit suicide to people who may be competent, incompetent, unduly influenced, and/or abused at the time of death. There is no distinction.[16]

Judge Hogan ruled that Measure 16 violated the United States Constitution and issued an injunction against its enforcement, stating that the law's "safeguards are inadequate to bar incompetent, depressed but treatable, judgment-impaired, or unduly influenced terminally ill patients from committing suicide."[15]

Judge Hogan's decision was appealed to the U.S. Court of Appeals for the Ninth Circuit. The court could have tackled the substance of the decision, setting up a determination by the Supreme Court as to whether states may legalize assisted suicide. Instead, it issued a procedural ruling, reversing Judge Hogan on the basis that the plaintiff's in the case did not have "standing" to sue because they were not suicidal.[16] This "Catch-22" ruling prevents the Oregon law from ever being judicially reviewed. Here's why: In order to seek a review of the law, a plaintiff must be terminally ill and suicidal. But potential suicidal plaintiffs won't want a review of the law. Thus, Measure 16 may have made history by becoming the first American law whose constitutionality is incapable of being judicially determined.

Gonzales v. Oregon

When Oregon voters legalized assisted suicide in 1994, state regulators had a problem. They wanted to authorize doctors to prescribe barbiturates and other narcotics as killing agents. But the federal government regulates the use of these drugs under the Controlled Substances Act (CSA).

The Drug Enforcement Administration reacted negatively to the prospect of Oregon doctors prescribing lethal doses of controlled substances to kill and issued an opinion claiming that using barbiturates to kill intentionally would violate federal law. Specifically, doctors can prescribe federally controlled substances only for a "legitimate medical purpose." According to the DEA, using these substances for suicide rather than as a medical treatment is not a legitimate medical use under federal law.

But that was not the last word on the subject. Attorney General Janet Reno overruled the DEA opinion in what is known as an administrative "interpretation" contained in a letter to Representative Henry Hyde (R-IL), in which she wrote that "Adverse action under the CSA may well be warranted…where a physician assists in a suicide in a state that *has not authorized the practice under any conditions*, or where a physician fails to comply with state procedures in doing so." But the Department of Justice would take no action against doctors in Oregon who prescribed federally controlled substances for the purpose of assisted suicide.[17] In other words, because Oregon had legalized assisted suicide, the attorney general in essence granted the state's doctors an exemption to the normal federal rules that would still be enforced in the other forty-nine states.

When President George W. Bush took office, Attorney General John Ashcroft decided to review the issue of controlled substances being prescribed for use in assisted suicide. Ashcroft instructed the Office of Legal Counsel to research the matter and determine whether the federal government had the right to sanction doctors who prescribed federally controlled substances for use in the intentional ending of life. The office's report, "Whether Physician-Assisted Suicide Serves a 'Legitimate Medical Purpose,'" concluded that using controlled substances to end life was not a "legitimate medical purpose" for these drugs under federal law.[18] This is not to say the memo suggested that the federal government had the right to overturn the Oregon law. Rather, the memo specifically advised that "methods of assisting in suicides" not involving the dispensing of federally controlled substances would entail "*no* violation of the CSA."[19]

A decision in the United States Supreme Court involving "medical marijuana" also apparently influenced Ashcroft's views. When California voters passed Proposition 215, which permits doctors to recommend marijuana for patients as a palliative medicine, Attorney General Janet Reno brought federal action to shut down medical marijuana distribution centers even though they were in compliance with California law. These enforcement actions resulted in a High Court ruling permitting the federal government to enforce the CSA's prohibition against using marijuana for any purpose—even though its use as a medicine is legal in California.[20]

Relying on the memo and the medical marijuana ruling, and no doubt motivated by his personal opposition to assisted suicide, Ashcroft reversed Reno's interpretation and determined that prescribing narcotics regulated under the CSA would indeed violate federal law. This interpretation was published in the *Federal Register* in November 2002.[21] Thus, contrary to some media reports and angry criticism by assisted suicide proponents, Ashcroft did *not* attempt to outlaw assisted suicide in Oregon. He was *not* attempting to violate "states' rights." And he most certainly did *not*, as some charged, seek to impose his Christian faith on the people of Oregon. Indeed, under the Ashcroft interpretation, assisted suicide remained legal in Oregon.

Predictably, Ashcroft's following of the law ignited a political firestorm. The State of Oregon and other assisted suicide advocates sued Ashcroft to prevent him from enforcing federal law on the grounds that it could preclude Oregon doctors from assisting suicides. Just as predictably, given the deeply political nature of this issue, the trial judge decided in *Oregon v. Ashcroft* that as a matter of law, Oregon had the exclusive right to regulate medical practice within its borders, even to the point that the federal government was precluded from applying a different legal standard with regard to the enforcement of federal law.[22] In other words, the Oregon decision was the opposite of that made by the United States Supreme Court regarding medical marijuana in California.

On appeal, the Ninth Circuit Court of Appeals ruled 2-1 that Ashcroft's directive "interferes with Oregon's authority to regulate medical care within its borders."[23] The dissenting judge disagreed, stating in part that "the Ashcroft Directive proscribes only one method of assisting suicide: prescription, dispensation, and administration of controlled substances.... Oregon physicians may continue to assist suicide by other means without risking" federal sanction."[24] Thus, the courts should defer to Ashcroft's determination.

Assisted suicide proponents cheered. But then, all bets were off as the Supreme Court agreed to hear the case.[25] As these words are written, lawyers on both sides of the issue are preparing briefs in *Gonzales v. Oregon* (the case's name was changed when Alberto Gonzales succeeded John Ashcroft as attorney general), which will finally determine whether the federal government's regulation of the CSA must defer to state views on assisted suicide's legality. The impact of the Supreme Court's ruling, while not determining whether assisted suicide can or should be legal, is likely to be a strong social influence on whether physician-hastened death comes to be perceived by society as an acceptable and legitimate medical practice in the United States of America.

Legalized Killing Comes to Oregon

In September 1997, the Oregon Death with Dignity Act went into effect. So how is the law working? It is impossible to know. As psychiatrist Gregory Hamilton, former president of Oregon's Physicians for Compassionate Care, says, "Rather than being an open experiment as promised by proponents, the actual practice of assisted suicide in Oregon is practiced in darkest secret," a bureaucratic stonewall opponents deride as "the iron shroud."[26] There are no independent investigations conducted by the state into actual assisted suicide deaths, nor are any attempts made beforehand to ensure that the guidelines are followed. Almost the only information the state receives is from the form filled out after a death by doctors who lethally prescribe—a source not likely to tell the state if the law is broken. Even the Oregon Health Department (OHD), which is ideologically behind the law, admits that it doesn't know if these physicians honestly or fully report on their activities.

According to the forms completed by lethally prescribing doctors up through 2004, 181 people are known to have legally committed assisted suicide since the law went into effect.[27] Euthanasia advocates claim that the information supplied by these death doctors indicates that the law is working well. But the little information that has come to light, which has not been controlled by the see-no-evil-hear-no-evil-speak-no-evil OHD bureaucrats, belies the stream of blithe assurances issued routinely by assisted suicide advocates.

In order to get voters to vote yes on Measure 16, advocates promised that physician-assisted suicide would be limited strictly to those rare cases in which patients were in "severe, unrelenting, and intolerable suffering" that could not otherwise be relieved.[28] Moreover, hastened deaths were supposed to take place only "in the context of a meaningful doctor-patient relationship," and then only after a deep and thorough discussion of all options between trusting patients and devoted physicians.[29]

But from the very beginning, that has not been the actual practice. Much is known about the first reported legal assisted suicide because the advocacy organization misnamed Compassion in Dying (CID) held a press conference shortly after her death to provide details. According to CID, "Mrs. A" had terminal breast cancer. She did not swallow physician-prescribed poison because of unbearable suffering and agony. Rather, in her own words, as played on audiotape posthumously at the CID news conference, she wanted to "be relieved of all the stress I have."[30] But stress caused by dying and growing debilitation, while certainly a very real and substantive medical issue that needs to be taken seriously by caregivers, is a treatable condition that does not require killing to alleviate.

A subsequent in-depth analysis of this case by medical and bioethics experts revealed a more detailed account of these troubling events. Upon receiving her terminal diagnosis, the woman asked her treating doctor to assist in her suicide. The doctor refused. She consulted with a second doctor, who also declined and diagnosed her as depressed. She then contacted CID, whose medical director, Dr. Peter Goodwin, spoke with her twice on the telephone, after which he decided that she wasn't depressed but merely "frustrated." Goodwin then referred her to Dr. Peter Reagan, a doctor with a close affiliation to CID who Goodwin knew would be willing to prescribe lethally.

Dr. Reagan referred her to a psychiatrist, who saw her only once, and to a second doctor to confirm the terminal diagnosis. He also conducted a "cursory" discussion with the patient about alternatives to assisted suicide. When she voiced fears of being kept alive by artificial nutrition if she did not kill herself, the death doctor failed to assure her that she had the right to refuse such care—perhaps a crucial factor in her decision to commit assisted suicide. The woman did not know her prescribing doctor well, and indeed, she died a mere two and a half weeks after their first meeting, at a time when she was not in pain and still looked after her own house.[31]

This was not careful medical practice. It was not killing as a last resort when nothing else could be done to alleviate suffering. It was *Kevorkianism*.

Then there was the case of Kate Cheney, reported in the (Portland) *Oregonian*, which provided a sickening glimpse of how easily supposedly protective guidelines are circumvented. [32] Cheney, age eighty-five, was diagnosed with terminal cancer and sought assisted suicide. But there was a problem: Cheney was probably in the early stages of dementia, raising significant questions about her mental competence. So, rather than prescribe lethal drugs, her doctor referred her to a psychiatrist.

Her daughter, Ericka Goldstein, accompanied Cheney to the psychiatric consultation. The psychiatrist found that Cheney had a loss of short-term memory and wrote in his report that while the assisted suicide seemed consistent with Cheney's values, "she does not seem to be explicitly pushing for this." He also determined that she did not have the "very high capacity required to weigh options about assisted suicide." Worse, the person who seemed most intent on Cheney's committing assisted suicide wasn't the elderly patient, but her daughter, Accordingly, the psychiatrist nixed the lethal prescription.

Advocates of legalized assisted suicide might, at this point, smile happily and point out that such refusals are of the way the law is supposed to operate to protect the vulnerable. But that wasn't the end of Kate Cheney's story. According to the *Oregonian* report, Cheney appeared to accept the psychiatrist's verdict but her daughter most explicitly did not. To circumvent the rejection of assisted suicide, Goldstein merely did what anyone in Oregon wanting assisted suicide can do if refused by one physician: she went doctor shopping.

Kaiser Permanente, Cheney's HMO, acceded to Goldstein's demand for another opinion. This time, the psychiatric consultation was with a clinical psychologist rather than an M.D. psychiatrist. Like the psychiatrist, this consulting psychologist found that Cheney had significant memory problems. For example, she could not recall when she had been diagnosed with terminal cancer. The psychologist also worried about familial pressure, writing that Cheney's decision to die "may be influenced by her family's wishes." Still, despite these reservations, the psychologist determined that Cheney was competent to commit suicide.

The final decision to approve the death was made by a Kaiser HMO ethicist/administrator named Robert Richardson, whom Cheney told that she wanted the poison pills not because she was in irremediable pain but because she feared not being able to attend to her personal hygiene. After the interview, satisfied that she was competent, he approved the lethal prescription.

It is important to reiterate that whatever protection that guidelines provide in Oregon end with the writing of the lethal prescription. At that point, no doctor was required to be at the patient's bedside. Indeed, the law does not require that anything be done thereafter to determine if the patient is competent when swallowing poison or to prevent the patient from being coerced into taking the pills. In short, once Kate Cheney received the prescription, under the law she was on her own.

What happened next in the Cheney case illustrates the potential for problems that can arise after the lethal prescription is issued. Cheney did not take the drugs right away. According to the *Oregonian* report, she first asked to die immediately after her daughter had to help her shower after an accident with her colostomy bag. But she quickly changed her mind. Then, Cheney was sent to a nursing home for a week so that her family could have some respite from caregiving.

The time spent in the nursing home may have pushed Cheney into wanting immediate death. As soon as she was brought home, she declared her desire to take the pills. Her grandchildren were quickly called to say their goodbyes and then Cheney swallowed her prescribed poison.

If Cheney was depressed when she swallowed the poison, there was no doctor available to diagnose it. If she was coaxed or pressured into taking the pills (which was not implied in the *Oregonian* story), there were no witnesses from outside the family to protest. Indeed, other than what family members told the *Oregonian* reporter, we don't know what happened at Kate Cheney's death since the Oregon guidelines do not require any independent assessment of assisted suicide deaths.

It appears that doctors may be issuing lethal prescriptions to patients who are not terminally ill under the terms of the law. In May 2004, psychiatrist N. Gregory Hamilton and his wife, Catherine Hamiltion, a social worker, presented a paper to the American Psychiatric Association meeting reporting on the case of Michael P. Freeland, who had been issued a lethal prescription nearly *two years* before he actually died of natural causes.[33] (Dr. Hamilton is the former president of Physicians for Compassionate Care, an organization dedicated to improving palliative care for the dying, which opposes Oregon's law.)

Even though assisted suicide had been legally permitted for more than six years when this case came to light, it was the first one—and to the best of my knowledge, remains the only one—in which the patient's medical records have been made available for review. And a sorry tale they tell: Not only was the patient apparently not terminally ill as defined by Oregon's law when he first received his lethal prescription, but he was allowed to keep his cache of suicide pills despite being diagnosed as having "depressive disorder," "chronic adjustment disorder with depressed mood," "intermittent delirium," and even after being declared mentally incompetent by a court.[34]

Michael P. Freeland was diagnosed with lung cancer in 2000.

He received a lethal prescription from Dr. Peter Reagan in early 2001. Euthanasia advocacy groups often refer suicidal patients to him when the patients' physicians refuse to go along with their requests for suicide drugs. (As noted earlier, Dr. Reagan wrote the lethal prescription for the first publicized legal assisted suicide in Oregon.)[35]

Freeland, as it happens, died naturally on December 5, 2002. Oregon law requires the patient to be reasonably expected to die within six months before receiving a lethal prescription. But Freeland's death occurred nearly two years after Dr. Reagan wrote the lethal prescription. Indeed, Freeland told the Hamiltons that Reagan contacted him after he didn't die in a timely fashion to reissue the prescription, so as to make sure his assisted suicide remained legal![36]

On January 23, 2002, more than a year after receiving Reagan's poison script, Freeland was admitted to Providence Portland Medical Center for depression with suicidal and possibly homicidal thoughts. A social worker went to Freeland's home and found it "uninhabitable," with "heaps of clutter, rodent feces, ashes extending two feet from the fireplace into the living room, lack of food and heat, etc. Thirty-two firearms and thousands of rounds of ammunition were removed by the police."

Freeland was hospitalized for a week and then discharged on January 30. The discharging psychiatrist noted with approval that the guns had been removed, "which resolves the major safety issue," but wrote that Freeland's lethal prescription remained "safely at home." Freeland was permitted to keep the overdose even though the psychiatrist reported he would "remain vulnerable to periods of delirium." In-home care was considered likely to assist with this problem, but a January 24 chart notation indicated that Freeman "does have his life-ending medications that he states he may or may not use, so that [in-home care] may or may not be a moot point."[37]

The day after Freeland's discharge, the psychiatrist wrote a letter to the court in support of establishing a guardianship for him, writing, "he is susceptible to periods of confusion and impaired judgment." According to the Hamiltons, the psychiatrist concluded that Freeland was unable to handle his own finances and that his cognitive impairments were unlikely to improve. He lived under supervision for a brief time, but was soon home alone with ready access to his suicide drugs.

Happily for Freeland, he had called Physicians for Compassionate Care for help, and as he neared his end, he had people surrounding him who were committed to helping him live his life, rather than committed to facilitating his death. Instead of dying alone by assisted suicide, he was cared for by the Hamiltons and by his friends—who assured the now dying man that "they valued him and did not want him to kill himself." Freeland was properly treated for depression with medication. He received good pain control, including a morphine pump. Best of all, he was reunited with his estranged daughter and died knowing she loved him and would cherish his memory.[38]

Based on their review of the facts and circumstances surrounding Freeland's receiving a lethal prescription, including his medical records, the Hamiltons reached important conclusions about the danger that legalization of assisted suicide poses to ill Oregonians with suicidal desires and about the law's discriminatory effect on patients and its impact on mental health professionals:

> The legalization of doctor-assisted suicide in Oregon has resulted in the introduction of competing paradigms—the traditional clinical approach [removing lethal means is central to the clinical treatment of suicide symptoms] and the assisted suicide competency model [providing lethal means]—for responding to suicidal thoughts and behaviors in seriously ill individuals.... These competing models appear to be based on incompatible underlying assumptions about the value of protecting life depending on predictions of how long a patient might live.... We conclude that the attempt to mix models is confusing to both clinicians and patients and endangers seriously ill patients, particularly those with a history of pre-existing mental illness.

Assisted suicide advocates, when faced with the examples cited above, simply point to the OHD yearly reports, claiming these validate their cause. But a close reading of these compilations of statistical data reveals that rather than providing assurance, the statistics actually justify the worries of assisted suicide opponents.

For many years, we have been told repeatedly by assisted suicide advocates that legalized mercy killing would be a "last resort," applied only when nothing else could be done to alleviate "severe, unrelenting and intolerable suffering."[39] Yet it appears that none of the Oregonians who reportedly committed assisted suicide during the law's first four years in effect were in that desperate condition. Pain was a factor in only a few cases. Indeed, rather than unbearable agony, the primary reasons for assisted suicide in the overwhelming majority of these deaths since the Oregon law commenced were:

- Losing autonomy: 87 percent.
- Decreasing ability to participate in activities that make life enjoyable: 84 percent.
- Perceived loss of dignity: 80 percent.
- Losing control of bodily functions: 59 percent.
- Being a burden on family, friends or caregivers: 36 percent.[40]

An independent study of assisted suicide (not limited to Oregon), published in 2005, found similar results. (Participants in the study were provided by assisted suicide advocacy groups, grief counselors and hospices.) The hastened deaths of 35 people were studied. Two-thirds decided to end it all due to worries about "sense of self." In 21 cases the issue was "desire for control." One patient was quoted as stating, "I will do things my way and the hell with everything and everybody else. Nobody is going to talk me out of a darn thing.... I will always be in control." Also in 21 of the 35 cases, current problems were not the cause of the desire to commit suicide but "fears about future quality of life and dying."[41]

These are all issues that certainly require loving attention—not suicide support—from caregivers, friends and relatives. As the authors of the 2005 report concluded, "These data confirm the recommendation, espoused by high-quality palliative care, that providers repeatedly assess the patient's concerns of losses and dying in order to understand and tailor end-of-life care to the patient's changing personal experience.... A patient's request for assistance with a hastened death should generate a thorough evaluation of the patient's motives and attempts at ameliorating the patient's suffering."[42]

In other words, rather than cold "choice," dying people need to know that their lives are cherished even if they can't, at the moment, value themselves, and treatment needs to be aimed at finding the cause of the suicidal desire so the problem can be treated.

In the words of the late Robert Salamanca, who lived for years with ALS before finally dying from the disease:

> Euthanasia advocates believe they are doing people like me a favor. They are not. The negative emotions toward the terminally ill and disabled generated by their advocacy is actually at the expense of the "dying" and their families and friends, who often feel disheartened and without self assurance because of a false picture of what it is like to die created by these enthusiasts who prey on the misinformed.
>
> What we, the terminally ill, need is exactly the opposite—to realize how important our lives are. And our loved ones, friends, and indeed society, need to help us feel that we are loved and appreciated unconditionally.[43]

Another significant problem with assisted suicide in Oregon, rarely explored by a compliant media, is the number of patients who barely knew their lethally prescribing doctors. As described earlier, the first woman to commit assisted suicide in Oregon had only a two-and-a-half-week relationship with the doctor who wrote her lethal prescription. Her case was more the rule than the exception. The yearly OHD reports have shown that many assisted suicide victims went to more than one doctor to obtain their lethal prescriptions and that many knew the prescribing doctors for only brief weeks before committing their deaths.

Assisted suicide proponents told us this wouldn't happen either. They gave assurances that assisted suicide would occur only after a deep exploration of values between patients and doctors who had long-term relationships. But we now know that in many cases, death decisions are being made by doctors the patients barely know, many being referred by assisted suicide advocacy groups after primary care physicians have refused to assist their patients' suicides. These "death doctors" are thus not chosen to treat the patients or to palliate their symptoms. They may not even specialize in treating the condition causing the patients' illnesses. They have one job: to write lethal prescriptions.

There are also material omissions in the reports that detract significantly from their empirical usefulness. The primary information about the people who committed assisted suicides comes from death-prescribing doctors—not necessarily the most reliable sources considering the brief relationships many had with their patients and their ideological predispositions. Treating doctors who did not participate directly in ending their patients' lives—who knew the patient longer and who could have provided accurate information on the patients' conditions and why assisted suicide was refused— were not interviewed. Nor were other doctors who refused to write lethal prescriptions. Family members were often not contacted either. Significantly, the investigators did not disclose whether any (or all) of the prescribing doctors were affiliated with assisted suicide advocacy groups, a matter of some importance if we are to judge whether the decisions to prescribe lethally were ideological. (Press reports indicate that at least some were.) Moreover, none of the patients were autopsied to determine whether they actually were terminally ill.

The OHD studies warn us that Oregon has started down the same destructive path that was blazed by the Netherlands. It is clear for those who want to see: Assisted suicide is not only bad medicine but even worse public policy.

Making Up Rights As They Go Along

Euthanasia advocates did not put all their advocacy eggs into a single legislation basket. They also sued, sued, and sued again, seeking to establish a federal and a state constitutional right to assisted suicide.

The most famous of these cases made it to the United States Supreme Court. In 1994, the assisted suicide advocacy group Compassion in Dying joined with three dying patients and five physicians to challenge Washington's law banning assisted suicide. Their record of success prior to reaching the High Court was mixed: they won in the trial court, then lost in the U.S. Court of Appeals for the Ninth Circuit, where a three-judge panel ruled that Washington's law was constitutional. But then the Ninth Circuit granted an *en banc* hearing by eleven judges, which by an 8-3 decision found that Washington's law against assisted suicide as it applied to the terminally ill was unconstitutional. The Supreme Court ultimately overruled that case.

Despite never becoming law, the decision of the *en banc* court, written by Chief Justice Stephen Reinhardt, is worth pondering.

First, the majority quickly and hubristically dismissed the court's obligation to apply the law as written and to depend on previous rulings: "We must strive to resist the natural judicial impulse to limit our vision to that which can plainly be observed on the face of the document before us, or even that which we have previously had the wisdom to recognize."[44]

Thus freeing themselves from the usual constraints that serve to limit the scope of judicial rulings by lesser judges, Reinhardt and seven of his colleagues, in effect, licensed themselves to create new constitutional rights from whole cloth: The wording of the United States Constitution, the binding nature of judicial precedent, and even the vote of the people of Washington only five years earlier that they did not want to legalize hastened death in their state carried little weight.

The Compassion in Dying case relies on opinion polls for justification; it blurs sensitive and vital distinctions; and the opinion is rife with factual error. For example, the eleven-judge panel found: "Unlike the depressed twenty-one-year-old, the romantically devastated twenty-eight-year-old, the alcoholic forty-year-old...who may be inclined to commit suicide, a terminally ill, competent adult cannot be cured." Yet, as noted earlier, no clear definition of terminal illness is medically or legally possible, since only in hindsight is it known with certainty when someone is going to die.

Judge Reinhardt also wrote: "While some people who contemplate suicide can be restored to a state of physical and mental well-being, terminally ill adults who wish to die can only be maintained in a debilitated and deteriorating state, unable to enjoy the presence of family or friends." But there are many experts who disagree with this despairing and nihilistic view of the process of dying. Dr. Ira Byock, a hospice physician with extensive experience in these matters, says: "Every life-stage has value, including the time of dying. Obviously, it can be wrenching and require an abrupt adjustment, but over time, if treated with respect, compassion and expertise, dying people often achieve a sense of mastery. It is an arduous time but a very personal and extraordinary time. It should not be dismissed as unimportant or not worth living."[45]

Factual inaccuracies are a minor problem compared with the rest of Judge Reinhardt's decision. Officially, the case stood for the now defunct proposition that there is a fundamental liberty interest in the Constitution in allowing citizens a "right to die." Unlike other constitutional rights, however, this "liberty interest" would not have been available to all people. Rather, deciding who possessed or did not possess it would have been done on a sliding scale. According to Reinhardt, the state had an interest in protecting the lives of the "young and healthy" against suicide, but not much interest at all in protecting the lives of people "who are diagnosed as terminally ill." So long as the dying were not coerced into choosing death and were mentally competent (extremely questionable propositions), Reinhardt and his seven majority opinion colleagues would have granted them an almost absolute right to choose to be assisted in their suicide by a doctor.

Judge Reinhardt shared the restricted view of many assisted suicide advocates about the state's obligation toward protecting its citizens. According to this view, the state isn't protecting lives by prohibiting assisted suicide, but in the words of Reinhardt, it is "forcing" people to stay alive. The state may engage in this totalitarianism against the young and healthy because "forcing a robust individual to continue living does not, at least absent extraordinary circumstances, subject him to 'pain...and suffering that is too intimate and personal for the state to insist on.'"

Note that if "extraordinary circumstances" exist, perhaps even young, healthy lives would not be protected. Moreover, if "suffering" is the primary issue justifying assisted suicide, if it is somehow "wrong" for the state to "force" suffering people to stay alive, Reinhardt's decision could be interpreted to permit members of an oppressed minority to petition for suicide assistance because they could no longer stand to live as victims of perpetual injustice. Indeed, to be logically consistent, the court would have to permit the killing if such a person demonstrated sufficient anguish that was "too intimate and personal for the state to insist on."

Judge Reinhardt's opinion was so extreme that some of his colleagues took the extraordinary step of trying to have all twenty-four active judges of the U.S. Court of Appeals for the Ninth Circuit rehear the case. When that failed, several justices filed dissents, which, among other criticisms, complained that Judge Reinhardt and his cohorts nullified "the public will" of Washington's voters, who in 1991 had voted not to allow assisted suicide. One judge, Diarmuid E. O'Scannlain, labeled the decision "embarrassing judicial excess" and a "shockingly broad act of judicial legislation."[46]

In the weeks following the Ninth Circuit's *en banc* decision in *Compassion in Dying*, the U.S. Court of Appeals for the Second Circuit, whose jurisdiction includes New York State, also ruled on the constitutionality of state laws that prohibit assisted suicide. The lawsuit had been filed by Dr. Timothy Quill, one of the nation's foremost euthanasia proponents, along with other physicians and terminally ill patients. The suit sought a ruling to declare unconstitutional New York's century-old law prohibiting assisted suicide. The trial court had dismissed Dr. Quill's suit as without merit. But the matter was appealed to a three-judge panel of the U.S. Court of Appeals for the Second Circuit.

The Second Circuit explicitly repudiated the Ninth Circuit's *en banc* decision by specifically ruling that assisted suicide is not a fundamental liberty interest founded in the Constitution. Unfortunately, the judges found a different constitutional justification to permit legalized suicide: equal protection of the law.[47]

The equal protection clause of the Fourteenth Amendment requires that similarly situated citizens must be treated alike under the law. Thus, requiring all six-year-old children to attend school treats similarly situated persons—six-year-old children—alike, whereas a law compelling six-year-old boys but not six-year-old girls to go to school would be to treat similarly situated persons differently, which would be an unconstitutional violation of the equal protection clause.

The Constitution does not require the law to treat matters that are not the same as if they were. Generally, the decision to decide what is a similar situation and what is not is up to lawmakers, requiring only that the distinctions made in law be "rationally related to a legitimate state interest."[48] In the example above, even though boys and girls are not exactly the same, the state would not be able to demonstrate a rational basis for allowing young girls and not young boys to stop attending school. But a law allowing seventeen-year-old minors to quit school would probably pass equal-protection muster, even though it treats some minors differently from others, the state having a rational basis for treating six-year-old minors and seventeen-year-old minors differently: In contrast, if a law restricts an activity deemed a fundamental liberty interest, such as freedom of speech (or in the Ninth Circuit's *Compassion in Dying* opinion, the right of an ill person to be killed by a doctor), the state can interfere with the activity only if it has a "compelling state interest," an extremely difficult legal standard to meet.

In the Quill court of appeals case, the court decided:

- Terminally ill patients who require life support and those who are dying but who do not require life support are similarly situated persons.
- Since it is legal for people to reject the medical treatment of life support, terminally ill people who are on life support and want to die can do so quickly by refusing such care.
- Terminally ill people who do not require life support are forced to stay alive, even if they want to die quickly, since rejecting treatment would not immediately accomplish that goal.
- Therefore, those who cannot die by refusing treatment should have the right to assisted suicide, to fulfill the requirement that the law treat them in a manner similar to their terminally ill counterparts who are on life support (in other words, by allowing patients to refuse life support, the state has created a right to die quickly that should apply to all terminally ill people).
- The state serves no rational interest in preventing the terminally ill from killing themselves, since their lives are all but over anyway.

Thus, according to the court, since similarly situated people—that is, the terminally ill—are being treated differently under the law, the assisted-suicide ban as applied to terminally ill people must fall before the equal protection clause.

As the United States Supreme Court would later rule, the decision exhibited faulty logic. Dying by natural processes is not the same thing as being killed. The former is what may happen if life support is terminated, whereas in assisted suicide, a death-causing agent intentionally induces the demise. Moreover, when life-sustaining medical intervention is withheld or withdrawn from a patient, the result is uncertain. Death may or may not come. In an assisted suicide, however, the patient's death is inevitable. It will occur immediately following the injection or ingestion of the poisonous agent.

Here are just two illustrations: Karen Ann Quinlan overdosed on drugs and alcohol and became permanently unconscious. After several years, her parents sued Karen's hospital to compel her doctors to stop the unwanted medical treatment of machine-assisted breathing. Eventually, the New Jersey Supreme Court properly approved their request, and Karen was taken off the respirator.[49] But Karen didn't die. Indeed, she lived for ten years, finally succumbing to an infection.[50]

Ron Comeau was diagnosed as being in a persistent vegetative state after he attempted to hang himself. His guardian *ad litem* petitioned the court to cut off his respirator, expecting that he would die. Instead, Comeau began to improve—and so his guardian, viewing Comeau's condition as still an unbearable life, decided to have him dehydrated. (Intervention by others, including relatives, ultimately saved Comeau's life.)[51]

The court of appeals decision in the Quill case also applied the wrong comparison. There is no analogy between a patient's right to refuse unwanted life-sustaining treatment and being killed by assisted suicide. It is freedom from treatment, not freedom from life, that has consistently served as the legal and ethical underpinning for cases about the right to refuse medical treatment, from Karen Ann Quinlan to Nancy Cruzan to numerous others. This distinction is rational and vital. It protects people from unwanted physical intrusions. It does not, however, create a right to be killed with all of the dangers and potential for exploitation and abuse that such a right would entail.

The Constitutional Issue Is Decided by the Supreme Court

In June 1997, the Supreme Court of the United States unanimously ruled that there is no right to assisted suicide to be found in the Constitution. The two contemporaneous decisions, *Washington v. Glucksburg* and *Vacco v. Quill*, were both thorough and far-reaching.[52] Chief Justice William Rehnquist penned both majority opinions. (There were also multiple concurring opinions.)

In Glucksburg, the Court determined that assisted suicide was not a fundamental right. First, the Court reviewed the laws surrounding suicide and assisted suicide during the last seven hundred years of Anglo-American jurisprudence, finding that assisted suicide is not a "fundamental liberty interest" protected by the "Due Process Clause."[53] That being so, all that the State of Washington had to demonstrate was that its ban on assisted suicide "be rationally related to legitimate government interests."[54] The decision stated that Washington had "unquestionably" accomplished this. The Court then set forth these interests over several pages of text:

- The State's "unqualified interest" in the preservation of human life, "even for those near death."
- Suicide is a "serious health problem," especially among "persons …in vulnerable groups." That being so, states have the right to pass laws, including laws criminalizing assisted suicide as a matter of suicide prevention.
- Those who commit suicide, including the terminally ill, "often suffer from depression or other mental disorders." Because depression can often be effectively treated—and its causes, such as pain, significantly ameliorated—"legal physician assisted suicide could make it more difficult for the State to protect depressed or mentally ill persons, or those who are suffering from untreated pain, from suicidal impulses."[55]
- The State has "an interest in protecting the integrity and ethics of the medical profession." Legalized physician-assisted suicide could "blur the line between healing and harming."[56]
- "Next, the State has an interest in protecting vulnerable groups—including the poor, elderly, and disabled persons—from abuse, neglect, and mistakes." If physician-assisted suicide were permitted, "many might resort to it to spare their families the substantial financial burden of end-of-life health care costs."[57]
- "The State's interest here goes beyond protecting the vulnerable from coercion; it extends to protecting disabled and terminally ill people from discrimination, negative and inaccurate stereotypes, and 'societal indifference.'… The State's assisted-suicide ban reflects and reinforces its policy that the lives of terminally ill, disabled, and elderly people must be no less valued than the lives of the young and healthy; and that a seriously disabled person's suicidal impulses should be interpreted and treated the same way as anyone's else's."[58]
- "Finally, the State may fear that permitting assisted suicide will

start it down the path to voluntary and perhaps even involuntary euthanasia."[59] In this regard, the decision made much of the experience in the Netherlands with termination without request and consent—an issue discussed at length in Chapter 4.

But what about the oft-made assertion by euthanasia advocates, adopted by the Second Circuit Court of Appeals, that assisted suicide is the legal equivalent to refusing unwanted life-sustaining medical treatment and that permitting one but legally prohibiting the other therefore violates the right to equal protection of the laws? Not so, the High Court declared in *Vacco v. Quill:* Refusing life-sustaining medical treatment and killing are not the same things at all. Noting that "when a patient refuses life-sustaining medical treatment, he dies from an underlying fatal disease," the Court ruled:

> [A] physician who withdraws, or honors a patient's refusal to begin, life sustaining medical treatment purposefully intends, or may so intend, only to respect his patient's wishes to cease doing useless and futile degrading things to the patient when the patient no longer stands to benefit from them.... A doctor who assists a suicide, however, must necessarily and indubitably, intend primarily that the patient be made dead. Similarly, a patient who commits suicide with a doctor's aid has the specific intent to end his or her own life, while a patient who refuses or discontinues treatment might not...[and, indeed] may instead fervently wish to live, but to do so free of unwanted medical technology, surgery, or drugs. [Citations omitted.][60]

In other words, the right to refuse unwanted medical treatment is not a "right to die" but a right to be free from unwanted bodily intrusions. Accordingly, the Court decided that New York's law prohibiting assisted suicide was perfectly constitutional.

Glucksburg and *Vacco* were devastating losses for the assisted suicide movement. (Euthanasia advocates did, however, successfully spin the media that their unanimous defeat was almost akin to a victory due to a comment by a concurring justice that states were free to continue to experiment with end-of-life issues.) It was now clear that any attempt to transform the United States into a suicide nation would require intense state-by-state political struggle rather than a sweeping declaration from the judiciary.

Or did it? Determined to prevail regardless of the laws or even the beliefs of the populace, euthanasia advocates also mounted legal challenges in selected state courts, claiming that privacy provisions in state constitutions preclude laws banning assisted suicide. Here too, however, the movement hit brick walls. First, Michigan refused the constitutional claim in a case involving Jack Kevorkian.[61] Then in 1997, the Supreme Court of Florida rejected claims that the Florida Constitution guarantees terminally ill patients a right to be made dead.[62] Finally, in 2001, the Alaska Supreme Court made a similar ruling.[63] The assisted suicide movement's dream of prevailing in one stroke via judicial fiat has all but evaporated.

The Struggle Continues

The years since the passage of Measure 16 have not generally been successful ones for the assisted suicide movement. It has repeatedly and unsuccessfully sought to pass legislation in many state legislatures to legalize assisted suicide. Jack Kevorkian was imprisoned for murder after he videotaped himself killing an ALS patient and then aired the killing on *60 Minutes*. In 1998, Michigan assisted suicide activists sought to pass an initiative legalizing assisted suicide in Kevorkian's home state and lost by an overwhelming 71-29 percent. In 2000, Maine, a state with demographics remarkably similar to Oregon's, rejected assisted suicide by 51-49 percent.

Why this stunning turnaround when assisted suicide threatened to sweep the country after Measure 16 went into effect? Here's what happened: Prior to Measure 16, the moral and legal struggle over euthanasia was largely—if inaccurately—viewed as a contest pitting religious conservatives and the pro-life movement against modernist rationalists. But with the passage of the Oregon law and the general applause granted Jack Kevorkian for his more than one hundred assisted suicides of mostly disabled people (approximately 75 percent of Kevorkian's victims were not terminally ill), a remarkable and robust alliance came together to combat the culture of death: disability rights activists, hospice professionals, religious groups, advocates for the poor, pro-lifers, and medical and nursing associations—people who disagree about other controversial issues of the day but agree that doctors should not be licensed to kill their patients. With such a diverse coalition, it has proved much easier to get the anti-assisted-suicide message across to the general populace.

Still, if euthanasia activists have proved anything it is that they never stop, never rest, never give up. They never cease their war of attrition against Hippocratic medical values and the equality-of-life ethic, which they hope to win by simply exhausting their opponents. Indeed, despite their many recent setbacks, the American euthanasia movement is today more powerful than it has ever been, now consisting of a plethora of local organizations and several national groups such as the Hemlock Society, Death with Dignity Education Center, and the Compassion in Dying Federation (CDF). Not only do they have committed activists to perform the daily tasks of trying to change a culture, they now have ample money to spend on advocacy, some being generously bankrolled by several notable foundations. For example, in 1997, CDF received $100,000 from George Soros's Open Society Institute, more than $300,000 from the Gerbode Foundation between 1995 and 1999, a $300,000, three-year grant in 1998 from the Columbia Foundation, and $50,000 from the Donald A. Pels Charitable Trust in the same year. Funding for the Death with Dignity Educational Center has also been generous, including grants from the Open Society Institute ($100,000 in 1997), the Gerbode Foundation ($544,900 since 1996), the Columbia Foundation ($200,000 since 1998), and the Walter and Elise Haas Foundation ($57,500 during 1996–97).[64] This level of giving seems to have continued to the present moment.[65]

These funds make for political and media clout. As Rita Marker, president of the International Task Force on Euthanasia and Assisted suicide, points out, "Influencing public opinion is an expensive endeavor. It requires a virtual nonstop public relations campaign, including frequent contact with the media, a lobbying presence in government centers, presence at policy-making forums, and an energetic public information component. It requires professional spokespersons to be available to be seen and heard. All of this is very costly, but very effective, often enabling assisted suicide activists to set the agenda."[66]

SIX

EUTHANASIA'S BETRAYAL
OF MEDICINE

IMAGINE A WORLD WHERE EVERYONE RECEIVES optimum health care, regardless of financial means. Imagine a world where all seriously ill or disabled persons are surrounded by a loving and supportive community of family, friends and professionals dedicated solely to their welfare, where elder abuse is a problem of the past and all are welcomed wholeheartedly as equal members of the human community. Imagine a world where family members are ever supportive and never pressure, intimidate, manipulate or abandon their loved ones. Imagine a world where everyone has altruistic motives. Imagine a world where depression is immediately recognized and treated. Imagine a world where disabled people are universally valued and are provided the services they require for full participation in the community. Imagine a world where health choices are all made with due deliberation and rational analysis, where people do not act in haste and are free of duress, menace, coercion or fraud.

Anyone who believes that such a world actually exists went to one too many Grateful Dead concerts. But don't tell that to death fundamentalists, because this is the environment in which they claim euthanasia would be practiced.

A Dysfunctional Health-Care Delivery System

Euthanasia advocates almost always ignore, or perhaps choose not to see, that the conditions under which they assert that euthanasia should be undertaken simply do not exist in our money-driven health-care system. They don't take into account the difficulties and stresses of family life, the vulnerability of people who are depressed or in pain to pressure and coercion, or, indeed, the reality of human nature when money issues such as inheritance or life insurance are involved. Nor do they acknowledge that it is likely that some physicians, perhaps those with a bias in favor of assisted suicide, may become (as in the case of the Netherlands and even in Oregon) death doctors whose primary "practice" devolves into the killing of patients.

Ironically, legal assisted suicide and euthanasia are not only unlikely to be intimate and compassionate affairs but, in fact, are likely to cause more misery and suffering than they would ever alleviate. This was the conclusion of the twenty-five-member New York State Task Force on Life and the Law, a permanent commission created by Governor Mario Cuomo in 1985. The task force spent more than a year intensely investigating whether assisted suicide should be legalized. Despite having some members who supported assisted suicide and euthanasia in theory before beginning their investigation, the group's recommendation was unanimous: euthanasia and assisted suicide should not be legalized.

The task force's report, *When Death Is Sought: Assisted Suicide and Euthanasia in the Medical Context*, remains highly relevant ten years after it was first published and is must-reading for anyone interested in the euthanasia debate.[1] One of the most striking features of the report is that it does not rely on abstract notions of religion, morality or philosophy, but rather focuses extensively on pragmatic and practical analysis of the world as it really is:

> In light of the pervasive failure of our health care system to treat pain and diagnose and treat depression, legalizing assisted suicide and euthanasia would be profoundly dangerous for many individuals who are ill and vulnerable. The risks would be most severe for those who are elderly, poor, socially disadvantaged, or without access to good medical care.[2]

When Death Is Sought effectively punctures the idyllic picture of assisted suicide put forth by euthanasia advocates. According to the task force, the "good case" in which all "safeguards would be

satisfied…bears little relation to prevalent social and medical practices."[3] In other words, despite the lip service they pay to high ideals,
the caring world rhetorically summoned by euthanasia advocates
simply doesn't exist—and will not exist in the foreseeable future.

Many social risks inherent in euthanasia were also cited by the
task force as a reason not to legalize the practice, among them the
following:

- Euthanasia would be practiced through the "prism of social
  inequality and bias that characterizes the delivery of services in all
  segments of our society, including health care."[4] This is the point:
  Racism, ageism, sexism, bigotry against disabled people, and
  issues of class and socioeconomic status would all materially affect
  killing decisions just as they do other issues in American life.
- "Most doctors do not have a long-standing relationship with their
  patients or information about the complex personal factors" that
  go into a request to be killed. Moreover, "neither treatment for
  pain nor diagnosis of and treatment for depression is widely available in clinical practice."[5] Yet untreated pain and depression are
  the primary reasons why dying patients request physician-assisted
  suicide.
- Medical killing based on "unbearable suffering" cannot logically
  be limited to the dying and, if legalized, would soon be available
  to anyone who claimed to be in agony.

Perhaps most important, the task force found that euthanasia
and assisted suicide are unnecessary to relieve suffering. "Contrary
to what many believe," the report noted, "the vast majority of individuals who are terminally ill or facing severe pain or disability are
not suicidal. Moreover, terminally ill patients who do desire suicide
or euthanasia often suffer from a treatable mental disorder, most
commonly depression. When these patients receive appropriate
treatment for depression, they usually abandon the wish to commit
suicide."[6]

Indeed, the Task Force noted that techniques to control pain,
treat depression and provide support for patients and families
already exist. The problem isn't with whether these truly beneficent
care practices work; if properly applied, they do in nearly every
case. Rather, society still must overcome the "numerous barriers"
that exist to their proper application, "including a lack of profes-

sional knowledge and training, unjustified fears about physical and psychological dependence, poor pain assessment…and reluctance of patients and their families to seek pain relief."[7] That will require dedicated effort and sustained energy, which too often are diverted from these important tasks to the struggle over legalizing euthanasia.

The New York State Task Force on Life and the Law was not alone in making these points. When Dr. Timothy Quill began his assisted suicide crusade, his colleagues at the University of Rochester Medical Center conducted a study of the issue. After more than a year's investigation, which included significant input by Dr. Quill, the University of Rochester Task Force unanimously recommended against legalization, for reasons similar to those detailed by the New York State Task Force, including the existence of "practical treatments and management techniques available at the present time which should prove adequate for palliation of suffering in virtually all clinical situations."[8] The Rochester report also noted that doctors have done an insufficient job of treating dying and suffering patients and recommended greater attention be paid to these vital care issues.

The conclusions of these studies are echoed by internal discussion within the medical profession, which has finally come to realize its partial responsibility for the fear and anxiety over suffering at the end of life felt by many of their patients, and the scandalous undertreatment of pain and depression—major sources of the energy driving the euthanasia movement.

For example, the *Journal of the American Medical Association* has stated that "inadequate treatment of pain continues to be a problem despite more knowledge about its causes and control and despite widespread efforts of governments and multiple medical and voluntary organizations to disseminate this knowledge…. All types of pain in all parts of the world are inadequately treated."[9] *American Medical News* editorialized, "Evidence suggests that there is a significant gap between the most effective pain treatment and what most patients actually get."[10] And the authors of a special report on pain control in the *New England Journal of Medicine* wrote, "Undertreatment of cancer pain is common because of clinicians' inadequate knowledge of effective assessment and management practices, negative attitudes of patients and clinicians toward the use of drugs for the relief of pain, and a variety of problems related to reimbursement for effective pain management."[11] Yet despite more than ten years of such intense pushing by the medical establishment, it is not an overstatement to say that "untreated and under treated pain is nothing short of a national scandal."[12]

If doctors in general currently do such a poor job of relieving the pain and depression of suffering people when doctor-induced death is illegal, what kind of job would they do if killing a patient were considered just another "treatment option," and a less expensive and time-consuming option at that? To put it another way, why would we trust doctors to kill us, when too often they don't do an adequate job of caring for us? With so many Americans uninsured, the "last resort only" scenario is a virtual impossibility.

Financial Incentives Would Promote Assisted Suicide

To assert that money drives the American health-care system is like stating that seals like fish. Doctors' fees generally amount to hundreds of dollars an hour. One day in the hospital alone can cost thousands of dollars, and that doesn't include the "extras" for which hospitals also charge, such as intensive care, oxygen, bandages and aspirin. Come down with a condition or sustain an injury that requires a few weeks of hospitalization followed by extended follow-up care and the tab easily rises into six figures.

This money imperative and the sheer cost of medicine in the USA makes euthanasia even more dangerous here than it is in the Netherlands. At last count, forty-four million Americans had no health insurance. Almost by definition, being uninsured means that one lacks sustained access to quality health-care services. Most doctors refuse to accept new patients who do not have health insurance, and most private hospitals will help uninsured ill people only when required by law to do so in a life-threatening emergency.

Being uninsured means that health care, when it is received, is generally delivered in a public hospital emergency room, where, after hours of waiting, the patient will meet with a harried doctor (often in training) who has been assigned to deal with the problem as quickly and cheaply as possible. Those with chronic conditions often face similar barriers to effective care, relying on free clinics or emergency rooms where the lack of consistent treatment can cause complications requiring an expensive emergency response later.

With the growth of for-profit hospitals and health-care financing systems, even this meager measure of care for the uninsured poor is now actively threatened. According to Bruce Hilton, director of the National Center for Bioethics, a study in Florida indicated that for-profit hospitals, which make up more than half of that state's health-care institutions, supply only 8 percent of the state's charity care.[13]

In this context, euthanasia would be a potential form of oppression against the uninsured, the working poor, divorced persons, minorities, the unemployed, the mentally ill and those lacking education who may not even speak English. For these people, the presumption that assisted suicide would be considered only after every other conceivable method of care has been tried is, to put it politely, unrealistic. Hospice, extended pain control, psychiatric treatments for depression—services essential to the "last resort" scenario—are usually inaccessible to the uninsured. If euthanasia advocates really believed that doctor-hastened death should be performed only if there is no other way to alleviate suffering, they would put their issue on the shelf until the structural flaws in American medicine are solved. To do otherwise is putting the cart before the horse.

In these circumstances, many who would want to live were they to receive proper care might, out of desperation, express a desire to die when they have difficulty obtaining it. Doctors might be tempted to follow the line of least resistance by going along with this desire. Such a scenario is not purely imaginary. In July 1996, Rebecca Badger, age thirty-nine, traveled from California to Michigan to become Jack Kevorkian's thirty-third known assisted suicide victim. In a KEYT-TV (Santa Barbara) television interview taped only days before her death, Badger, who believed she had multiple sclerosis and who lost her private health insurance after a divorce forced her onto Medi-Cal (California's Medicaid program), complained bitterly about five-hour hospital waits to see a doctor and explained that the reason she was going to Kevorkian was her constant, unrelieved pain. Badger also said that if only her pain were relieved, she would want to live.[14]

But Badger's autopsy report showed that she did not have MS at all. Dr. Ljubisa J. Dragovic, a neuropathologist with specialized training in detecting neurological conditions and thus an expert in identifying MS, performed Badger's autopsy. He told me, "Rebecca Badger had no sign of the disease. The findings are completely negative. The problem with MS is that a lot of conditions can simulate MS and MS can simulate a lot of conditions."[15]

What Badger did suffer from was diagnosed depression and abandonment by the health-care system just when she most needed compassionate treatment of her ailments. According to her daughter, Badger, a recovering alcoholic who was addicted to prescription medications, had lost faith in the medicine and believed that her maladies would never be taken seriously. In despair, she took her final, fatal trip to Michigan for a rendezvous with death.[16]

HMOs and Euthanasia: A Deadly Combination

Recent changes in the economics and financial incentives of American medicine have made euthanasia especially hazardous. Our health system has evolved from one based on "fee for service" to one dominated by HMOs and managed care, in which money is made not by providing services but primarily by controlling costs. In the former system, an insured seriously ill person generally made profits for hospitals and physicians. Today, such a person may represent costs. This change turns the traditional presumptions about health-care financing and the delivery of medical services inside out.

The cost-cutting agendas of managed care are an intrinsic part of private and publicly financed health care. HMOs are ubiquitous. Payments to physicians who treat recipients of Medicaid (the federal and state-funded and state-administered health insurance for the poorest of the poor) and Medicare (the health insurance plan for the elderly and some disabled) are increasingly being squeezed to the point where there is nothing left to give. Indeed, Medicare now pays doctors so little in compensation for their services that many physicians now refuse to take on Medicare recipients as new patients.[17]

Now, consider these intense pressures to cut costs in the context of legalized euthanasia. If killing patients because they are seriously ill or disabled becomes viewed as merely another "treatment," the lives of patients who require expensive depth of care will be endangered. Remember, for HMOs, profits come not through providing services but from limiting costs, which in real life often means reducing services. Imagine the money that could be saved—and thus profits earned—by HMOs in not treating cancer, AIDS, MS or quadriplegic patients because they "choose" instead to be killed.

As Dr. Daniel P. Sulmasy of the Center for Clinical Bioethics at the Georgetown University Medical Center has written in *Archives of Internal Medicine,* we may be heading toward a health-care system where cost control and the killing of patients go hand in hand:

> As providers of managed death, many physicians will be sincerely motivated by respect for patient autonomy, but the cost factor will always lurk silently in the background. This will be especially true if they are providing managed death in a setting of managed care. A perilous line of argument might then emerge:... 1) Too much money is spent on health care; 2) certain patients are expensive to take care of (i.e., those with physical disabilities and the elderly); 3) these patients appear to suffer a great deal, lead lives of diminished dignity, and are a burden to others;... 4) recognizing the diminished dignity, suffering and burdens borne by these persons and those around them, their right to euthanasia or assisted suicide should be legally recognized; and 5) the happy side effect will be health care cost savings.[18]

Lending credence to Dr. Sulmasy's warning is the intense cost-cutting pressure already placed on doctors at the clinical level. One of the hallmarks of HMO care is the dual role of the plan member's primary care physician (PCP). First, the PCP—usually an internist, family care specialist or, for children, a pediatrician—is the plan member's personal doctor, in charge of preventive care, managing chronic conditions, providing inoculations and the like. The PCP also serves a function on behalf of the HMO as cost-cutting "gate-keeper," the person in charge of controlling the cost of each patient's care.

It is the gatekeeper function that has so many physicians and consumer advocates worried about financial conflicts of interest between doctors and their patients. Doctors in many HMOs are paid individually (or as part of a small group) on a capitation basis. This means that the PCP (or the group) receives a flat monthly fee for each patient, regardless of how much care the patient requires. (HMO defenders point out that some patients rarely see the doctor and so the capitation system evens out, with the doctor compensated for care he or she is never called upon to provide.)

That a doctor receives no extra compensation for additional effort isn't the primary worry about capitation. The real concern is that some companies impose a capitation system in which the PCP is *personally held financially responsible* by the HMO for any referrals made outside his or her group, to specialists or for tests. In such contracts, the PCP receives a higher-than-usual capitation payment, perhaps forty dollars per month per patient, but in return must personally pay for each patient's lab tests, consultations with specialists, and emergency care, up to a maximum per patient that may be as high as five thousand dollars, after which the HMO takes over.[19] In a system where doctors lose money every time they refer a patient out of house, they may be reluctant to allow their patients to consult specialists, including pain-control experts or psychiatrists, who are crucial to the proper care of many dying or chronically ill patients. Without such treatment, these patients might turn in despair to a death doctor—or ask their PCP to become one—in search of relief.

These and other financial pressures placed on doctors in clinical practice by HMOs may already be having life-and-death repercussions. Take the case of the Christie family of Woodside, California. In 1993, Katherine and Harry Christie joined an HMO known as TakeCare Health Plan. They chose the Palo Alto Medical Clinic as their primary medical group (a group of doctors of varying specialties who would be responsible for the family's medical care). At the time, Carley, the Christies' nine-year-old daughter, was having significant kidney problems. According to a Petition to Assess Civil Penalties filed by the California Department of Corporations (the agency in charge of regulating HMOs in the state), Carley's PCP, Dr. Susan Smith, referred her for consultation to Dr. James Bassett, a Palo Alto Medical Clinic colleague, despite the fact that Dr. Bassett had little experience in pediatric urology.[20]

Dr. Bassett diagnosed Carley with a rare and life-threatening cancer known as Wilms' tumor. Having no experience in treating Wilms' tumor, and knowing that he was not the doctor to care adequately for Carley, Dr. Bassett suggested that the Christies take Carley to Dr. Michael Link, a pediatric urologist with extensive experience in treating Wilms' tumor, which often requires surgery, chemotherapy and radiation. Dr. Link and other members of his specialized multidisciplinary team were not part of the Palo Alto Medical Clinic group practice.

Under the HMO contract with the Christies, any out-of-group referral needed the go-ahead of Carley's PCP, Dr. Smith. Refusing to abide by what the Department of Corporations called "good professional practice," Dr. Smith refused to authorize a referral to Dr. Link and instead insisted that her colleague Dr. Bassett, with no experience in Wilms' tumor surgery or treatment, perform the surgery.[21] Adding to the outrageousness of this decision was the worry that Dr. Bassett may have worsened Carley's condition previously during a biopsy by "causing spillage of the tumor [into other parts of her body]. This spillage triggered an additional nine months of painful chemotherapy...."[22]

The Christies were in a dreadful bind: Their daughter needed immediate surgery to save her life, yet they faced paying for it themselves unless they permitted an unqualified doctor to provide the care. As the clock was ticking toward the time when surgery would have to be performed, the Christies transferred Carley's care to the experienced medical team. The surgery was successful. Carley's life was saved.

TakeCare soon informed the Christies that it would not pay for Carley's treatment, "in retaliation," according to the Department of Corporations, "for the Christies' choosing a qualified pediatric surgeon to remove Carley's tumor."[23] The HMO also refused to pay for the cost of hospitalization, which represented $47,000 of the $55,000 total cost of Carley's care, despite the fact that the same hospital would have been used regardless of which doctors treated Carley. Thus, in addition to worrying about their daughter's recuperation, the Christies were now facing pronounced financial difficulty.

The Christies entered the contractual grievance process of the HMO. (Owing to a binding arbitration clause, they were unable to sue.) They obtained an arbitration award recovering their medical expenses and arbitration fees, but not their legal fees. They then filed a complaint with the Department of Corporations, alleging that the HMO had violated the California Health and Safety Code. The Christies were not after a monetary settlement for themselves, but rather hoped the DOC would fine the company to set an example for all of the state's HMOs. An administrative fine of $500,000 was levied against TakeCare, which was upheld on appeal.

The California Department of Corporations contends that a primary reason why Carley was refused referral to a qualified specialist was the HMO's capitation agreement with Palo Alto Medical Clinic, which required the physicians' group to pay for Carley's surgery out of its own funds if it was performed by nongroup physicians—money that would have been saved by keeping her care in-house.[24] The HMO denied the charge.

The Christie family story was not a tale of euthanasia, of course. But if a capitation-based financial conflict may have put at significant risk a nine-year-old girl with a good chance of recovery, imagine what these financial incentives would mean to elderly cancer patients, disabled persons requiring long-term specialized care, or dying people who require intensive and perhaps costly pain control. In order to save their own money, PCPs might deny expensive specialized care to their most needful and vulnerable patients, leading to unrelieved suffering and resulting despair. This in turn could propel patients toward euthanasia. Indeed, the doctor could legally recommend the killing as a "treatment option." This is an especially worrying scenario considering the depth of trust and hope that seriously ill patients place in their physicians.

What would it be like to know that the doctor who was licensed to kill you also benefited financially from the act? Or to know that a doctor who recommended suicide for your spouse could be financially punished for providing him or her with "too much" care? What would happen to the trust between you and your doctor? How would potential financial gain affect your doctor's attitude toward your care if you developed a problem that required specialized treatment? Would you have ready access to pain control, psychiatric treatment, hospice, and other care opportunities that would be more expensive than euthanasia? Moreover, if killing the weak and sick became a profit center in the immensely powerful health-care industry, what would happen to medical ethics overall? And would legalized killing change society's attitudes toward the value of the lives of people deemed eligible for hastened death: the dying, the ill, the elderly and the disabled? With HMOs becoming the norm, these questions must be answered before we embrace euthanasia or take seriously the "last resort" scenarios spun by death fundamentalists.

The potential for the development of an HMO/assisted suicide nexus was illustrated vividly in 2002 when an executive at Kaiser Permanente Northwest, an Oregon HMO that permits its doctors to assist the suicides of Kaiser Plan Members, sent an e-mail memo to Plan doctors requesting volunteers to assist the suicides of people who were not their own patients. The memo revealed that to the apparent chagrin of the memo writer, few Kaiser doctors were willing to participate in assisting the killing of their own patients. Hence, the executive solicited any Kaiser doctor willing to act as "Attending Physician under the law for members who ARE NOT your patients" to contact administrators. (Emphasis in the memo.)[25] Since "attending physicians" write the lethal prescriptions under the Oregon law, this Kaiser executive clearly wanted plan doctors to agree to end the lives of patients they had never even treated.

Most euthanasia advocates don't like discussing these financial-moral issues. But a rare few are quite candid about the money agenda behind the euthanasia movement. Indeed, Derek Humphry, godfather of the euthanasia movement, admits that saving money is the "unspoken argument" in favor of legalizing physician killing of patients. In the book *Freedom to Die*, which Humphry co-authored with pro-euthanasia attorney Mary Clement, the authors write:

> A rational argument can be made for allowing PAS [physician-assisted suicide] in order to offset the amount society and family spend on the ill, *as long as it is the voluntary wish* of the mentally competent terminally and incurably ill adult. There will likely come a time when PAS becomes a commonplace occurrence for individuals who *want* to die and feel it is the right thing to do by their loved ones. There is no contradicting the fact that since the largest medical expenses are incurred in the final days and weeks of life, the hastened demise of people with only a short time left would free resources for others. Hundreds of billions of dollars could benefit those patients who not only *can* be cured but who want to live. [Emphasis in the text.][26]

Humphry and Clement assert that "economic necessity" will "continue to drive the right to die movement largely because of its appeal to common sense." They then add, "Economic realty, therefore, is the main answer to the question [about the emergence of the euthanasia movement], 'Why now?'"[27] For perhaps the first and only time in his death-purveying career, Derek Humphry has it exactly right. In the end, legalized assisted suicide and euthanasia—at least in the United States—would not be about compassion and altruism; it would be about money.

The Silent Epidemic: Medical Malpractice

Another disturbing truth about our health-care delivery system that is routinely overlooked in euthanasia advocacy is the "silent epidemic" of medical malpractice.[28] According to Charles Inlander, president of the People's Medical Society, one of the nation's largest patient advocacy groups with more than 100,000 dues-paying members, "Between 136,000 and 310,000 people a year are injured or killed due to medical mistakes by their doctors," a figure Inlander called "conservative."[29]

An authoritative study published by the Harvard Medical Practice Study Group, conducted at Harvard's School of Public Health and one of the most comprehensive and objective investigations of medical malpractice ever performed, found that more than 98,000 patients in hospitals located in New York State suffered "adverse events," injuries from medical care rather than disease, in one year, 1984. Twenty-seven percent of these adverse events were the result of medical negligence, causing 6,895 patient deaths in the state's hospitals that year.[30] Projecting these figures nationwide, the study's authors suggested that at least 80,000 people are killed in hospitals each year by medical malpractice, more than deaths caused by suicide, homicide and AIDS combined. These figures only represent deaths in hospitals—and don't reflect the potential for a significant worsening of the situation in recent years caused by nursing staff cuts and other cost-cutting measures that have hit the hospital industry like a perfect storm under the pressure of managed care economics. They also do not measure misdiagnoses, failure to properly alleviate pain or depression, or other failings in the clinical setting that bear on the euthanasia issue. A study released in 2005 reached a similar conclusion, finding that 98,000 deaths per year were caused in the United States by medical errors.[31]

Between 5 and 15 percent of the physician population are believed to be "incompetent or dangerous," and these doctors would be as entitled as any other physician to kill patients if euthanasia were legalized.[32] Indeed, some might be attracted to euthanasia "practice," as legalization proposals provide civil and criminal legal immunity to doctors who kill their patients. Legalizing killing by doctors could even become a way for a few very unscrupulous doctors to cover up their malpractice or limit damages from lawsuits, by killing the victims they have injured in the name of "death with dignity" and the "right to die."

A euthanasia case that occurred in San Francisco several years ago illustrates how easy it would be for a doctor to kill a patient as a means of covering up malpractice. In March 1995 a nine-year-old girl was admitted into the University of California Medical Center for elective surgery to realign her jaw. The surgery, which required that her jaws be wired shut, went well, but afterward her jaws were not unwired when she became nauseated. The girl aspirated her own vomit and was left with severe brain damage.[33]

The girl had been unconscious for a few weeks when a pediatrician specialist, an employee of the hospital who was not the cause of the girl's aspiration-caused injury, undertook her care for a couple of hours while on duty. A different doctor had previously convinced the girl's mother to suspend life support, but the girl hadn't died. After being removed from a respirator she began to breathe spontaneously, after which, apparently, the hospital refused to support the girl nutritionally. A few hours after the decision to cut off food and fluids, the employee-doctor injected the child with potassium chloride, which paralyzed the girl's heart and killed her. (A legal dispute later arose over whether the girl's distraught mother had asked the doctor to administer the lethal injection.)

This intentional killing of a child did not result in criminal prosecution. Nor, as far as is publicly known, did the California Medical Board discipline the doctor, although one source told me the case is still being investigated. However, three nurses who blew the whistle on the doctor were initially suspended without pay, allegedly owing to their supposed delay in reporting the incident. (The nurses' suspension was overturned on administrative appeal, but one of the lawyers in the case told me that they were all reassigned to other duties, prompting at least one nurse to quit her job and move to another city.) The employee-doctor, however, only had her hospital staff privileges suspended and did not lose pay.

The killing doctor claimed, in anonymous interviews, that her decision to inject the girl was motivated solely by a "compassionate" desire to end the girl's suffering at the request of the mother.[34] Perhaps. But what if her motive had actually been venal, to reduce the malpractice legal exposure of her hospital in the case, or to protect a physician friend who had actually injured the girl? What if she had been the original malpracticing doctor (which she was not) and her motive was self-protection? Who would know? She could claim that she was acting as an angel of mercy to provide "death with dignity" when her actual motive was to reduce the monetary damages to be paid out of the malpractice case.

The malpractice civil suit brought by her mother involving the girl's post-surgery injury and subsequent killing was settled quickly for an undisclosed amount. If the terms of the settlement were those usually employed in legal settlements of this kind, the hospital and doctors involved did not admit liability or wrongdoing. (My request to the University of California Medical Center for an interview with the killing doctor was refused, nor would it release the name of anyone involved.)

Euthanasia advocates often use cases such as this to support their contention that euthanasia is common. In fact, there is no reliable information on the frequency or infrequency of euthanasia in the clinical setting. No one knows whether, or how often, doctors actually kill their patients.

Surveys taken of doctors about this issue tend to rebut the claim that euthanasia and assisted suicide are common occurrences. For example, in the wake of the passage of Measure 16, Oregon doctors were surveyed by the *New England Journal of Medicine* to determine their attitudes and experiences with assisted suicide. Only 7 percent of the responding doctors had ever written a lethal prescription for use in a patient's suicide—187 out of 2,761 doctors surveyed.[35] A similar study published in the same journal in 1994 found that only 9.4 percent of physicians had taken action to "directly" cause a patient to die (not necessarily euthanasia or assisted suicide), and only 3.7 percent had provided information that would cause a patient's death.[36] The polling also suggests that physicians, while reflecting society's deep divisions about legalizing assisted suicide, are generally quite worried about its application in the real world. The Oregon poll found that more than half of Oregon physicians would be unwilling because of moral objections to prescribe an overdose. Adding to their unease was the fear felt by more than 90 percent of the doctors that their patients would seek hastened death so as not to be a burden on others. This fear was borne out once legal assisted suicide began in Oregon, as we saw in the last chapter.

The results of the *New England Journal of Medicine* study were so significant that one of its authors, Diane E. Meier, changed her position from supporting legalization before she began her research to opposing it once her study was completed. Whereas she had viewed legalization as a way to regulate a supposedly common clinical practice, once it became clear to her that doctors do not commonly kill patients, she opposed legalization out of fear that it would "become a cheap and easy way to avoid the costly and time-intensive care needed by the terminally ill."[37]

Meier's opposition to the legalization of assisted suicide and euthanasia echoes the official positions of almost all professional medical organizations and other health-care groups. The American Medical Association opposes euthanasia and assisted suicide. So does the National Hospice Organization, which certainly understands the issues involved with end-of-life care. The American Nurses Association is also staunchly opposed.

Refusing Wanted Treatment

So far, we have seen that euthanasia advocates largely appeal to patient autonomy to promote their wider agenda. So too has the dehydration of cognitively disabled people been justified as a matter of respecting the personal values and decision making of patients or their surrogates. In a culture steeped in individualism, there is no question that such appeals resonate with many who cherish personal autonomy and the right of "choice."

This raises an interesting and important question: Do these purveyors of assisted death really believe in "choice"? For example, what if the seriously ill or disabled patient or his surrogates wish to continue treatment that many in bioethics and among the medical intelligentsia believe should be stopped? What if the patient's personal value system holds that it is right and proper to fight for life until death can no longer be held at bay?

As a matter of consistency, one would expect that decisions to resist dying—even with the use of heroic measures—would be deemed as sacrosanct as the decision to seek death or refuse life-sustaining medical treatment. But consistency and autonomy are not necessarily the point. Now that the "right to die" has sunk its hooks into the culture, those who assert the concomitant "right to live" are increasingly being told that autonomy has its limits.

While society and the media have focused on assisted suicide and the right to refuse unwanted treatment, little attention has been paid by the media to concurrent efforts promoted in bioethics to disregard patient autonomy when dying and profoundly disabled patients want their lives sustained. This is the emerging bioethical debate over "futile care" (sometimes called "inappropriate care"), in which many bioethicists, academics, members of the medical intelligentsia and social engineers argue that life-sustaining treatment requests can and should be disregarded by physicians if the quality of the patient's life is deemed not worth living.

Futile care advocates—sometimes called "futilitarians"—sometimes act as if the struggle against medical paternalism over the last twenty years never happened, when certain patients want life-sustaining treatment that the doctor believes is "futile." "The decision about futile therapy cannot and should not be abdicated by the physician to the patient, family, surrogate, court, or society in general," says Allen J. Bennett, M.D., vice chairman of the Committee on Bioethical Issues of the Medical Society of the State of New York. "To abdicate a decision about the futility of a procedure or medical treatment is to abdicate professional responsibility for the patient.... Futility decisions should be left to physicians."[38] More succinctly, the California Healthcare Foundation, in a written objection to legislation that would have prevented California hospitals from imposing futile care theory on unwilling patients and their families, stated: "The provision of medical care must be left in the hands of treating providers to do what is best for patients.... Decisions to provide or withdraw care *must be made by the appropriate medical personnel* on a case-by-case basis and not limited or extended by law." (Emphasis added.) [39]

Futile care theory proposes that the old, the dying, those on the margins and the profoundly disabled can be pushed out of the lifeboat in order to allow others in or, indeed, to keep the boat afloat. Thus, futile care theory can be accurately described as a first cousin to euthanasia in that it rejects the equality-of-human-life ethic in favor of a subjective value system that determines whose lives are worth protecting and whose lives are not.

In brief, futile care theory goes something like this: When a patient reaches a certain stage of age, illness or injury, any further treatment other than comfort care is futile and should be withheld or stopped. That the patient may *want* the treatment anyway, because of deeply held values or a desire to improve in medical condition, is not decisive; the doctors involved have the right to refuse treatment unilaterally based on their autonomy or professionalism.

At this point, let me make it clear that I am not talking about treatment that is truly and objectively "futile." If a patient requests a medical intervention that would provide no physiological benefit, the doctor can and should refuse. To use an extreme example to illustrate the point, if a patient afflicted with a simple ear infection requested an appendectomy to cure it, the doctor could and should refuse to perform the surgery because it would have no effect on the earache.

But this is not what futilitarians are promoting. Rather, they espouse a radical view of health-care decision making that would allow the values of health-care professionals or health insurance company executives, or even community "consensus" over what should be done to and for the patient, to take precedence over patients' own wishes for their care.

Futile care theory has quietly gained momentum for the last several years. Mandatory treatment guidelines have already been drafted by bioethics think tanks and are beginning to be implemented in hospitals around the country. These are not rules intended to define minimum allowable standards (which are desperately needed in this age of HMOs), but rather to serve as guidelines and procedures for denying wanted life-sustaining care.

The first targets of what developed into the futile care movement were patients diagnosed with persistent unconsciousness. For example, in 1994, Dr. Marcia Angell, then executive editor of the *New England Journal of Medicine*, editorialized that current presumptions in favor of life as they apply to the permanently unconscious must be changed so that "demoralized" caregivers won't have to provide care that they believe is futile—or that wastes "valuable resources."[40]

Dr. Angell offered three proposals that would permit care to be withdrawn. The first would be to broaden the definition of death to include diagnosis of permanent unconsciousness. (This approach is also seen by some in bioethics as a way to increase the supply of transplantable organs.)[41]

There are currently two primary and appropriate definitions of death in use: brain death, meaning the total cessation of all measurable electrical activity in the brain, and complete cessation of heartbeat and respiration.[42] Dr. Angell's radical suggestion would be to take living people with functioning bodies, including brain systems, and pretend that they were deceased for utilitarian purposes. Demonstrating the illogic of the suggestion, Dr. Angell, noting that these "patients do not 'look dead,'" admits that "it would, paradoxically, be necessary to withdraw life-sustaining treatment, including artificial feeding, to stop the cardiopulmonary function." In other words, the "dead" patients would have to be made actually dead so that their treatment could cease.

Dr. Angell's second proposal would allow legislatures to pass laws prohibiting life-sustaining medical treatment for the unconscious after a specified period of time. Under this approach, the decision to make a person die by withholding nutrition would be made in advance by society without regard to any individual case. Thus, according to Angell, the family who wanted care to continue could at least be comforted by the knowledge that the decision to terminate their loved one's life was not personal. This is an example of futilitarianism.

The third and "less sweeping" proposal, favored personally by Dr. Angell, would create a legal presumption that persons who are unconscious would not want treatment after a specified time. In that way, a family that held the "idiosyncratic" view that their loved one should not be dehydrated to death would have to prove that the patient had expressed a specific desire to be treated under these specific circumstances. In other words, the current (weak) presumption in favor of life for the profoundly cognitively disabled would be changed to an explicit legal presumption in favor of death.

Dr. Angell and many others who agree with her assert that *their* personal beliefs that unconscious patients do not have lives worth living should trump the values of patients or families who see unconscious people as fully human and worthy of love and care. Ironically, their reason for stopping the "treatment" of food and fluids would not be because the treatment was failing but because it was succeeding in keeping patients alive—to futilitarians, an unacceptable outcome. Or to put it another way, in futile care theory, it isn't the treatment that is actually dismissed as futile; it is the *patient*.

Recall from the second chapter that if a patient wants to be dehydrated to death when cognitively disabled, or if the family request this, it is now supposedly done out of a deep and abiding respect for the patient's autonomy. But under futile care theory, if the same family should instead rebel against the prevailing medical value system and desire to keep their unconscious loved one alive, then autonomy is suddenly the enemy.

Note, too, the values expressed in Dr. Angell's editorial. It seems that we "have lost the virtue of caring for people simply because they are people," remarks Thomas Marzen of the National Center for the Medically Dependent and Disabled, a legal advocacy group for the profoundly disabled.[43] Indeed, nowhere in her editorial does Dr. Angell speak of unconscious patients as people. Rather, they are viewed as problems that "demoralize" caregivers and waste resources.

There is another flaw in Dr. Angell's thesis. She gives short shrift to the fact that people diagnosed by doctors as permanently unconscious often are not actually unconscious. According to a growing body of medical literature, misdiagnosis of the persistent vegetative state is common. For example, a study published in the June 1991 *Archives of Neurology* found that of eighty-four patients with a firm diagnosis of PVS, forty-nine (58 percent) recovered consciousness within a three-year period. Studies also show that researchers have been unable to identify objective "predictors of recovery," to differentiate between those who may awaken and those who most likely will not. Moreover, some "unconscious" patients who later awaken report that they were not unaware as is supposed, but rather had "visions" or "out-of-body experiences" or were aware and emotionally responsive to everything going on around them but unable to communicate.[44] A study in Great Britain revealed that perhaps 40 percent of patients diagnosed with PVS are actually conscious.[45] If these and other similar studies were accurate, Dr. Angell's proposed ethic, if accepted, would likely cause the deaths of some people who would have recovered consciousness given sufficient time. It also means that those dehydrated to death on the assumption that they were completely unaware and hence unable to suffer could die in a most agonizing manner, whether or not they or their families wanted that outcome.

Unconscious patients aren't the only ones threatened by futilitarianism. So too are the elderly, physically disabled people and others with serious chronic conditions. The influential bioethicist Daniel Callahan offered several rather vague definitions of futility in his 1993 book, *The Troubled Dream of Life*. It exists, he wrote, when:

- "there is a likely, though not necessarily certain, downward course of an illness, making death a strong probability"; or,
- "successful treatment is more likely to bring extended unconsciousness or advanced dementia than cure or significant amelioration"; or,
- "the available treatments for a potentially fatal condition entail a significant likelihood of extended pain or suffering"; or,
- "the available treatments significantly increase the probability of a bad death, even if they promise to extend life."[46]

In such cases, Callahan urged that a presumption against medical treatment, other than comfort care, be created and that people who insist on these futile treatments be required to pay for it themselves.

Forcing people off wanted life-sustaining treatment isn't a fantasy scenario. A few futile care cases have already reached the courts.

The first such case occurred in 1990–91 and pitted the husband of Helga Wanglie, an elderly woman in a permanent coma with multiple organ failure, against her doctors and hospital. Helga was dependent on a ventilator for her continued life. Her doctors received permission from her husband to place a "do not resuscitate" (DNR) order on Helga's chart but he refused to permit them to withdraw the ventilator. As a consequence, he was sued.

According to Steven Miles, a physician and bioethics consultant who became the public spokesman for the hospital, there were three reasons why Helga's doctors wanted to stop her treatment. "The palliative aspects of her care would not work because she was incapable of feeling the benefit of having the ventilator relieve air hunger; the continued provision of the respirator would not keep open the possibility that she would return to any type of minimally rational life; and, the use of the respirator would not allow her to have a relational life in the present."[47]

I asked Miles whether her continued life, in and of itself, was considered a benefit to her. "Yes," he replied, "but we did not have a way to help her acquire a quality of life that she herself could value."

Mr. Wanglie's position was that his wife valued life for life's sake and that she would want to remain alive under these conditions. The question presented to the court: Whose ultimate moral values should prevail, the husband/wife's or those of the medical professionals?

Dr. Miles brought a court case to have Mr. Wanglie removed as his wife's medical decision maker. (Miles told me he became the petitioner after Helga's treating physician was forced to withdraw due to a death in the family.) The trial was to be held in two parts: first, to determine who should make decisions about Helga's care, Mr. Wanglie or an independent person to be selected by the court as a guardian *ad litem*; and second, to decide whether Helga's physicians had to continue her treatment according to the desires of Mr. Wanglie, were he named by the court as his wife's medical decision maker.

After a hearing, the court refused to oust Mr. Wanglie as his wife's medical surrogate, ruling that as her husband of many years, he was the best person to make Helga's health-care decisions.[48] The ruling settled only the first part of the case. Still to be decided was whether the doctors had to continue to treat Helga with a respirator despite their view that the treatment was futile. This issue was never adjudicated because Helga died and the matter was dropped.

A similar scenario unfolded in Flint, Michigan, in 1993, where Baby Terry was born prematurely at 23 weeks gestation. (The normal gestation for a human infant is 38 to 40 weeks.) Baby Terry, weighed 1 pound 7 ounces at birth and was desperately ill. Deprived of oxygen, his brain had been damaged and he required a respirator to stay alive.

Doctors at Hurley Medical Center advised Terry's parents, Rosetta Christle, age twenty-one, and Terry Achtabowski, age twenty-two, that Terry's life support was futile. But Christle and Achtabowski disagreed. They weren't ready to give up. Their baby had gained a pound and successfully resisted a bacterial infection and they wanted him to have every opportunity to fight for his life.

The parents' refusal to accept termination of treatment was unacceptable to Baby Terry's doctors and the hospital administration. They called in the Michigan Department of Social Services, which quickly brought court action to strip the young parents of their right to make decisions over their son's medical treatment. (Such drastic action is usually taken only when parents *refuse* needed medical treatment for their children.) A hearing was convened and testimony elicited. The physicians were unanimous in their desire to terminate care, testifying that Terry was in pain, although relieved by morphine, that his bodily systems were slowly breaking down, and that he had no chance of long-term survival. The Hurley Hospital ethics committee weighed in on August 9, 1993, opining that the parents' insistence on continued treatment "would be contrary to medical judgment and to *moral and ethical beliefs of physicians* caring for the patient." (My emphasis.)[49] In other words, when it came to choosing between the values of Baby Terry's parents, based in large part on their religious faith, and the values of doctors and the hospital, the state argued that only the latter opinions mattered.

Solely on the basis of their refusal to permit treatment to be ended, Judge Thomas Gadola of the Genesee County Probate Court found Christle and Achtabowski unfit to make proper health-care decisions for their baby and stripped them of their rights as parents. He then awarded temporary custody of Baby Terry to his maternal great-aunt, who had previously stated her willingness to obey the doctors and cut off life support.

Legal wrangling continued. Before the case concluded and a final decision was made as to who should have final authority over the care of Baby Terry—his parents or his doctors—the infant died in his mother's arms, age two and a half months. Lawyers for Christle and Achtabowski still wanted a formal court decision overruling the trial court, but the court of appeals dismissed the case as moot.

Another family was forced to go to court to obtain wanted treatment in a more recent case in Winnipeg, Manitoba, in Canada. Andrew Sawatzky, seventy-nine, had late-stage Parkinson's disease and had experienced debilitating strokes. His doctors decided to place a DNR order on his chart over the objections of Sawatzky's wife, Helene. When she could not get the doctors to remove the DNR order from the chart, Helene sued. The court granted a temporary court order removing the DNR, pending further investigation as to whether the doctors' values or those of the Sawatzkys would determine Andrew's level of care. The case became moot when Andrew's condition improved so much that he was able to return home.

In England, the courts sided with doctors in a futility case when parents sought similar relief, with very frightening implications for the most weak and vulnerable members of British society. David Glass, age twelve, is a mentally retarded boy who is blind and quadriplegic. He is also greatly loved by his parents and siblings, who cherish him as an integral part of the family.

In October 1998, David was admitted to St. Mary's Hospital in Portsmouth with a respiratory failure. Instead of trying to save his life, doctors unilaterally withdrew curative treatment and injected him with a palliative agent, telling the parents that their son was dying and that nature should be allowed to take its course.

The parents refused to stand by and watch their abandoned son die because doctors did not perceive his life as worth living. They instituted resuscitation on their own and saved David's life. One doctor later testified that he objected strenuously to the parents actions because they had "prevented him from dying."[50] Clearly, if family members could save David without the expertise of formal treatment, the refusal of care was more a matter of physician bias than of compassionately allowing nature to take a sad but inevitable course.

David's parents sued to prevent such an awful abandonment from being repeated. Unexpectedly, they lost. The trial and appeals courts both ruled that doctors, not parents, have the ultimate say over David's life and death. This ruling is in line with a recent ethics opinion published by the British Medical Association, which established an ethical protocol granting doctors the ultimate power to determine when and if treatment will be terminated.

FOR OBVIOUS REASONS, HOSPITAL PUBLICISTS do not hold press conferences to announce that they have granted themselves permission to refuse wanted life-sustaining treatment. Thus, nobody really knows which hospitals have adopted futile care protocols and which have not, or indeed whether protocols are actually being applied against patients and their families. But it does appear that the futile care agenda is spreading. A very disturbing survey published in the fall 2000 edition of the *Cambridge Quarterly of Health Care Ethics* reported that 24 out of 26 California hospitals that were surveyed "defined nonobligatory treatment" in terms that were not "physiology based." Twelve of the hospitals surveyed prohibited treating people diagnosed with permanent unconsciousness (other than providing comfort care), on account of these patients' supposed inability to know they are being treated. Only seven of the hospitals left the final decision about whether to continue treatment in the hands of the patient or the family.[51]

A primary purpose of these futile care protocols is to block families and patients who sue to receive wanted treatment. The idea is to present judges with the protocols as a defense against lawsuits demanding treatment, in effect telling the courts that the bioethicists and doctors have already worked things out, that futile care theory is ethical and widely accepted, and that the patient received due process via the administrative process established by the futility protocols. At that point, the $400–per-hour lawyer for the hospital would argue, "Judge, how can you, a mere lawyer, gainsay what the medical profession has carefully considered over several years and determined to be medically appropriate?" Futilitarians expect that judges would respond positively to this argument and allow treatment to be withdrawn.

Unfortunately, that's probably a pretty good bet. For as the authors of the *Cambridge Quarterly* study put it, "Hospitals are likely to find the legal system willing (and even eager) to defer to well-defined and procedurally scrupulous processes for internal resolutions of futility disputes."[52]

But is this approach something that the people—who, after all, are the very ones who would be most affected by medical futility—support? Since so little has been written and broadcast in the mainstream press about futile care theory, that is hard to know. However, the rise and fall of a futile care think tank, the Colorado Collective for Medical Decisions (CCMD), provides an important clue.

CCMD's former director, Dr. Donald J. Murphy, hoped the work of CCMD would empower doctors, hospitals, nursing homes and health-care financing entities all over the country, including for-profit HMOs, to refuse "futile" medical treatment, even when the care was desired by the patient. According to the group's published preliminary guidelines, "futile care" would have included food and fluids and other forms of life support for persistently unconscious people. CPR would have been denied—even when wanted by, for example, family members—to the "frail, institutionalized elderly"; to people with a "terminal illness" where there is "less than a 5% chance of surviving to discharge after CPR"; to patients who are "receiving hospice care"; and in cases where more than "7 minutes pass from the cardiac arrest before CPR can be initiated"—to name a few conditions.[53]

The stated purpose behind CCMD futilitarianism was to save health-care resources for those whom "society" deems more worthy of consuming them. The advocates of such changes maintain that such quasi rationing would better promote overall "health," a concept that Dr. Murphy asserted includes broad community matters of "education, transportation, and recreation, as well as medical care."[54] If that meant sacrificing the ill, the elderly, even people who would have a "5, 10, or even 20 percent chance of surviving," according to Dr. Murphy, that difficult decision would just have to be made.[53]

CCMD's idea was to develop the guidelines and then introduce them at a series of community forums for approval. But a funny thing happened on the way to futilitarianism: When the public learned that CCMD wanted permission to impose its values upon ill patients and their families, futile care theory fell flat on its face.

Here's the story: Murphy approached the Colorado Trust, a philanthropic foundation dedicated to funding projects designed to promote "accessible and affordable healthcare programs." The trust granted CCMD $1.3 million to develop its guidelines. "It was a unique grant," said Nancy Baughman Csuti, senior evaluation officer for the Colorado Trust. "It was not done in response to a Request For Proposals. Dr. Murphy just came in as the leader of his organization and made a strong presentation asking for the money."

CCMD used the Colorado Trust's donation to convene community focus groups intended to determine—and hopefully to mold—the public's attitudes toward end-of-life care. Murphy's purpose was to generate so much public agreement with CCMD's proposed guidelines that hospitals, HMOs and physicians would be emboldened to immediately begin the widespread withholding of "inappropriate" care. But to Murphy's chagrin, "the community" generally rejected futile care theory. "It became clear that people believe that they should be in control of their own care," Csuti told me.

Seeing the handwriting on the wall, the Colorado Trust ceased funding CCMD and used the information gleaned from the focus groups to help craft a new Palliative Care Initiative by which the trust hopes to promote better and more humane medical treatment at the end of life—a program *not* based on a coercive model. Why the change? Csuti says: "Our foundation believes that the community must buy into new approaches to medicine. It became clear that the guidelines would not fly. So, the Foundation is now pursuing a different path."

In an ironic postscript to the story, demonstrating how groups that live by philanthropy can also die by philanthropy, the loss of the Colorado Trust's funding dealt a deathblow to CCMD. The organization is no longer active and Dr. Murphy has moved on to new endeavors.[56]

But the Colorado victory seems to be the exception. As an increasing number of futile care protocols have been quietly promulgated in hospitals around the country, bioethicists and physicians are boldly beginning to force people off wanted life-sustaining care. Texas doctors and bioethicists are taking the lead because of a 1999 law that explicitly permits hospital ethics committees to impose futility decisions on patients. Once it has been determined that treatment will be refused, under the Texas law, patients or families only have ten days to find another hospital—or the patient almost surely dies.

As is usually the case in such matters, the first victims have been on the far margins. Thus, in Houston, Sun Hudson, a five-month-old infant born with a fatal form of dwarfism, was taken off a ventilator over his mother's objections. Sun died in March 2005.[57]

In another Houston case, with echoes of Terri Schiavo, the wife of Spiro Nikolouzos *wanted* tube-feeding for her persistently unconscious husband, based on his previously stated desire to live. But contrary to the Schiavo case, Nikolouzos' personal values were not deemed determinative: A hospital ethics committee voted to discontinue his tube-supplied food and water and his ventilator support. He would have died, but unexpectedly a San Antonio hospital agreed to provide the care. Then, its ethics committee also decided to cut off care, but Nikolouzos was transferred to a nursing home. So, as of this writing at least, Nikolouzos is being allowed to stay alive. But notice that the final decision about the matter isn't his wife's: under futile care theory, it belongs to bioethics committees or doctors.[58]

Follow the Money

A primary purpose behind futile care theory—as with the rarely stated but clear impetus driving assisted suicide—is to save medical resources for patients who are considered to have a greater claim on them or to help pay for expanded access to health insurance.

But the belief that the health-care system will be destroyed unless we cease spending so much money on dying people is fundamentally misguided. End-of-life care takes up only 10 to 12 percent of the entire health-care budget. So, unless we refuse to treat every patient as soon as the terminal diagnosis is given, savings from futile care theory would not be significant.[59]

Dr. Joanne Lynn, professor of community and family medicine at the Center for the Evaluation of Clinical Sciences, Dartmouth Medical School, testified before the Senate Finance Committee in 1994, saying:

> There is a widespread myth that enormous resources are wasted on the dying. The evidence for this is actually quite frail. About one-quarter of payments under Medicare are directed at the care of those who die during that year. This seems to be a reasonable proportion—after all, persons are commonly quite sick in the year before they

die.... Very few dying persons now have resuscitation efforts or extended stays in intensive care.[60]

"The Economics of Dying," an article published in the *New England Journal of Medicine* in 1994, is even more to the point. Its authors, Drs. Ezekiel Emanuel and Linda Emanuel, reviewed studies of the cost savings that could be achieved by Medicare if more people signed advance directives (such as durable powers of attorney for health care; see pages 237-238), if there were broader use of DNRs ("do not resuscitate" orders), if futile care guidelines were enacted and the like. Although the studies were not definitive, the Emanuels concluded:

> The amount that might be saved by reducing the use of aggressive life-sustaining interventions for dying patients is at most 3.3 percent of total national health care expenditures. In 1993, with $900 billion going to health care, this savings would amount to $29.7 billion.... We must stop deluding ourselves that advance directives and less aggressive care at the end of life will solve the financial problems of the health care system.[61]

Even rationing advocates admit that there is little money to be saved by forcing people out of desired end-of-life treatment opportunities. Dr. Murphy of the late, unlamented CCMD admitted to me that applying futile care protocols would not save the health-care system a lot of money. So why try to impose them upon a reluctant society? Permitting doctors to refuse "futile" care is only the first step in the proverbial thousand-mile journey. In the end, many futilitarians hope to arrive at a rationed health-care system where "community consensus" determines the parameters of medical treatment. Indeed, Dr. Murphy told me that the next step after futile care would be to "restrict marginally beneficial care," where, he claimed, "greater resource savings are to be found."[62] What would be an example of marginally beneficial care? According to Dr. Murphy, "mammograms for women over 80" or medical treatment that the community finds inappropriate for some people because of, say, age or state of health, but acceptable for those it deems more deserving of care.[63]

Considering the similar value systems at play in both assisted suicide and futile care theory, we shouldn't be surprised. For many activists and advocates involved in these end-of-life issues, patient autonomy in end-of-life decision making is not the ultimate goal; the death of certain patients is. If patient autonomy achieves that end, well and good. But if patients or families want to "rage against the dying of the light," as Dylan Thomas put it, then the theory of futile treatment will be applied. Clearly, assisted suicide and futile care theory have no place in a moral, compassionate health-care system.

Destination "Duty to Die"

Futile care theory's implicit message is that some people have lives of such poor quality and meaninglessness, that regardless of their desires unequivocally expressed, the only acceptable answer is to stop sustaining their lives. Thus, we see that a foundation is being laid for what might be called a "duty to die."

Is this too harsh a judgment? I wish it were. Not only does the bioethics movement broadly support futile care theory, but some have gone even farther arguing that some patients have an explicit duty to die.

The premier advocate for the "duty to die" is John Hardwig, a philosophy professor at East Tennessee University. Hardwig's ideas were featured in a 1997 cover story in the world's foremost bioethics journal, the *Hastings Center Report:*

> A duty to die is more likely when continuing to live will impose significant burdens—emotional burdens, extensive caregiving, destruction of life plans, and yes, financial hardship—on your family and loved ones. This is the fundamental insight underlying a duty to die. [64]

While Hardwig believes the duty should not be mandated legally due to the importance of autonomy, he told me that someone with a "duty to die" should seriously consider suicide. [65]

Other bioethicists have also weighed in on establishing a duty to die. University of Utah philosopher Margaret P. Battin, for example, has argued that global egalitarianism may one day require people in richer countries to forgo expensive life-sustaining treatment or even commit suicide to promote "the interests of justice in health care," which would be "reflected in more nearly equal health prospects and life expectancies around the globe."[66] Not surprisingly, Battin is an enthusiast for legalizing euthanasia.

Judith Lee Kissell, a professor from Georgia, believes that the duty to die is "an authentic, full-fledged, moral imperative."[67] She asserts that "the duty should be inculcated at an early age." For instance, children born into families that include disabled persons "can be led to realize early the wisdom of terminating lifesaving or life-preserving treatment of disabled siblings. Such self-sacrifice from a young member of their household would provide an invaluable lifelong example of love, devotion, and true family values."[68]

One of the more candid proponents of euthanasia, Baroness Mary Warnock, a member of the English House of Lords, argues that ill and elderly people who are burdening their families should "creep off and get out of the way." In a recent interview with the *Times* of London, she explained:

> I know I am not really allowed to say it but one of the things that would motivate me is I couldn't bear hanging on and being such a burden on people. When I say that, people throw up their hands in horror, "This is just [the attitude] we dread if [euthanasia] becomes permissible by law; people will feel they have to do it for the sake of their family." But I don't see what's so bad about that. In other contexts sacrificing oneself for one's family would be considered good. I don't see what is so horrible about the motive of not wanting to be an increasing nuisance.[69]

Lest we become complacent because such views are, at present, out of the mainstream, we should recall that in the 1980s, bioethicists and other members of the medical intelligentsia were arguing that "biologically tenacious" people should be made to die by dehydration via the removal of feeding tubes. As we have seen, withdrawing sustenance became commonplace during the 1990s. In the 1990s, bioethicists began to promote futile care theory. Now, in the mid 2000s, we see this policy beginning to be imposed, which itself would establish an implicit duty to die. If the current trends continue—especially if futile care theory and euthanasia become institutionalized in health law—is it not foreseeable that by, say, 2020 the "duty to die" will be considered an obligation of citizenship?

SEVEN

EUTHANASIA AS AN
ENEMY OF THE DISABLED

I N HUMAN HISTORY, INVIDIOUS DISTINCTIONS have been based on race, nationality, tribe, religion, age, gender, sexual orientation, ideology and disability, just to name a few. Now, perhaps we will have to add state of health or happiness to this woeful list.

In particular, disabled people feel that they are in the cross hairs of the euthanasia movement, which views them as potential "beneficiaries" (in the words of Ninth Circuit Court of Appeals judge Stephen Reinhardt) of the right to be killed by a doctor. Rather than seeing euthanasia as a guarantee of "liberty," they view legalization as a dire threat and a form of bigotry against disabled people, which sends the loud message that their lives are worthless.

Paul Longmore, a nationally respected disability rights activist, writer and associate professor of history at California State University at San Francisco, describes the long trail of discrimination that might lead some disabled persons to "choose" to be killed:

> Current euthanasia activists talk a lot about personal autonomy and choice. Well, for people with disabilities who have opted for assisted suicide, it was a spurious choice. These are people who have been denied the ability to choose about virtually every other option in their lives: They have been segregated out of society; they have been denied the right to work; they have been discriminated against in getting an education; they have been blocked from expressing themselves romantically and sexually; they have been penalized for marrying by having public benefits shut off, including desperately

193

needed health insurance; they have been shunned by loved ones and friends. In virtually every case in which a person with a disability has sought legal assistance in ending their lives, they have been discriminated against in most if not all of these ways.[1]

The late Evan Kemp, a political conservative who served as chairman of the Equal Employment Opportunities Commission under former President Bush, would have disagreed with Longmore on many points, but he shared Longmore's worries about the likely targets of the euthanasia culture. "Euthanasia," he stated bluntly, "is nothing more than human beings—often doctors—killing disabled, ill, or elderly people."[2] During his last years, Kemp worked assiduously to oppose assisted suicide.

Diane Coleman explains how public perceptions have made people with disabilities especially vulnerable:

> The widespread public image of severe disability as a fate worse then death is not exactly a surprise to the disability community. Disability rights activists have fought against these negative stereotypes of disability for decades in the effort to achieve basic civil rights protections. What has been a surprise for many advocates is the boldness with which these stereotypes are asserted as fact by proponents of assisted suicide, and the willingness of the press and the public to accept them, without even checking them against the views of people who themselves live with severe disabilities…. These stereotypes then become grounds for carving out a deadly exception to longstanding laws and public policies about suicide prevention.[3]

Coleman is founder of Not Dead Yet, the noted disability rights organization that campaigns against assisted suicide and other forms of anti-disability discrimination.

"Disability has supplanted death in people's minds as the worst thing that can happen," says the psychologist Carol Gill, a disability rights activist and head of the Chicago Center for Disability Research. "These prejudices are sometimes shared by physicians, ethicists and others in the health-care hierarchy. That can be frightening. If a doctor doesn't think that a life with disability is tenable, they think they are doing a [disabled] patient a favor by advocating an end to treatment [so death will occur]."[4] As detailed in the last chapter, such refusals of care are becoming systemic via futile care theory. If active euthanasia were legalized, such pressures could only increase.

Early in Jack Kevorkian's killing spree, a disability rights journal remarked that:

> Kevorkian and other "death with dignity" proponents are broadening the definition of "extreme human suffering" to encompass mental and physical disabilities that leave individuals unable to live life unassisted. Activists fear that such thinking will reinforce society's acceptance of health care rationing and the denial of adequate funding for assistive technology and personal assistance services. One activist attending a recent meeting on disability and euthanasia scoffed, "Dignity my eye! All that concern about dignity boils down to society's contempt for people who need help to go to the bathroom!"[5]

These prejudices seep into the delivery of health care that those of us who are able-bodied take for granted. Examples of such biases are routinely reported in disability rights literature. The following excerpt from an article in the disability health and wellness journal, *One Step Ahead's Second Opinion,* is typical of the impediments placed in the paths of disabled people:

> Robert Powell has lived with partial paralysis since childhood and learned two years ago he has a heart condition.... [The] hospital staff repeatedly asked him how much he wanted done to save his life should his condition fail to respond to routine treatment. Having barely reached middle age, he assured them he wanted aggressive measures to save his life. Staff continued to question him about his decision. They finally requested a psychiatric consult because they felt he was "having trouble accepting death."[6]

Facing and overcoming this type of prejudice is difficult enough in a health-care system whose official ethics still value all lives equally. But now, with the equality-of-human-life ideal under attack from the euthanasia agenda, from bioethics and by society's prejudice against people with disabilities, many in the disability rights movement are very concerned that they will be victimized by legalized euthanasia. One prominent disability rights activist, a disabled person who is extremely alarmed by society's apparent acceptance of euthanasia, told me, "I don't expect to die a natural death."

Disability rights organizations such as Not Dead Yet work tirelessly to stop the legalization of assisted suicide. "Not Dead Yet is declaring war on the ultimate form of discrimination, euthanasia," says Diane Coleman. "We've watched over the last decade as our brothers and sisters have been denied suicide prevention that nondisabled people take for granted. We've watched as families have been allowed to withhold food and water from their disabled children. We are acting before it is too late."[7]

Activists of Not Dead Yet engage in demonstrations and other educational efforts around the country to alert the general public to the threat that euthanasia poses to disabled people. Fittingly, the organization's first demonstration, in June 1996, was in front of the house of Jack Kevorkian, whom Not Dead Yet considers a bigot on the basis of his disdainful statements about the value of the lives of disabled people and because he has helped so many depressed disabled people kill themselves.

Not Dead Yet next targeted a medical ethics conference where a keynote presenter advocated limiting medical treatments for certain disabled people as futile "exoticare." Rather than endure the adverse publicity of people in wheelchairs demonstrating against discrimination, the ethicists invited representatives of Not Dead Yet to address the convention. "We asked the ethicists how many of the hospital ethics committees had disabled people as members," Coleman recalls. "Only two out of forty or fifty of the people raised their hands. When we asked if the disabled people who were represented had knowledge and experience in independent living, no one raised their hands. Yet, these committees continually make decisions about life and death based on the perceived quality of disabled people's lives."[8]

Members of Not Dead Yet also were present in Jack Kevorkian's last trip to court. As "Dr. Death" faced trial for murdering Thomas Youk, a man disabled by the terminal illness ALS, members of the organization sat daily in the public section of the courtroom, bearing witness against Kevorkian's bigotry against their community.

The Robert Latimer Case

Few events illustrate the anti-disability attitude that afflicts society better than the reaction of much of Canada to the murder of twelve-year-old Tracy Latimer, who had a severe case of cerebral palsy. Her father, Robert, killed Tracy one Sunday in 1994 when the rest of the Latimer family was at church. After the family had left, Latimer carried Tracy to the garage, put her inside the cab of the family pickup truck, turned on the ignition, and closed the garage door. He then walked away leaving his daughter to die alone, choking on carbon monoxide fumes.

Robert Latimer was arrested, convicted of second-degree murder and given a sentence of life in prison, of which he would have to serve a minimum of ten years. The Latimer case caused a national uproar, but not against the father. Rather, his conviction and jail sentence outraged many Canadians. Rather than occasion for revulsion, the case turned into a cause célèbre for legalizing euthanasia. One columnist asked, "Where were the doctors when Robert Latimer needed them?" and advocated that "a committee to make life and death decisions" be formed when "life becomes intolerable and death may be the most compassionate thing."[9]

Supporters donated tens of thousands of dollars to the Latimer legal defense fund and the pro-Latimer uproar was crucial in obtaining Robert Latimer's release from prison, pending appeal. One judge, dissenting from an early court of appeals decision affirming Latimer's sentence, even included in the text of his dissent letters from outraged citizens demanding that Latimer be freed rather than punished for his "act of love."[10]

Within months of Tracy's death, an American parent, Susan Smith, killed her two sons by pushing her car into a lake with the boys firmly buckled into their car safety seats. Like Tracy, the Smith children died alone as their parent watched from only a short distance away. But unlike Tracy, the Smith boys attracted the entire country's sympathy. While Robert Latimer was widely hailed as a loving father, Susan Smith was branded a monster and had to be protected from an angry crowd.

Why the difference? There is only one explanation: Smith's children were able-bodied and pleasant to look at, and therefore they had a right to their lives. Tracy Latimer was disabled and unphotogenic, and therefore she was seen by many as better off dead. That was certainly the message received by another Canadian youngster who took the killing of Tracy and the popular support for Robert Latimer quite personally. His name was Teague Johnson. Teague and Tracy had a lot in common. They were about the same age. Both had severe cases of cerebral palsy. Both were quadriplegic. Both were often in pain and required various treatments to alleviate their discomfort. Both had great difficulties in communication. Unlike Tracy, Teague had learned facilitated communication techniques that allowed him to express himself to his close relatives and friends.

"I remember Teague was very distressed by the idea that a father could take it upon himself to choose death for his disabled daughter," recalls Teague's father, Larry Johnson. "And he was distressed that so many Canadians reacted with sympathy for the man who killed a daughter who differed from Teague only in the fact that five or six people in Teague's life had been able to help him say his own words and clarify his own wishes."[11]

Teague was so anguished by Tracy's murder and the widespread approval of it by his fellow Canadians that he wrote an opinion column, which was published in the *Vancouver Sun* on December 9, 1994:*

> My name is Teague. I am 11 years old and have really severe cerebral palsy. The Latimer case…has caused me a great deal of unhappiness and worry…. I feel strongly that all children are valuable and deserve to live full and complete lives. No one should make the decision for another person about whether their life is worth living or not….
>
> I have to fight pain all the time. When I was little life was pain. My foster Mom Cara helped me to learn to manage and control my pain. Now my life is so full of joy. There isn't time enough in the day for me to learn and experience all I wish to do. I have a family and many friends who love me. I have a world of knowledge to discover. I have so much to give.
>
> I can't walk or feed myself but I am not "suffering from cerebral palsy." I use a wheelchair but I am not "confined to a wheelchair." I have pain but I do not need to be "put out of my misery."
>
> My body is not my enemy. It is that which allows me to enjoy

---

*This and other writings of Teague Johnson quoted herein are copyrighted by Larry Johnson and are reprinted with his permission.

Mozart, experience Shakespeare, savor a bouillabaisse feast, and cuddle my Mom. Life is a precious gift. It belongs to the person to whom it was given. Not to her parents, nor to the state. Tracy's life was hers "to make of it what she could" [quoting the Latimer trial judge]. My life is going to be astounding.[12]

Teague's loved ones helped him communicate his values of love, mutual connectedness and universal equality to people all over the world on the Internet. In a letter to a friend dated April 4, 1994, facilitated by Teague's foster mother, "Ca," Teague wrote:

I am really working hard these days to be strong and healthy. I really want to live a long, long time because I have so much to do. There is so much I want to learn and many people who need me. My Ca loves me and really needs me to be her foster boy. That's right, I used to think that I needed my Ca but she really needs me. I thought really I was a burden to my Ca. But really, I discovered that the best place for my Ca to be is living with me. My Ca needs me to be really happy. My L. [Larry, Teague's father] needs me to really help him with his master's thesis. Really, without me these grownups would actually stop learning new things. And I have lots to teach the world. I am going to be an important teacher.[13]

Another note from Teague:

I am working on helping the world understand that children with disabilities are really the same as other children and need love and a good education. Really people shouldn't make assumptions on what someone is like based on what they look like. I hope [to show] people that those assumptions about people based on religion and race and sexual orientation are really wrong too. I am doing this by talking to people, and making speeches, and writing articles for newspapers. This is really my mission. And really if one segment of the population, like…people with disabilities, are considered second class citizens, then that makes it easier for people to start treating other segments of the population too.[14]

Facilitated communication is a matter of some controversy. Some experts contend that the disabled person isn't doing the actual communicating, but rather, that well-meaning facilitators are unconsciously supplying words and thoughts that are not really there. Other experts accept facilitated communication as genuine. Whatever the case, the sentiments expressed by Teague are important and meaningful. For, as Paul Longmore says of the Tracy Latimer case, "One of the serious dangers to all disabled people is that there is an ideal, a standard, a norm, against which people with disabilities are measured. The further you depart from the ideal, the less human you are deemed, until you get to people who are nonverbal and quadriplegic, where many see the disabled person as literally non-human. That appears to be driving the public attitudes in the Tracy Latimer case."[15]

Teague Johnson died in his father's arms from natural causes at age twelve. "Teague never doubted that his own life was worth living," Larry Johnson says. "He was excited about the future, and he continually made plans to advance his education and to engage in new and exciting projects. He lived to communicate his thoughts to the people and to help them understand that peace, love and joy were possible for every human being."[16]

As for Robert Latimer, who had a different view about the value of his daughter's life, he remained free on bail for several years while his case was on appeal. He was granted a new trial because the prosecution asked jury members about their feelings toward assisted suicide before the trial, which is not permitted under Canadian law. Once again he was convicted. That case finally went to the Supreme Court of Canada, where it was affirmed. He is now doing his ten years. Even after all this time, there are Web sites and continual petition gathering and political agitation by Latimer's many supporters to obtain clemency for him.[17]

It now appears that the public's reaction to Latimer may have increased the number of developmentally disabled children being killed by a parent in Canada. This is the conclusion of Professor Dick Sobsey, director of the JP Das Developmental Disabilities Centre at the University of Alberta. Sobsey reviewed homicide statistics in the United States and Canada involving the killing of developmentally disabled children.

> After correcting for population Americans with developmental disabilities were 2.5 times as likely to be killed by the parents as Canadians [before the 1994 Latimer killing]. From 1994 to the present [the end of 2001] we found 21 cases in Canada and 101 cases in the United States. [The U.S. has ten times the population of Canada.] This

means that suddenly Canadians with developmental disabilities were 84% more likely than Americans to be killed by their parents.

Another way to look at this is that in the United States the percent of homicide victims with developmental disabilities did not change significantly since 1994—less than 1%. In Canada, it increased 88.5% since 1994.[18]

Elizabeth Bouvia

Few cases enrage disability rights activists more than that of Elizabeth Bouvia. In the early 1980s, Bouvia was suicidal after undergoing one devastating emotional crisis after another within two years: Her brother died; she was in deep financial distress; she left graduate school because of discrimination; she had a miscarriage; and her marriage dissolved. She checked herself into a psychiatric hospital and declared her desire for pain-control medications that would assist her in committing suicide by self-starvation.

Normally, such a request would have been rejected out of hand; it would have been interpreted as a cry for help, and medical professionals and other compassionate and involved persons would have attempted to help Bouvia find a reason to go on living. But some thought this case was different. Why? Bouvia's stated reason for wanting to die was that she had cerebral palsy and was quadriplegic.

Ignoring the profound emotional blows that Bouvia had recently experienced, blows that individually or collectively could produce a desire for suicide in almost anyone, the American Civil Liberties Union took up her cause. The lead ACLU attorney in the case, Richard Scott, had been the first legal counsel of the Hemlock Society. The expert mental health professional testifying in support of her dying was Faye Girsh, later the executive director of the Hemlock Society.

The trial court refused Bouvia's request. She left the hospital, and after an unsuccessful trip to Mexico to seek aid in dying, she began to eat again. Her suicidal impulse seemed to have abated, but it later returned. She again checked into a hospital and stopped eating, and attorney Scott returned to court. To keep her alive, the hospital put in a feeding tube.

The second trial judge refused her request for assisted suicide.

The ACLU appealed the decision. But a new era was about to arrive on the food-and-fluids front, and consistent with the emerging ethic, the California Court of Appeals judge saw Bouvia's case in a different light. It decided that this was not a matter of assisted suicide but of refusing medical treatment. In language dripping with the pervasive societal prejudice that death is better than disability, Judge Lynn Compton of the California Court of Appeals wrote:

> In Elizabeth Bouvia's view, the quality of her life has been diminished to the point of hopelessness, uselessness, unenjoyability, and frustration. She, as the patient, lying helplessly in bed, unable to care for herself, may consider existence meaningless. She is not to be faulted for so concluding.... We cannot conceive it to be the policy of this State to inflict such an ordeal on anybody.[19]

On the surface, Judge Compton's thesis may sound reasonable. But it really expresses the insidious abandoning philosophy of "rational suicide." After all, *anybody* who wants to commit suicide believes that his or her life is "meaningless," "useless," and "hopeless," forever to be without joy. Otherwise, the person would not want to die. Yet when the cause of such despair is the end of a love affair, the death of a child, loss of reputation and so on, no court would rule (at least not yet) that the suicide wish should be accommodated because it is wrong for the "state to inflict such an ordeal on anybody." Solely because Bouvia's stated reason to die was her disability, the court viewed her differently: Of course she wanted to die. Who wouldn't? She was disabled; thus, her hopelessness and despair were perceived as permanent conditions, unlike feelings caused by the loss of a career or the death of a loved one.

The late Mark O'Brien, who was a quadriplegic from his early childhood because of a severe case of polio, lived for the last forty-four years of his life in an iron lung. He not only graduated from the University of California at Berkeley but also was a published poet, a journalist and an author. O'Brien said of the court's reasoning: "It is false to say quadriplegics can never have a meaningful life. [Bouvia] had more mobility than I do. To link disability with worthlessness and uselessness, as too many people do and as the court of appeals did, is pure superstition. These attitudes are based on fears and false presumptions held by people who aren't disabled."[20]

Bouvia's life was clearly not foreordained to uselessness. She had lived on her own in an apartment and had attended San Diego State University.[21] She once volunteered as a social worker and might well have continued in that field to a paying position had she not quit college in a dispute over her studies, after which the college refused to readmit her.[22]

Paul Longmore, who has written extensively on the Bouvia case, agrees with Mark O'Brien's assessment. "When we [in the disability rights community] tried to point out that Elizabeth's depression was caused in large part by society's unwillingness to give us the assistance that would allow us to live independently, to work, to be free from discrimination, we were contemptuously dismissed by the court and in the media. Yet, in the end, everything we said was right and everything the ACLU said was wrong."[23]

Longmore's point is this: Elizabeth Bouvia didn't die. Instead of killing herself, she chose to go on, and now, many sometimes-difficult years later, she is living independently, with the help of a personal assistant, in California. Ironically, her lawyer, Richard Scott, was the one who ended up committing suicide.

Larry McAfee

The Bouvia case was not unusual in its reasoning or its result. Other disabled people have asked successfully for court help in committing suicide by starvation, usually because their aspirations for independent living have been blocked, not because of their physical limitations. Joseph Shapiro, in *No Pity*, wrote about a young man named Larry McAfee, disabled in a motorcycle accident, who wanted to die because "every day when I wake up, there is nothing to look forward to."[24] The court agreed that his disability made his life hopeless and not worth living and sanctioned pulling his feeding tube in 1989.

Shapiro convincingly demonstrates what the court seemed unable to grasp: McAfee felt useless because he was "being handled like a piece of radioactive waste," forced unnecessarily to live in nursing homes solely because of his quadriplegia while denied life-enriching opportunities for independent living.[25]

For reasons quite relevant to this discussion, McAfee's story had a happy ending. After his case made headlines, McAfee received assistance—not in dying but in living. He was given a computer, which he worked by using his head and which allowed him to pursue his interest in architecture and engineering. Then, when he finally had the opportunity to have attendants to assist him, people he could hire and fire, his spirits rallied and he decided that he definitely wanted to live. He was able to leave the nursing home and he lived for several more years in a shared living arrangement with other disabled young men. He died from natural causes in 1996.

WHAT IF EUTHANASIA AND ASSISTED SUICIDE were legalized for disabled people like Elizabeth Bouvia and Larry McAfee, who request "rational suicide" out of despair caused in large measure by societal discrimination and disdain? What if, rather than having to go through lengthy court proceedings, Bouvia and McAfee had been required only to wait fifteen days from their request before being given a lethal injection or poisonous potion? In such a world, both of these people would have been dead and buried long before their spirits rebounded and they moved on to the next phase of their lives.

A review of the professional literature supports the contention of disability rights activists that disability is more of an emotional problem for the general community than it is for most disabled individuals. One study, which compared the attitudes of disabled people with those of medical professionals, found that 86 percent of high-level quadriplegics with spinal cord injuries rated their own quality of life as average or better than average, while only 17 percent of the doctors and nurses surveyed thought they themselves would have an average or better-than-average quality of life if they became disabled.[26] Interviews and tests administered to 133 persons with severe mobility impairments revealed no differences between them and the nondisabled norm on psychosocial measures. Another study found no significant difference between persons with severe disabilities and persons without any disabilities on quality-of-life measurements.[27] Hospital personnel consistently overestimated their disabled patients' level of depression, whereas self-rating of depression by these patients found levels similar to those of the general population.[28]

We must thus ask ourselves: Would legalizing assisted suicide and euthanasia for disabled people—too many of whom are cared for in medicalized or nursing home settings that devalue their lives, and in a health-care system increasingly concerned about cost of care—truly be "compassionate"? Or would it be an expression of the general community's own fears, prejudices and—in Mark O'Brien's apt term—superstitions about disability? If it were indeed the latter, as many in the disability rights community strongly assert, wouldn't the facilitation of disabled persons' deaths actually be to abandon them? Calling it an exercise in liberty or death with dignity would not change that reality.

The extent to which society accepts the belief that death is better than disability is aptly illustrated by the case of Dr. Gregory Messenger, a Michigan dermatologist whose son, Michael, was born prematurely at twenty-six weeks. Fearing that Michael would be disabled and suffer, Dr. Messenger took him off a respirator with the intent that the boy should die. He acted unilaterally, even though Michael had not been examined, the necessary diagnostic tests to determine his likely prognosis had not been conducted, his wife's doctor estimated the chance of Michael's survival before the emergency birth at 30 to 50 percent, and a substantial number of babies born at twenty-six weeks survive, many without significant impairment. Michael Messenger died at age eighty-two minutes.[29]

Everyone can sympathize with Dr. Messenger's grief, worry and fear about his baby. But did that give him the right to end his baby's life before his son had a chance to fight for his own survival? According to the jury, apparently so. After only four hours' deliberation, they acquitted Dr. Messenger of manslaughter charges, a verdict that some delighted bioethicists called a victory for parental rights.[30]

The Messenger case also has about it the noxious odor of the euthanasia advocate Peter Singer's theory that parents and doctors should have the legal and ethical right to have doctors kill unwanted disabled infants, a right that currently exists in the Netherlands. Singer states in *Rethinking Life and Death* (a reiteration of the same thoughts that he has presented in other forums):

> Both for the sake of 'our children' [other healthy children, whether or not they have yet been born], then, and for our own sake, we may not

want a child to start life's uncertain voyage if the prospects are clouded. When this can be known at a very early stage of the voyage…we can still say no, and start again from the beginning.[31]

The Antifamily Values of Euthanasia

Even the most loving and supportive families are plunged into emotional crisis when a family member becomes catastrophically ill or injured. Sadly, too many families approach health crises or tackle long-term care challenges without adequate information about services and products that would materially assist them. For example, many people who care for elderly parents are unaware of the many social-service options that exist to help them, such as respite centers, adult day care, hospice, group homes, support groups and more.

The national culture can also be a barrier to effective caregiving. Caregivers report that many people look askance at their friends and neighbors who sacrifice personal pursuits in order to give sick and dying loved ones the care they need and deserve. This sad truth was illustrated by Lucette Lagnado in a *Wall Street Journal* article titled "Mercy Living," in which she wrote about the reactions of her friends and acquaintances when she brought her elderly and disabled mother home rather than keep her in a nursing home. Noting that "mercy killing is increasingly de rigueur," Lagnado wrote, "In the two years I cared for Mom at my home, if friends didn't make me feel that I was somehow mishandling—even wasting—my life, then the 'professionals' did…. Forced to rely on a battery of neurologists, cardiologists, gastroenterologists and pulmonologists…. I learned to steel myself for that cold look, the shake of the head that meant there was not much hope for her, so why bother?" One doctor even yelled at Lagnado. "What was I doing keeping a sick mother at home, he thundered. Posing a question as loaded as it was insidious, he asked: 'Is she really alive?'"[32]

Lagnado's experience is not unique. Increasingly, caring for people who are elderly, profoundly disabled or seriously ill is seen by many as a burden or an affliction that wastes time and resources that would be better spent "productively." This subversive message is delivered throughout society, in personal conversations, in the attitudes of the youth culture, in the media, sometimes even in advocacy for the "right to die," in which dependency and disability are commonly equated with a lack of dignity and human worth.

This milieu of fractured communities, of societal indifference, of isolation, of many families shredded by dysfunction, of widespread ignorance about the ins and outs of caregiving, of ill or disabled loved ones receiving inadequate treatment for pain or depression, of patients worrying about being burdens—this is the milieu in which families would face "rational" decision making about euthanasia and assisted suicide. Even in the best of families, those with only loving and altruistic motives, such "crisis atmospheres" would not be conducive to reasoned decision making about killing as a perceived answer to difficulty. If legalized euthanasia were brought as a "solution" into a family crisis among people who are not loving or mutually supportive, or where there was substantial money at stake, the lethal danger to the ill and vulnerable would be hard to overstate.

Myrna Lebov

The tragic assisted suicide of the author and editor Myrna Lebov is a case in point. Disabled by multiple sclerosis, Myrna committed suicide on July 4, 1995, at the age of fifty-two, with the active assistance of her husband, George Delury, a former editor of the *World Almanac*. He was soon charged in her death.

As soon as the news broke about Delury's arrest, many in the death-on-demand movement rushed to his support. The Hemlock Society created a legal defense fund for him. William Batt, chairman of the New York chapter, expressed confidence that Lebov had not been coerced, since most people would want to die if they were in her condition.[33] The case was widely seen within the assisted suicide movement as a breakthrough that would move their cause forward. (These advocates supported Delury even though there was no indication that Lebov was terminally ill.)

Initially, the media reported on the assisted suicide in the facile and breathless manner it usually brings to such cases. Most reports accepted at face value Delury's claim that he was merely a compassionate husband doing what his totally debilitated and suffering but courageous wife desperately wanted. The *Charleston Daily News*, for example, under the headline "Writer Wanted Relief," reported:

"She knew her future was without hope. Instead of withering in a nursing home, Lebov, fifty-two, swallowed pills and died in her Manhattan apartment."[34]

Delury became an instant "victim-celebrity." He made numerous television appearances, gave a speech in front of the American Psychiatric Association, and signed a book deal. Far and wide, he was acclaimed as a dedicated husband willing to risk jail to help his wife achieve her deeply desired end to suffering. He was allowed to quickly plead guilty to a minor crime and served only four months.

But a few months later, the *Forward,* a Jewish weekly, reported that all was not as Delury wanted it to seem. For example, Delury repeatedly claimed publicly that Lebov's life had been reduced to the merely "biological" by her disease. Yet the *Forward* reporter discovered that only a week before she died, Myrna swam twenty-eight laps with the help of a therapist.[35] The paper also discovered that Delury had convinced Lebov to accept a buyout of her monthly disability insurance payments by taking a check for fifty thousand dollars, which he then cashed against her express wishes.[36] Lebov's sister, Beverly Sloane, appalled at the sympathy and support she perceived her former brother-in-law was receiving among the public and in the press, publicly countered Delury's characterizations of Lebov's final months, describing her sibling as engaged in life, albeit struggling against depression caused, in part, by an emotionally unsupportive husband.

The lid blew off Delury's claim of selfless altruism when the New York district attorney's office released the contents of his diary. It revealed that Lebov did not have an unwavering and long-stated desire to die, as he had alleged. Rather, as often happens in people struggling with serious illnesses, her moods waxed and waned. One day she would be suicidal but the next day Delury's diary revealed his wife wanting to engage in life. Moreover, the diary clearly demonstrated that it was Delury, *not* Lebov, who had the unremitting suicide agenda.

Delury admitted that he encouraged his wife to kill herself, or as he put it, "to decide to quit." He researched her antidepressant medication to see if it could kill her, and when she took less than the prescribed amount, which in and of itself could cause depression, he used the surplus to mix the brew that ended her life. But he went further than that. He helped destroy her will to live by making her feel worthless and a burden on him. Beverly Sloane says, "There was definitely psychological coercion involved [in Lebov's death]. He was telling her in front of others, including my daughter…that she was exhausting, she was a burden, that in two years he would be dead [from taking care of her]."[37]

Delury's own diary supports Sloane's recollections. On March 28, 1995, Delury wrote in his diary of his plans to tell his wife the following:

> I have work to do, people to see, places to travel. But no one asks about my needs. I have fallen prey to the tyranny of a victim. You are sucking my life out of my [sic] like a vampire and nobody cares. In fact, it would appear that I am about to be cast in the role of villain because I no longer believe in you.[38]

Delury later admitted on the NBC program *Dateline* that he had shown Lebov this very passage.[39]

That Delury wanted Lebov to kill herself is beyond dispute. On May 1, he wrote:

> Sheer hell. Myrna is more or less euphoric. She spoke of writing a book today. [Lebov was a published author, having written *Not Just a Secretary* in 1984.] She's interested in everything, wants everything explained, and believes that every bit of bad news has some way out…. It's all too much. I'm not going to come out of this in one piece with my honor. I'm so tired of it all, maybe I should kill myself.[40]

On May 27, Delury wrote:

> Myrna's mood was erratic today. Subdued in the morning, focused and realistic in the afternoon, rather more assertive in the evening— all definitely forward looking and without any indication that she wants to die. On the contrary, this evening she suggested that I was the only one who wanted her to die.[41]

On June 10, Delury's diary entry described an argument with Lebov that started after she left a message to her niece that "things are looking splendid":

> I blew up! Shouting into the phone that everything was just the same, it was simply Myrna feeling different. I told Myrna that she had hurt me very badly, not my feelings, but physically and emotionally. "Now

what will Beverly think? That I'm lying about how tough things are here." I put it to Myrna bluntly—"If you won't take care of me, I won't take care of you."[42]

July 3, the day before Myrna's death, Delury wrote:

> Myrna is now questioning the efficacy of solution, a sure sign that she will not take it [the overdose] tonight and doesn't want to. So, confusion and hesitancy strike again. If she changes her mind tonight and does decide to go ahead, I will be surprised.[43]

Finally, on July 4, Delury got what he wanted: his wife's death. After postponing an earlier suicide date that her husband had advocated, the couple's anniversary, Lebov swallowed the overdose of antidepressant medicine that her husband had prepared for her and died. George Delury did not wait for her death by her bedside, but according to his diary, went into another room and went to sleep. The next morning he wrote, "Slept through the alarm. It's over. Myrna is dead. Desolation."[44]

In an interview with *Dateline*, Lebov's swimming therapist disclosed that she had indeed discussed suicide during their therapy sessions, although she subsequently told the therapist that she had decided to live. Lebov's stated reason for planning to self-destruct on July 4, Independence Day, was that she wanted to give her husband the freedom from her that he so fervently desired.[45] As one police official put it, George Delury put Myrna Lebov out of *his* misery.

And how was this man—a man who emotionally abandoned his disabled wife, a man who did nothing to seek treatment for his wife's intermittent suicidal thoughts but instead helped push her into choosing an early grave—treated? Delury became something of a hero within the euthanasia movement, often speaking at assisted suicide conventions. He had a book published, *But What If She Wants to Die?*[46] Despite the abandonment revealed by Delury's own diary and the disclosure made in his book that he had put a plastic bag over his wife's head to make sure she died, Susan Cheever, the reviewer for the *New York Times*, described Delury as a loving husband and the history of the marriage a "love story."[47]

Myrna's sister remains appalled by the widespread support for Delury. "People were quick to accept George's excuse for ending

Myrna's life," she told me. "But in my opinion, he used the assisted suicide controversy as an alibi for intentional homicide. Her disease did not change the essence of Myrna. She was a loving, intelligent, warm, compassionate, sensitive, giving human being. She was a joy to talk to and be with. She was making plans for the future. She was not in pain. She was not terminally ill. She should still be alive enjoying the love of her family and he should still be in jail."[48] (Sloane and other family members sued Delury for the "wrongful death" of Myrna Lebov. The case settled, with Delury promising to pay approximately $14,000 plus interest.)[49]

Gerald Klooster

Similar dynamics can be seen at work in a case that made national headlines and was featured on *60 Minutes*. Dr. Gerald Klooster was a retired physician from Castro Valley, California, who had Alzheimer's disease. When Klooster's son, Gerald (Chip) Klooster II, learned in August 1995 that his mother was about to take his father to Jack Kevorkian, he immediately flew to Florida, where his parents were visiting friends, and quickly whisked his father to safety. Chip then moved Gerald into his own home in Michigan, and after a psychiatric examination showed that Gerald was medically incompetent, he sent the finding to Kevorkian through his attorneys, pleading, "Please do not harm my father, he definitely does not want to end his life."

Chip then obtained temporary guardianship in his home state of Michigan and sought permanent custody of his father in a court battle that pitted him against his mother and siblings. Michigan judge Richard Mulhauser heard five days of testimony: Gerald's wife, Ruth, took the Fifth Amendment, and testimony was presented that Gerald was not in pain, that he enjoyed his family, and that he had years left to live. Moreover, according to witnesses, Gerald repeatedly expressed a desire to live, not die, a statement he repeated on *60 Minutes* on February 25, 1996.[50]

At the end of the five-day trial, Judge Mulhauser granted temporary custody of his father to Chip, ruling that "there is overwhelming evidence in the record of this case that Ruth intended to pursue the ending of Gerald Klooster's life through either the use of fatal drugs...or by taking him to Dr. Kevorkian in Michigan"; that

"Ruth's children, except son 'Chip,' proved incapable of protecting Gerald"; that "it must be presumed that Ruth still intends her husband's suicide"; that "Ruth was on a mission and that mission was the end of her husband's life because she believed it was the right thing to do"; and that "Chip likely saved his father's life."[51] In other words, according to the judge, Gerald's hastened death was Ruth's agenda, not Gerald's. She was the one who contacted Kevorkian and made arrangements to bring her husband to him, a visit that would probably have been a one-way trip.

The Klooster case soon turned into a bitter interstate custody struggle between Chip, in Michigan, and his siblings and mother, in California. In Alameda County, California, Judge William McInstry, who had not heard the evidence presented to Judge Mulhauser, granted custody of Gerald to Chip's sister, Kristen Hamstra, and ordered Gerald returned to California, threatening Chip with jail and a $500-per-day fine. Meanwhile, Chip was ordered by Judge Mulhauser to keep Gerald in Michigan. The interstate battle soon ended in federal court, where a mediator helped the family reach a settlement, in which Gerald was returned to his home in California after Chip's mother and siblings specifically agreed in writing that Gerald would not be euthanized or assisted with suicide, even if such practices became legal. Ruth also agreed to counseling to help her cope with her husband's ailment. Chip's sister, Kristen Hamstra, was named as her father's conservator.

Gerald lived with Kristen for several months. Then, over Chip's strenuous objections, Judge McInstry allowed Gerald to live with Ruth, who solemnly promised there would be no attempt to hasten the death of her husband.

A few months later, Chip's worst fears were realized. Gerald lay in a hospital near death from an overdose of alcohol and sleeping pills. The police treated the case as an "attempted suicide with suspicious circumstances," in part because Ruth had attempted to prevent resuscitation by paramedics after she called 911 and because of the family history.[51] After a hearing, Judge McInstry returned custody of Gerald to Kristen, ignoring Ruth's pleas that she "would never hurt Gerald."[52]

Gerald recovered from the overdose. On February 7, 1997,

Judge McInstry granted Ruth's request that her husband live with her after she hired a live-in helper and took other court-requested actions designed to protect Gerald's safety. (The police investigation was unable to determine whether there was wrongdoing involved in Gerald's near-fatal overdose.)

Gerald Klooster eventually died of natural causes. After having repeatedly accused Chip of being in the case for the money, Ruth Klooster sold the rights to her story and it was turned into a made-for-television movie.

Judith Bement

Susan Randall, the distraught daughter of Judith Bement, asked her stepfather, John Bement, an excruciating question. "When you put the [plastic] bag on mom's head, was she awake? I mean, did she know you were doing that? I just need peace of mind."

Bement did not realize that Susan was cooperating with a police investigation into her mother's death or that she was taping their conversation as well as conversations with her sister, Cynthia, who had been present for part of the assisted killing. Bement replied, "I don't know. I don't know. She was not totally out but she wasn't conscious."

The tape transcript reveals that years previously, when Judith was first diagnosed with ALS, John Bement promised to assist his wife's suicide. He claimed that placing a plastic bag over his Judith's head after she took twenty Seconals was simply the keeping of that promise.

But Susan didn't see it that way. She had been with her mother on the night of her death and Judith was happy. She said, "But when I left, we were joking around and everything was fine and it was a split second and everything just went to hell. Do you know what happened?"

"Well, what she wanted was the pills.... I read that book and...

"What book?"

"*Final Exit.*"

"I never saw it."

"It's a book this guy wrote. So he says whenever you take these drugs that after the person is unconscious, you slip the bag over their head—kind of like insurance because, you know, somebody could survive."

Bement then rationalized his actions: "She wasn't going to get any better. If it wasn't then it would be a month later, two months later."[53]

Susan is convinced that her mother was not suicidal on the night she died and that she had not given up on life. "My mother had made plans for the future," she told me. "Her moods fluctuated, sure, but they were dictated by the quality of care she was receiving. When she felt valued and loved, she wanted to live. When she was made to feel like she was a burden, she grew despondent. She was not going to die soon. She had not qualified for hospice care because they said she would not die within six months. What mom needed was quality care and to know that she was loved, not a plastic bag over her head to suffocate the life out of her."

What shocked Susan was not only the manner of her mother's death but her stepfather's actions in its aftermath. "John began to date immediately after mom's death. His entire lifestyle changed. When mom was alive and needed him, he would often not come home at night, he said, because of his job as a local truck driver. I know because I stayed with her. As soon as she died, suddenly he started coming home every single night. I would drive by her house and his vehicle was always there."

Even worse for Susan, the townsfolk of Springville, New York, in her words, "were conned into believing his sad story of acting out of love for his wife. Before and during John's trial, all their sympathy went to him, even though he never took the stand in his own defense. I was ostracized for a while and only because I tried to stand up for my mom."

Had Judith ever expressed a desire to die? "Yes," Susan says. "When she was first diagnosed, a neurologist in Buffalo told her, 'You are a lost cause. You might as well go home, sit in a chair and wait to die.' She became despondent after that. Who wouldn't? For two years, she gave up on life. But then my daughter was born, and she started seeing things differently. She had an active life again. Sure, she sometimes got depressed, but she would bounce out of it and get on with life."

Bement was convicted of second-degree manslaughter, yet the

local media and public opinion generally supported John, as did, apparently, the judge. Despite his never having testified either at his trial or at the sentencing hearing—which would have allowed the district attorney to challenge his motives on cross-examination— Bement was sentenced to only two nonconsecutive weeks in jail.

Susan is bitter. "With that sentence, the law confirmed what that awful doctor told my mother. Her life had no value. Her death wasn't worth worrying too much about. That was an insult to my mother and to all sick people. I hope that if I ever get into a position where I am vulnerable like mother was, that there is a law that protects my life and prevents others from getting rid of me and then saying it was okay because it was all about compassion."[54]

EIGHT

HOSPICE OR HEMLOCK—
THE CHOICE IS OURS

EUTHANASIA IS JUSTIFIED BY CLAIMS OF compassion, appeals to raw emotionalism and paeans to "choice." But in light of the consequences that could flow from the legalization and legitimization of euthanasia, we should all think deeply about what accepting the values of the death culture would really mean for our country and the world.

Social libertarians argue that the state has no interest in preventing suicide, because each person's body is exclusively his or her own, and we must be free even to destroy it if that is what we want. But do we really want to live in a society that accepts the abandoning premises inherent in "rational suicide" and whose public policies would require authorities to stand back and watch deeply depressed persons jump off a bridge or shoot themselves in the head?

That being said, suicide per se is not the issue. Jumping off a bridge or turning on a car engine in a closed garage to kill oneself by carbon monoxide poisoning is an individual act. Being killed by a doctor or committing physician-assisted suicide is a joint endeavor between two or more people, conspiracy if you will, to commit a form of homicide. The point at issue is not the propriety of suicide itself, but whether we should have the legal right to have ourselves killed by another person. Looked at from another angle, the question before us is whether the broad prohibition against killing by private persons—except in self-defense or in defense of others—should be discarded so as to permit third parties to collaborate and participate in the deaths of sick and disabled people and those who are incompetent, and this on the basis of beliefs that certain lives are not worth living.

This question is of monumental importance. If we remain the society of "ordered liberty" envisioned by the Founders, a nation created to promote the greatest common good while allowing for as much individual liberty as practically consistent with this broader purpose, we will reject euthanasia and assisted suicide as a danger to vulnerable persons, as a threat to basic institutions, and as a dangerous frayer of the social fabric. If, on the other hand, our nation is above all else a radical personal-autonomy state, existing primarily to maximize individual behavioral license regardless of the overall impact such conduct has on the whole—if indeed the state's primary *raison d'être* is merely to prevent one autonomous individual's proverbial fist from punching another autonomous individual's proverbial nose—then legalized euthanasia makes sense.

But, as Charles Krauthammer of the *Washington Post* has warned, if choosing to be killed by others is a matter of individual liberty, then what "private" activity is there that can be proscribed? If individuals cannot be prevented from arranging their own killing, then how can we logically outlaw a pregnant woman's taking crack cocaine? What could possibly be more personal than what one chooses to put into one's body? What is more intimate than one's chosen state of consciousness? Similarly, if we accept euthanasia as a basic liberty interest the state cannot proscribe, would the laws that prohibit the selling of human organs for transplants fall too, perhaps as an adjunct to legalized assisted suicide?

Such a policy could easily fit into the "choice" category as well as into the increasing commercialism of our culture; it is also likely that such a policy would create a marketplace in human organs, leading to the catastrophic exploitation of the poor and to a medical system where transplants would go to the highest bidders.

Not surprisingly, some of the most notable physicians and bioethicists in the organ transplant community already envision just such a scenario. Robert W. Arnold and Stuart J. Youngner wrote hopefully about the possibility in the influential bioethics publication *Kennedy Institute of Ethics Journal*:

> If active euthanasia—e.g., lethal injection—and physician-assisted suicide are legally sanctioned...patients could couple organ donation

with their planned deaths; we would not have to depend only upon persons on life support. This practice would yield not only more donors but more types of organs as well, since the heart could be removed from dying, not just dead, patients.[1]

In a very real sense, how we decide the euthanasia controversy will determine the kind of society we live in and the one we will create for our children. The issue transcends what may be good or bad, right or wrong for individuals. It literally defines who and what we are as a society, a culture and a people.

Change isn't necessarily progress. As the victims of the French and Russian revolutions discovered, change can be violent and culturally destructive. Since we are dealing with the most fundamental issue, life and death, we should not make changes lightly or base them on emotionalism or sound-bite slogans and rationales. Legalizing euthanasia would cast aside 2,500 years of accumulated wisdom, ethics and morality, and would dramatically burden our culture with foreseen and unforeseen consequences. We should risk such consequences only if it is rational to do so.

I propose a three-pronged test to judge the rationality of creating a "right to die":

- Is there a deep and abiding need for this proposed revolutionary change that cannot be met through other means?
- Are the expected benefits of the change worth the foreseeable risks of the change?
- Would the change be progress?

Is There a Deep and Abiding Need to Legalize Euthanasia?

Pain Can Be Controlled
The most emotionally compelling argument in favor of euthanasia is that it is needed to help relieve human suffering caused by illness and to prevent people from dying in agony that cannot be controlled. But this is a false premise. Yes, too many patients die in unrelieved pain: But this isn't because we *can't* provide relief; rather, it is because we *don't*.

The difference between "can't" and "don't" is a vital part of this analysis. If relief form agonizing pain and suffering is the overarching purpose for legalizing assisted killing, and if medical science

has the wherewithal to relieve pain and significantly reduce suffering, then there is no real need to legalize euthanasia. Rather, there is
a need to improve the delivery of proper medicine by making the
currently available relief universally accessible.

This is fact: Nearly all pain can be effectively treated and controlled, including pain associated with arthritis, cancer, AIDS and
multiple sclerosis. Regardless of the cause of pain, severity of condition, or type of disease or affliction, with proper medical treatment
nearly every patient can exercise "power over pain," adding tremendously to the quality of his or her life and even its length. The
beneficent potential of pain control and relief through palliative care
of other symptoms such as itching, constipation and nausea cannot
be overstated.

Of course, some conditions are more difficult to palliate than
others. For example, one of the most painful diseases known to medicine is bone cancer. The pain can be excruciating, unbearable. Bones
grow brittle and break easily. The patient may be unable to bear simply being touched. But even this pain can be significantly relieved. It
isn't easy. It takes multiple strategies and hard work and concerted
effort by dedicated doctors.

Dr. Robin Bernhoft, a Washington surgeon, has seen such an
effort succeed in his own family. That is one of the reasons he
opposes euthanasia. Dr. Bernhoft told me the following story:

> People who say bone cancer pain cannot be relieved are mistaken. My
> brother died of multiple myeloma [a bone-marrow cancer] when he
> was forty-one. His cancer destroyed his spine and ribs. He had frac-
> tures all over his chest that moved when he breathed. It was as
> painful a case of cancer as I have seen since I became a surgeon in
> 1976. But Larry was lucky. He was at the Mayo Clinic, where doctors
> knew how to take care of such horrible pain, even back in 1981.
> Throughout his illness, he remained very comfortable, and very alert,
> because they knew how to treat such pain. Pain can almost always be
> controlled—and without putting people into a drugged stupor. Pain
> medicine—even morphine—goes straight to the pain. If the dosage is
> properly controlled, the patient will not feel drunk or drugged, and
> most importantly will not be in pain.[2]

The bad news, of course, is that too many patients are not
given the quality of treatment that Larry Bernhoft received. We have

a choice: Do we improve the training of doctors in the areas of pain, depression, disability and the needs of the dying, and demand that their professional performance meet the highest standard? Or do we lower our medical standards, in Dr. Bernhoft's provocative words, to "veterinary levels" and allow doctors off the hook by permitting them to kill?

If we want the former, we have a lot of work to do. When it comes to pain control, doctors are notorious underachievers. In the United States alone, tens of millions of people—cancer patients, AIDS patients, MS patients, rheumatoid arthritis patients and others—receive inadequate pain relief, causing unnecessary suffering and giving impetus to the euthanasia movement. According to medical literature, there are several reasons for this failure of modem professional medicine:

• *Too many doctors did not receive sufficient training in pain control* in medical school and have not pursued the subject since graduation. As a consequence, they don't even know about the newest pain-control techniques, thus depriving their patients of relief that should be theirs.

Too many doctors fear that pain medicine will cause drug addiction. This is a false fear. When used appropriately for pain control, and when applied properly, narcotic agents are virtually never addicting. That means that narcotics can be used liberally to relieve pain and suffering, without adding to the country's drug-abuse problem.

• *Patients also fear becoming addicted,* sometimes leading to refusal of readily available pain control. I have faced this problem with my own family, when my father was dying of colon cancer. I came to visit him in the hospital after surgery to clear his bile duct of a tumor. The surgeon had botched the job; Dad was lying in bed, writhing in pain, an ice pack held against his wound.

"Didn't they give you something for the pain?" I demanded.

"They did, but I refused."

"WHAT? Why?"

"I don't want to become addicted," he replied in the firmest voice he could muster.

Dad had been a top sergeant in the army before receiving battlefield promotions to captain during World War II. He prided

himself on being strong. But this was a false bravado that was causing him unnecessary suffering. I said, "Dad, you're a tough guy. You
won't get addicted. But even if you do, I know you're strong enough
to beat it. For goodness sake, take the [bleeping] pain medicine!"

Dad looked up at me gratefully. "Okay," he said sheepishly.

Apparently my father had just needed permission to take
strong drugs. We called the nurse into the room and he was soon
comfortable. For the remaining months of Dad's life, he never had
problems with pain.

• *Pain control is often an innocent casualty of the war on drugs.*
Many state laws designed to curb drug abuse make it difficult or
inconvenient for doctors to treat their patients' pain effectively. But
this is beginning to change. Several states have passed laws explicitly setting forth that aggressive pain control is a proper medical
act—even if it leads to the accidental death of the patient. As a consequence, morphine use in these states has soared. For example,
after Iowa passed such a law in conjunction with a new state law
banning assisted suicide, morphine use increased 136 percent from
1998 to 2001. Rhode Island passed a similar law and saw morphine
use increase 164 percent over the same period.[3]

• *Too many doctors do not take the time or effort to reevaluate their
patients' pain on a regular and continuing basis.* Some doctors never
even ask patients about their pain.[4] Patients too, are often reluctant
to tell their doctors that they hurt. There are several reasons for this:
Some patients believe that the presence of pain means that they are
going to die or that their illness has worsened—which isn't necessarily true. Some believe that "good patients" don't bother their
doctors by reporting pain. In fact, the opposite is true. Good patients
let their doctors know what is going on. Otherwise their doctors
may be hindered from providing optimal care.[5]*

---

* For readers interested in learning more about pain control, see *Power over Pain: How
to Get the Pain Control You Need*, which I co-authored with Dr. Eric M. Chevlen, a brilliant pain-control specialist. The book is a consumer's guide to obtaining quality
medical care for pain. It is written in a highly readable and approachable format and
is intended to help you and your doctor work together to ensure that you receive
optimal pain-controlling care. For more information, go to www.poweroverpain.com
or contact the International Task Force on Euthanasia and Assisted Suicide at 800-
786-3839.

Hospice Care Already Provides "Death with Dignity"

Many dying people who consider assisted suicide are afraid of future pain, abandonment or a "medicalized" death hooked up to machines in a cold, sterile institutional setting. While some patients do still die this way, dying does not have to be so impersonal and burdensome.

Over the last few decades, the hospice movement has slowly reversed the over-medicalization of death. Hospice is less a place than a concept. According to the *Harvard Health Letter,* "The hospice philosophy is that dying should be accepted as a unique part of life, not resisted with every weapon in medicine's armamentarium. When nothing more can be gained from [curative] treatment, hospices focus on making people as comfortable as possible."[6]

The goal is to provide whatever care patients need to enable them to die naturally, in peace and with dignity. This means that no efforts are made to extend the patient's life. Instead, the focus is on providing whatever treatment is necessary to control pain and alleviate symptoms, while at the same time providing emotional support for the patient and the family.

A typical team includes a physician (such as the hospice physicians interviewed for this book, Drs. Eric Chevlen, Ira Byock and Gary Lee); hospice nurses who make house calls to check on patients and provide needed medical services; social workers who are available to assist the patient and family and assess their needs; and psychological therapists and bereavement counselors to provide valuable grief counseling and emotional support. Volunteers work creatively to fill caregiving niches for the benefit of patient and family. Respite care is also available to aid families needing a short break from the intense effort of caregiving. Since most hospice care occurs in the home (although there are hospice facilities), once a patient enters hospice, usually when the prognosis is life expectancy of six months or less, he or she can say goodbye to impersonal hospitals and being "hooked up to machines" that so many of us fear during the dying process.

The beneficence of hospice, for those patients who desire to cease curative or life-prolonging medical treatment and transition peacefully into death, cannot be overstated. "Hospice is often misunderstood as limited to controlling a dying person's symptoms," says Dr. Ira Byock. "Symptom control is the first priority of hospice, but it is not the ultimate goal. The fundamental purpose of hospice is to enhance the quality of life for the dying individual and the family, to give the opportunity for the patient to live as fully as possible in community with his or her friends or family, to get affairs in order, to deepen and complete relationships. Hospice is about the completing of a life, and in that context it is…wonderfully human."[7]

Euthanasia advocates usually give lip-service support to hospice but contend that hospice providers should also be in the business of hastening their patients' deaths—a combination that the euthanasia advocate Lonny Shavelson calls "hospice and hemlock."[8] This idea is anathema to most hospice professionals, as it is the antithesis of the hospice philosophy.

The message of hospice is that each patient is valuable and important, and that dying is a basic stage of life that is worth living through and growing from—until death comes through natural processes. Or, as Dame Cicely Saunders has recently written, hospice asserts on behalf of the dying patient his or her "common humanity and personal importance" until the moment of natural death.[9]

The euthanasia philosophy is just the opposite. By definition, euthanasia is a statement that life is not worth living and not worth protecting. Worse, the euthanasia philosophy claims that the answer to dying, disability or other "hopeless illness" is to induce death artificially and "get it over with." No wonder the world's most notable hospice professionals disagree with the hemlock approach.

Dr. Carlos F. Gomez, assistant professor of medicine at the University of Virginia School of Medicine and a hospice physician of national repute, firmly opposes mixing hospice with hemlock as an easy way out of truly caring for dying patients. He told a congressional committee looking into the assisted suicide issue: "We now have it well within our technical means to alleviate, to palliate and comfort and control the worst symptoms of those of our fellow citizens who are terminally ill. The question before…the country at large is whether we have the heart, the courage, and the will to make it so, or whether we will opt for expediency and call it mercy."[10]

Dr. Gary Lee also strongly opposes mixing hospice with hemlock. "I am there to take care of the patient," he says. "You can't move the line in hospice to allow the killing of patients. It would destroy the line." Dr. Byock puts it even more succinctly: "The hospice focus is on life and the alleviation of suffering," whereas "the goal of assisted suicide and euthanasia is death."[11]

From this perspective, euthanasia threatens the hospice movement. "Hospice commits to the patient and the family that we will take care of them, to nonabandonment," says Dr. Lee. "But if euthanasia became a standard of practice, too many times there would be a real incentive to do it. There are some patients whose proper care requires time and effort, professional services that aren't necessarily paid for by insurance companies. I might say, 'There has to be an easier way.' I could too easily find myself seeing euthanasia as the simple answer; one that is less time-consuming and the least expensive. If accepted, euthanasia could very easily take the place of proper patient care."[12]

The Dutch experience with hospice lends credence to Dr. Lee's concerns. Studies show that hospice-style palliative care is stunted in the Netherlands. There are very few hospice facilities, very little in the way of organized hospice activity, and few specialists in palliative care, although some efforts are now under way to jump-start the hospice movement in that country. One reason for the lack of hospice opportunities in the Netherlands is the general-practitioner style of medical delivery, in which doctors make house calls and care for citizens from birth until death—a hands-on approach to medicine that the hospice movement is reintroducing to American health care. However, the widespread availability of euthanasia in the Netherlands may be another reason for the stunted growth of the Dutch hospice movement. One Dutch doctor is reported to have asked, "Why should I worry about palliation when I have euthanasia?"

This demonstrates the falsity of the argument often made by assisted suicide advocates that killing is a "compassionate" answer to the problem of human suffering. The root meaning of compassion is to "suffer with." But assisted suicide isn't about suffering with. It is about terminating the problem with cold efficiency.

Hospice exists because of the dedication and compassion of its founder, Dame Cicely Saunders, who in the wake of World War II was inspired to create the hospice concept while caring for a dying war refugee named David Tasma. As Saunders and Tasma spoke of his impending death, she had an epiphany that the compassionate approach to caring for the dying was to treat "the total patient." In pursuit of her dream, she went to medical school at the age of thirty-three. After becoming an M.D., Saunders worked for nearly twenty years to establish the hospice concept. St. Christopher's Hospice opened in London in 1967, with in-home care beginning in 1969. In 1971, she introduced the concept to America.[13]

Almost everyone over the age of ten has been touched in some fashion by Saunders' compassionate concept. I certainly have. My father fought the good fight against colon cancer for about two years until the day he sat on a hospital bed contemplating a bile drainage bag that doctors had inserted to prevent jaundice. He looked at me and sighed deeply, his shoulders sagging. I knew then that his fight to remain alive had ended.

Dad entered hospice. His last several months were peaceful, pain-free and nurtured. He spent hours sitting on a bench in his back yard overlooking his beloved cactus garden, contemplating the ultimate issues raised by human mortality. Dad died peacefully in a Veterans Hospital hospice unit in Los Angeles, leaving me an invaluable lesson in how to die.

I also reflect upon the death of Frank, my childhood best friend's father and my "second dad." In 1997, he also died of colon cancer. Unfortunately, it was difficult for his family to get his doctor to agree to hospice care, causing him much unnecessary suffering. But once admitted to hospice, Frank's life changed from one dominated by pain and suffering, into a relaxed, peaceful and pain-free ending surrounded by his family, with his favorite opera playing on the stereo.

On April 1, 2005, my wonderful friend Julia died of breast cancer at the too-young age of fifty. Julia had three young children and she was determined that they would always know that she didn't leave them lightly or easily. For nine years she fought with grit and determination against her spreading disease.

Julia's spirit was willing but finally her body gave out. She and her husband, Colin, decided the time had come for hospice. Julia received excellent in-home hospice care for the remaining months of her life, during which time she remained vitally involved with her family and friends. Her symptoms were managed as she slowly weakened. In fact, she received such good care that my wife and I enjoyed a leisurely lunch with Julia and Colin at a restaurant near their home a mere four days before she died.

There is a direct through-line of true compassion and love from David Tasma in 1948 to my father in 1984, Frank in 1997, Julia in 2005—and to the millions of others who have benefited from hospice care since 1967. Hospice properly applied is the true, compassionate death with dignity.

Dying isn't death; it is part of living. Assisted suicide proponents miss this crucial point. That is why Dame Cicely Saunders is an adamant opponent of allowing end-of-life care to devolve into end-of-life killing.

Independent Living Eliminates Despair by Empowering Disabled People
As we have learned in these pages from people such as Paul Longmore, Diane Coleman and Carol Gill, disabled people usually seek out assisted suicide because they have suffered the kind of life crisis that can afflict anyone—divorce, the death of a loved one, career crisis, financial collapse and the like—or because their desire to live freely and independently has been needlessly stymied, leading to feelings of despair and hopelessness. As with untreated pain and undesired medicalized dying, this need not be so. Increasingly, the disability rights and independent-living movement works on behalf of disabled people and their families to help overcome hurdles that needlessly interfere with the living of full and productive lives. The movement provides disabled people with personal assistants who help them learn independent-living skills and help perform tasks that their disabilities prevent or make difficult. It also provides other forms of peer counseling and deals with issues of housing advocacy, disability rights advocacy, transportation and, most important of all, information and referral. By law, the centers for independent living must have at least 51 percent control by people with disabilities, ensuring that the perspective of disabled people is amply considered in decision making. There are independent-living centers all around the country.

Independent living makes a tremendous difference in so many lives. Take the late Mark O'Brien, the journalist-poet described earlier in the book. O'Brien contracted polio at the age of six and was a complete quadriplegic for forty-one years. The polio so profoundly disabled his musculature that he was dependent on an iron lung for the rest of his life, rarely leaving the machine except for a few hours a month when he was able to survive in a supine position on a ventilator, allowing him to be wheeled outside for an hour or so and to make personal appearances at lectures near his home in Berkeley. Otherwise, from the age of six to his death just before his fiftieth birthday in 1999, Mark spent his entire life inside his yellow iron lung, which dominated the living room of his one-bedroom loft apartment.

Jack Kevorkian has said that those among us who have significant physical impairments, people such as Mark O'Brien, are "certifiably pathological" if they are not in despair.[14] Nothing could be more wrong. While he faced some considerable challenges, Mark enjoyed his life and lived it to the fullest—in large part because of the independent-living movement. "Before I lived on my own," O'Brien told me, "I was afraid my life wouldn't amount to anything, that I couldn't do anything, that I would never be able to contribute to society. But because of independent living, I now have my own career, work at it, and live my own life. Because of independent living, I paid income taxes for the first time in my life. Most disabled people could achieve at least partial self-sufficiency with the appropriate services made available to them."[15]

O'Brien strongly believed that "the idea of disabled people being stuck in nursing homes for life is not only wasteful of resources, it is wasteful of people and little better than slavery. We know how to assist people to live independently; it is cheaper than warehousing people; we are just not doing it sufficiently to be of assistance to most disabled people. I consider the cause of independent living to be the moral equivalent of the civil rights movement of the 1960s."[16]

Another example of the difference that independent living can make for even the most profoundly disabled was brought to my attention by an attorney named Beth Roney Drennan, of Baraboo, Wisconsin. Drennan was appointed guardian *ad litem* for David W. Domenosky, a young man whose brain was injured in an auto accident. Domenosky awakened from a six-month coma with total quadriplegia. He was shocked to learn that, although his medical records showed that he had no intellectual impairment, and although he was able to communicate by blinks and stares, doctors had discussed withholding antibiotics from him in the event he developed an infection. His parents refused to authorize discontinuing treatment for their son.

When Drennan asked about this, one of Domenosky's nurses nonchalantly admitted that the idea was for him to die if he should ever develop pneumonia.[17] When Drennan asked a supervising nurse at a different facility (where she was thinking of placing Domenosky) her views on this matter, the woman asserted that she too believed treatment should be withheld from Domenosky because he "is no longer experiencing life." The nurse then asked Drennan, "Do you want your tax dollars supporting people like this forever?"[18]

Appalled at what she considered a cavalier attitude about Domenosky's life on the part of some of his professional caregivers, worried that "David would be killed without his mother being consulted" (not an unreasonable fear, as we have seen), and believing firmly in her client's right not only to live but to thrive, Drennan spent more than a year, in her words, "fighting blindly" to get Domenosky out of the nursing home and into a better placement.

Eventually, Drennan's care for Domenosky and her innate tenacity led her to a disability rights group committed to the independent-living concept. With their help, she has overcome "budget cuts, recalcitrant bureaucrats and overburdened case workers," and has placed David in his own apartment.

Domenosky's release from the nursing home was only the beginning of Drennan's plans for her friend and client. "David will get communication therapy," Drennan told me excitedly in 1995. "He will receive vocational training so he can work or otherwise involve himself in projects, plus he will receive physical therapy to improve his physical abilities." According to Drennan, Domenosky is almost as charged about his upcoming new life as she is. "He is most excited about 'getting back into the culture,'" Drennan says. "He can hardly wait to listen to his own style of music, watch current movies on video, create a new life for himself outside of a nursing home setting."[19]

In May 2002, I decided to see whether Drennan's plans for

Domenosky were panning out. "It all turned out better than we even thought it would be!" Drennan told me. "All our work was a complete success: David did move into a beautiful new home right after your book [the first edition of *Forced Exit*] came out. He was always positive that getting into his own place would be the key to his happiness and he was right. He is so happy, and it has been several years now. He was given a similarly challenged roommate his own age right at the start and that has worked out fine. He has fabulous caregivers and his cheerful attitude wins everyone over. He communicates excellently by blinking. He has gained a little weight and looks adorable. He is about thirty now and still has a little 'tail' of long hair in back of his head to keep the cool look. Best news: He is eating now by mouth! The tube is used only for medications. All those years he couldn't even taste food and now, last time I saw him he was eating a cookie—and laughing at the same time. He has a new van and a busy social schedule, his caregivers tell me. He went to one of his caregivers' college graduation, he goes shopping, all kinds of things."[20]

Compare Drennan's understanding of human compassion to the mindsets of so many others—doctors, euthanasia advocates, well-meaning relatives of disabled people—who proclaim that some lives are simply not worth living, that for the good of the patient, to ease the burden on the patient's family and relieve society of a financial burden, disabled people like Domenosky can ethically be dehydrated to death, assisted with suicide or, indeed, fatally injected. To this, Drennan responds:

> In our culture, I think that many people see affection as something that occurs *post hoc, ergo propter hoc* [after something and therefore because of it]. They believe there must be a "cause" for affection; that the cause comes first. If there is enough cause, then the effect follows; that if the person is deserving or has certain attributes, then that is a cause for having affection for them. But I believe that real affection for each other is inherent in our natural state, and that if we do nothing to block that affection, it will flow through us toward others, at least in some degree. No cause is required, no attributes of mind or body; it's not earned by conditions, but not lost by them either. Not even old age, loss of teeth, loss of hair, loss of physical beauty or ability to move the body due to quadriplegia can make the affection go away.

Those of us who have affection for David, see the beauty and infinite value of his life—and that affection is not conditioned on the state of David's body. David is wonderful, just as and because he is.[21]

Is the Expected Benefit of Euthanasia Worth Its Considerable Risks?

At this juncture in the debate, death fundamentalists will usually say, "But what about the few who, despite the best of care, would still want euthanasia rather than to await a natural death or live a life with the limitations of disability or chronic disease? Shouldn't they be given the opportunity to have their lives ended as they choose?"

Again, that depends on what one believes the purpose of society to be, as expressed through its public policy. Should the morality, ethical concepts and laws that protect and benefit the many be cast aside because a relatively small group of people does not want to abide by them?

Certainly, there are times when the rights of even one person override the views of the rest of society. But the genius of our system is that at such times, special legal niches can be created to accommodate and protect the rights of small groups. For example, the law in most states requires universal education to age sixteen or so. Yet Amish parents have the legal right to remove their children from public school years before they reach sixteen, owing to the special nature of the Amish subculture.

The niche created to accommodate the Amish has little if any impact on the general society. Nor does it endanger non-Amish children. The same cannot be said of euthanasia. As we derive rights from our community, so too we bear responsibilities to it. That is what it means to be part of a community. Even though a few people would undoubtedly wish to hasten their deaths despite receiving the best medical care that exists, asking to be killed should be viewed in the same way as threatening to jump off the Golden Gate Bridge: as a request for help. The compassionate answer must be to render assistance, not give the suicidal person a "helpful" push off the rail.

Moreover, what message would be sent to others with similar

illnesses as people who are being assisted in suicide? One day when I went to visit my hospice friend Bob, who eventually died of ALS, he was so angry he was spitting nails. The year was 1997, and the United States Supreme Court was about to hear arguments as to whether the Constitution provided a "right" to assisted suicide.

The media was all over the story. *Nightline* presented the case of a Rhode Island man with ALS who claimed to want assisted suicide. Bob believed that the entire program had been biased in favor of allowing the man to be killed. "How do you think that makes *me* feel," he demanded. "That my life isn't worth protecting or living." Bob was so incensed he wrote an opinion article published in the *San Francisco Chronicle* entitled "I Don't Want a Choice to Die," saying:

> Euthanasia advocates believe they are doing people like me a favor. They are not. The negative emotions toward the terminally ill and disabled generated by their advocacy is actually at the expense of the "dying" and their families and friends, who often feel disheartened and without self-assurance because of a false picture of what it is like to die created by these enthusiasts who prey on the misinformed.
>
> What we, the terminally ill, need is exactly the opposite—to realize how important our lives are. And our loved ones, friends, and indeed society, need to help us to feel that we are loved and appreciated unconditionally.[22]

Bob was right. Legalization would not increase compassion or equal treatment toward dying people. It would be a step backward, sending the loud message that certain lives just are not worth living.

Would the Change Be Progress?

Legalizing euthanasia would not be a step forward for society but rather a giant leap backward in our desire to serve and assist those among us whose lives have been impacted by a terminal diagnosis, disability, chronic pain, the debilitation of advanced years, the despair of depression—indeed, anyone and everyone experiencing what euthanasia advocates call "hopeless illness." It would be to countenance their killing, in essence to legalize murder. It would inevitably lead, as it has in the Netherlands, to involuntary euthanasia. This is especially dangerous for those among us who are less powerful: African Americans and other minorities who too often receive lower standards of health care, such as the poor and the uneducated, those with little understanding or ability to assert their rights to quality health care in an increasingly commercialized medical milieu. It would be to make a virtue out of abandonment and accelerate the country's tendency to isolate those most in need of community.

This last point was brought home to me in a forceful manner recently in my work as a hospice volunteer. I turn once again to the wisdom of my hospice friend Bob. I visited Bob once a week for almost two years. During that time, we spent many hours discussing his feelings about dying, about becoming disabled, indeed, about the purpose and meaning of life. Our many conversations were deep, profound, inspiring and rewarding.

Bob's experience made vividly clear the isolation faced too often by dying and disabled people. "For the first two and a half years after my diagnosis I wanted to kill myself," Bob told me early in our relationship. "It was not the illness so much that depressed me but the reaction of the people around me. First they stopped visiting, then they stopped calling to speak to me, and then they stopped calling. I found myself completely isolated. I felt like a token presence in the world."

Jack Kevorkian was first making headlines during this time and Bob took acute notice. He told me that he listened to the newscasts carefully and that they definitely impacted his thinking about suicide. "During my worst moments, the idea of a quick demise had an appeal," he recalls. "I didn't want to be a burden and I figured it would be the best thing for everyone."

Suicide thoughts and Bob eventually parted company as he, his wife and their children pulled together and kept on going through the difficulties caused by his inability to work and the distress caused by his weakening condition. When he joined the Mormon Church, he found a new community whose members rallied to his side. Church members visited Bob every day. Two and a half years after his diagnosis he "came out of the fog," as he put it. He discovered that he deeply wanted to live for as long as nature permitted.

Bob lived nearly five years longer than expected He spent his final days happy to be alive, relishing each day. He wrote a novel. He invested on the Internet and used the computer to collect art. He was especially proud of a Dali lithograph he purchased at an on-line auction. "Believe me, this time has been a blessing," he once told me, "I have grown. I have come into my own. I know myself better than I ever thought I would. I understand more about life than I ever thought I could. I am living more intensely than I ever have. I wouldn't have missed the last several years for anything in the world."

Had Bob requested assisted suicide during his years of depression, death fundamentalists would have considered the request "rational." They would have labeled his illness "hopeless." They would have believed, on the basis of their own fears and prejudices, that the quality of his life was not worth living. They would have readily granted his request for a hastened death, thinking they were being oh so compassionate. (In fact, ALS has become something of the poster disease for the entire euthanasia movement.) What they would not have considered was that by acceding to his suicidal desire, they actually would have been robbing him of some of the best and most important years of his life. And no one would ever have known, because those years would have been lost to Bob forever.

Recent studies verify Bob's experience. One of the primary reasons that dying people seek euthanasia, according to a study published in *The Lancet* in August 2001, concerns the loss of social ties, a sense of "existential isolation."[23] Another study, conducted by the Bioethics Institute of New York Medical College in 2001, supported this finding. Dr. Daniel P. Sulmasy followed fifty-eight patients hospitalized for serious illness such as cancer, dementia and AIDS. The patients' doorways were videotaped for twenty-four-hour periods. Sulmasy found that they spent "the vast majority of their time in solitude, with few visits from medical personnel or family members."[24]

The answer to the problems of isolation and abandonment clearly isn't validating the sense of worthlessness that loneliness and boredom engenders. Rather, it is to reintegrate the dying patient into the community, restoring a sense that the patient is "us" and not "them."

In this regard, the words of Dennis Brace of Youngstown, Ohio, should also be heeded. Brace, forty-two, was told more than four years ago that his inoperable colon cancer would kill him within a few months. Several doctors told him there was virtually no point in fighting, since his cancer had spread to his muscle tissues.[25] He felt abandoned and alone.

According to Brace, one of the greatest emotional burdens he faced in combating his malady was the attitudes expressed by euthanasia proponents, who in their different ways send the message that his life was as good as over. "What am I supposed to think when the government or the courts or society says it is okay to snuff out people like me because we are sick?" Brace asked. "If you wanted to push me into giving up, that is how to do it. Any kind of negativism from the outside is devastating to a person in my position. This euthanasia stuff is the opposite of compassion and support. It is saying to me that no one cares."

Like Bob, Dennis Brace lived fully to the last. He cared for his roses, appeared in a video called *Euthanasia: False Light,* and did volunteer work. He died a pain-free and dignified death, thanks to the quality hospice and palliative care he received from his friend and doctor, Eric M. Chevlen.

Creating a Culture of Compassion

Rejecting the death culture does not mean we should accept the status quo. Euthanasia, like a fever, is a symptom, not the underlying disease. We should cure the underlying unhealthy conditions that lead advocates to demand it.

We Must Overcome Our National Death Phobia

"People routinely think that doctors know how to prognosticate, how to mitigate pain, and generally how to serve dying persons," Dr. Joanne Lynn told the Senate Finance Committee. "Nothing could be further from the truth. This culture has been so thoroughly death-denying that we have not even described our course to death nor developed professional skills in service of the dying, except for the development of hospice services…. We do not know how to see to it that most that die get excellent care, shaped to their needs, and responsive to their symptoms."[26]

"By any standard one chooses," it has been observed, "medical schools in the United States fail to provide even adequate education in the care of the dying."[27] Only 5 of 126 medical schools in the United States offer a separate required course in the care of the dying. According to the AMA, as of 1995 only 26 percent of residency programs offered a course on the medico-legal aspects of end-of-life care as a regular part of the curriculum. A national survey of accredited residency programs in family medicine and internal medicine/pediatrics, the specializations from which primary care physicians come, revealed that 15 percent of these programs offer no formal training in terminal care and that residents in the majority of these programs coordinated the care of ten or fewer terminally ill patients throughout the course of their studies. Only 17 percent of these programs use hospice rotations, despite the widespread availability of hospice programs that could be served by the residents and that could teach them. The report summarized this and other data in asserting that the evidence reveals a "well-established pattern of neglect of medical education in the care of the dying."[28]

People who are dying, disabled or seriously ill are often abandoned by friends and are isolated by a culture that celebrates youth and vitality and that often places cosmetic values ahead of human values. We treat those among us with disabling conditions as unwelcome reminders of our ultimate lack of control over life and of the fact that someday we too will come face to face with our own mortality. This needs to change.

And in fact, calls for more humane treatment of dying people are finally being heard. For example, the Ethics Committee of the American Geriatric Society has produced a nine-point plan to improve the care of the dying, including renewed focus on respecting patient values in treatment decisions; the creation of multidisciplinary teams to treat dying people; more attention to the relief of symptoms with emphasis on pain control; better reimbursement policies for providers of palliative care; and education of doctors and patients on the desirability of a peaceful and natural death when this is desired by the patient rather than a drive for curative care until shortly before death. Those are good suggestions, and hopefully the medical profession will listen and act upon them.

We should strive to ensure that no one is left to face death alone. Rather than shy away from dying people, as many of us do, we should embrace them, letting them know that we love and care for them, and that we will be with them to the end. We need to stop avoiding visits to those we know who are ill or dying, and we should volunteer with hospice or other beneficent organizations that succor the ill and assist the needy.

To give ourselves peace of mind about our own end-of-life care, every adult should create an advance directive stating our preferences about desired medical treatment should we become incapacitated. A caveat is in order here. Advance directives should not be taken lightly. As we have seen, once you fill one out, you may get what you ask for—even if later on you have a last-minute change of heart. Too often, people wait until a hospital admissions clerk gives an advance directive form to them before considering these important issues. Federal law requires that every new patient to a hospital or nursing home be provided an advance directive form to sign, if the patient so desires.

There are two primary kinds of advance directive, generally known as the "living will" and the "durable power of attorney for health care" (sometimes called a health-care proxy). Living wills negate informed consent. Since no one knows the future, advance instructions for care or the withholding of care must be written in general terms. If an incapacitation occurs, the patient's feelings and desires about this *specific* circumstance may not be known. The living will therefore puts tremendous power into the hands of doctors, who are authorized to decide whether and when the living will takes effect, when treatment should be withdrawn or withheld. Moreover, the decision regarding the type and extent of medical intervention to be withheld is the doctor's. And this power is not restricted to withholding "extraordinary care" such as ventilators to assist with breathing; it may include anything from not treating a curable bacterial infection to withdrawing food and fluids so that the patient starves and dehydrates to death. Thus, with a living will, the check of informed consent is surrendered to medicalized decision making—especially dangerous in HMO settings where doctors may have potent financial incentives to withhold care.

With a durable power of attorney for health care (DPAHC), in contrast, the right to informed consent is substantially retained.

Why? Rather than appoint a doctor as decider, the DPAHC appoints an "attorney in fact" to be the patient's health-care decision maker should he or she become incapacitated. The attorney in fact, also known as an agent or a proxy, for all intents and purposes steps into the shoes of the patient and decides issues of treatment or nontreatment as the patient would were he or she able to do so. Like the patient, the proxy can ask questions, request second opinions, disagree with the doctor's recommendation and so on. The DPAHC also permits people to opt in favor of life-prolonging care, an option often unavailable in the language of living wills.

In a world of assembly-line medicine, where many patients have little interaction with their doctors, isn't it better to eschew a doctor-empowering living will in favor of a patient-empowering durable power of attorney? It's not as catchy a name, but it is a much better document, one that may spell the difference between suffering a premature death and receiving personal decision making for health care, which everyone deserves.

If people are to become confident in the use of advance directives, laws need to be drafted to avoid the problem of denying people requested care if they become technically incompetent, in cases where they have previously written an advance directive in which they refuse care. Michigan already has just such a law. "Under Michigan statutory law, the benefit of the doubt is given to providing lifesaving treatment if there is any expressed desire to receive it," says attorney John Hess, who represented Michael Martin's mother and sister and saved the disabled man's life (as described in Chapter Two). "Even if you are incompetent and, secondly, even if you are unable to participate in general with your own health care decisions, as long as you have the ability to communicate a desire to live, it must be honored under the law, regardless of what a previously executed writing says."[29] The Michigan statute is a good model for the rest of the country.

Those who view advance directives as a vehicle for ending the lives of seriously ill or disabled people sooner rather than later might squawk that such a law interferes with the purpose for which these legal documents were created. But the purpose of advance directives is not to get sick people to take an early checkout, but rather to give them a tool to control their own destinies. People are far more likely to prepare advance directives that request nontreatment (assuming that is their desire) if they know that, in the event they change their minds, there won't be a futilitarian or an HMO executive opposing their newly expressed desire to fight to live.

One last point about advance directives: Most advocacy about signing these important documents stresses refusing care. That doesn't mean you have to go along with the nontreatment agenda. When preparing your advance directive, it is important to remember that you can opt for continued treatment.

Exert Better Control over HMOs

Health care isn't just another industry, like manufacturing and selling cars, computers or shoes. While the forces of the "invisible hand of the marketplace" might be the best way to ensure the manufacture of quality goods at fair prices, it is not necessarily the best way to ensure access to quality health care, and it can be extremely dangerous for patients—especially if euthanasia and futilitarianism become legal.

This book has only touched upon the dangers facing patients in the emerging profit-driven HMO health-care financing system. In the long run, a system that is open and accessible to everyone, whether through government involvement or the private sector, is a moral and ethical imperative. However that is to be done—I suspect it will be a hybrid private/public approach—the system must be founded on the equality-of-life ethic that protects the lives and upholds the moral worth of patients who are expensive to care for properly.

At best, these necessary reforms are years away. For now we are stuck with the managed-care system, where profits are made from cutting costs rather than from providing care. In such a milieu, we must not permit the weakest and most vulnerable among us to be sacrificed to the bottom line of corporate medicine, whether through assisted suicide or through the quasi rationing of health care promoted by advocates of futile care theory.

Here are some ideas that I believe can help:

• Prevent insurers and HMOs from giving bonuses and other financial incentives to doctors and nurses for withholding care, improperly limiting hospitalization, refusing referrals to special-

ists, not writing needed prescriptions, etc. It is especially imperative that capitation contracts requiring doctors to pay for
patient-specialized care out of their own pockets be banned.

- Require safe staffing levels at all health-care facilities.
- Provide whistleblower protection for doctors, nurses and other
  HMO employees, along with contract service providers and other
  HMO-affiliated caregivers, so that they can report abuses without
  fear of job sanction.
- Prohibit mandatory arbitration clauses that bar wronged HMO
  members from taking their cause to the courts.
- If a physician commits malpractice as a result of pressure from
  HMO policies, allow the HMO to be a defendant in the case.
- Guarantee patients full access to information about their medical
  care by prohibiting gag rules that prevent doctors from telling the
  truth about their financial arrangements with a patient's HMO,
  from criticizing the HMO, or from discussing care that the HMO
  might not wish to pay for.
- Create nonprofit, HMO-member-controlled consumer advocacy
  groups to serve as HMO watchdogs.
- Set a standard of care such that ninety cents out of every health-
  care dollar is spent on patient care rather than on HMO
  bureaucracies, marketing, profits or bonuses.

The civil justice system should also be used to deter improper
HMO practices. The fear of loss of money can be a great deterrent to
improper behavior. If HMOs could be sued for punitive damages
(money above and beyond the actual level of damages caused) in
cases of egregious and willful wrongdoing, the likelihood of their
intentionally sacrificing patients to the bottom line would be greatly
reduced. Federal legislation may be required to overcome a U.S.
Supreme Court decision that prohibited beneficiaries from collecting
punitive damages against wrongdoing by health insurance companies if the employee received the insurance as an employment or
union benefit.

Consumers and business or union executives in charge of nego-
tiating health insurance contracts for employees or members need to
use the power of consumerism to punish "bad" HMOs—those that
sacrifice quality of care for profits or put the desires of investors
before the needs of patients—by withholding their business. On the

other hand, "good" HMOs that put patient care first should be rewarded with patronage, even if the premiums cost a bit more.

(Much is made in the media about the problems associated with HMOs—and properly so. But publicly funded health care is not necessarily a panacea—as demonstrated vividly by Oregon's Medicaid rationing scheme. The sad truth is that government-funded health-care systems that struggle with inadequate resources present many of the same dangers to the weak and vulnerable as does the HMO economic model. For example, because of a financial crunch, the Ontario Medical Association admitted in April 2002 that 900,000 Ontario citizens do not have a primary care physician despite having a legal right to a doctor, and that, due to funding issues, Ontario loses two hundred doctors a year.[30] Imagine if the people of Canada ever come to see assisted suicide as the answer to their health funding dilemma. The "right to die" could easily morph under social pressures into a "duty to die.")

Make Pain Control More Accessible

If we want to create a truly humane health-care system that cares for people rather than kills them, pain control must be made universally available. Toward that end, physicians who treat patients in the clinical setting should be required by medical associations and state law to educate themselves on pain-control techniques and other palliative protocols. For pain that average doctors cannot overcome, all HMOs must be required to make referrals to board-certified pain-control experts readily available to plan members without arbitrary restriction, on an as-needed basis. In that way, suffering people such as Rebecca Badger, Jack Kevorkian's thirty-third victim, who stated in a pre-suicide television interview that she would prefer to live if she could escape the pain, would be able to obtain relief without resorting to death peddlers.[31]

We also need to stop making pain sufferers the victims of the war on drugs. Too many states place obstacles in the way of doctors aiming to provide adequate pain treatment. For example, many states have rules that require triplicate prescription forms for the dispensation of certain medications, and some state authorities even harass physicians deemed to be too liberal in prescribing certain controlled substances.

One suggestion that requires reasoned consideration is the legalization of marijuana for medicinal purposes. (Several states have legalized "medical marijuana," but in 2001 the Supreme Court of the United States ruled that such laws do not prevent the U.S. government from enforcing federal laws prohibiting all use of cannabis.) Supporters of legalizing cannabis for medicinal purposes claim that the drug smoked in its natural state (instead of taken as a pill) can ease the suffering of patients with AIDS, cancer, glaucoma, MS and other afflictions. Since morphine and other drugs are legalized for medicinal purposes, there is little reason to ban marijuana from being prescribed—assuming, of course, that it actually alleviates suffering.

Improve Hospital Ethics Committees
Hospital ethics committees have tremendous power in today's health-care delivery system. Yet their membership is anonymous and their meetings are held in secret, leaving tremendous potential for abuse and decision making based on prejudice or incomplete information, as occurred in the Michael Martin and Robert Wendland cases.

"There are no unified standards and no regular performance reviews applied to ethics committees," says Lance K. Stell, M.D., Ph.D., a medical ethicist with the Department of Internal Medicine at the Carolinas Medical Center in Charlotte, North Carolina. Dr. Stell observes, "It is amazing how often ethics committees make judgments without even seeing the patient or discussing the patient with all concerned parties, including the nursing staff and other caregivers. More than once I have seen a decision made to stop treating a patient, and then when I have gone to see the person I have been appalled."[32]

Dr. Stell tells of one case he personally witnessed where a daughter requested that her mother be taken off a ventilator. Yet when Dr. Stell went to see the patient, she "vigorously nodded her head" upon being asked whether she wished to continue indefinitely with assisted breathing. "It turned out the daughter had financial problems and needed money and so she decided the time had come to get her mother out of the way," Dr. Stell told me. "If our ethics committee had been a rubber stamp, and if the surgeon hadn't vigorously opposed the idea, the patient's life might well have been ended. Some ethics committees are rubber stamps, and some doctors are very compliant in these cases."[33]

This concern is especially acute in view of the power some futile care protocols are placing in hospital ethics committees. For example, in 2000 the Mercy Health Systems in Philadelphia published their futile care policy, which empowers a hospital ethics committee, called an Institutional Interdisciplinary Review Board (IIRB), not only to say no to wanted medical treatment deemed "inappropriate" by a patient's doctor, but also to prevent a different doctor from providing the treatment to the patient after a transfer of care.[34] When such policies give anonymous committees the power of life and death, it is imperative to prevent ethics committee deliberations from becoming star chambers.

With so much potential for abuse of vulnerable (and expensive) patients, it is time to think seriously about the proper workings of these committees, their makeup, and the limits that should be placed on their power to impose a health institution's will upon patients and families. For example, what kind of training should ethics committee members receive? (It should definitely be broader and better rounded than "right-to-die" seminars funded by health-care foundations!) Should certifications be required? Should committee deliberations continue to be confidential? Should the proceedings of the committees be formalized, recorded and subject to review? These are important thoughts for future consideration.

There is something that can be done now. Every ethics committee should take the advice of Diane Coleman, an expert on independent living and a disability rights activist: Hospitals, HMOs and other health-care organizations should make every effort to have on their ethics committees substantial representation of people who are disabled and who are knowledgeable about the independent-living movement and other care options for disabled people, which have such power to improve lives. In that way, fear, prejudice and ignorance about life with disability will be far less likely to be the basis of ethics committees' decision making.

Losing Our Ubuntu?

Once, when I was recounting some of the events I have written about in this book to my best friend, Arthur Cribbs, he shook his head and said to me, "Man, we are losing our *ubuntu*." Art, an African American, explained to me that *ubuntu* is a Zulu word he picked up from a friend who has traveled extensively in Africa. The concept of *ubuntu* has no exact English counterpart—the term "soul" is inadequate—but can be roughly translated as "humanity toward others," an essential aspect of the exquisite spark that makes humankind special and unique in the known universe.

When we shrugged as Jack Kevorkian was "facilitating" the deaths of desperate and depressed people whose suffering could have been substantially alleviated with proper medical treatment and humane care, we were losing our *ubuntu*. When the euthanasia policies of the Netherlands are perceived by many as an "enlightened" model for our own health-care system—even though they include infanticide and involuntary killing—we are losing our *ubuntu*. When we stand by and watch desperately needed health-care dollars transferred from health-care delivery into the pockets of profiteers, threatening the well-being of patients, we are losing our *ubuntu*. When "philosophers" such as Peter Singer explicitly equate the moral value of the life of a fish with the moral value of the life of a human infant and receive prestigious appointments to a tenured chair at Princeton University, we are losing our *ubuntu*. When courts send messages through their rulings and decisions that death is preferable to disability and that the lives of dying, chronically ill and disabled people are not as worthy of state protection as are the lives of those among us who are young, healthy and vital, we are losing our *ubuntu*. When the "right to die" has more resonance among much of the public than protecting the right to live, we are, without doubt, losing our *ubuntu*.

And yet...our *ubuntu* is not yet lost. We remain a caring and compassionate people. Indeed, death fundamentalists exploit these very attributes. But it will be these attributes that, in the end, will restore us to a more humane and enlightened course.

A good step toward reclaiming *ubuntu* is the Missoula Demonstration Project, the brainchild of Dr. Ira Byock, in Missoula, Montana. Under the direction of its executive director, the gerontologist Barbara K. Spring, Ph.D., the project is actively restoring community to people approaching the end of their lives. "People who are dying tend to become isolated," Dr. Byock says. "We are changing that. We are committed to restoring a sense of belonging."[35]

The project is involving the whole city in a nonmedical approach to these important issues. Workers set up intergenerational programs such as combining day care for children with care for the elderly. Discussions are held in schools, in churches, among civic groups and in health-care facilities to teach people that dying is a natural part of living and that caring for terminally ill people is a life-enhancing experience.

Dying people also receive the message that they are important members of the community. Their life histories are recorded and the tapes are available in the local library. They are helped to come to terms with their fears through support groups and innovative approaches such as art therapy.

"The intent behind the project," Dr. Byock says, "is to show America what truly 'dying well' can mean and to demonstrate that one's life is not over because a terminal prognosis is given. Dying is a very scary, extraordinary time of life that requires adjustments and changes in expectations. But so do other times of change, such as marriage, having a child, or losing a spouse. What I have seen and know to be true is that people can exert a sense of mastery over this stage of life."[36]

Can dying really be a meaningful time in life, as Dr. Byock asserts? Dr. Maurice Victor certainly believes that such a time of life has tremendous potential. "Once pain and depression are treated," he says, "there is gratification to be obtained simply from living. I have talked with survivors of concentration camps who experienced as extreme suffering as can be imagined. One woman put it very well: "Life matters. Just to have the opportunity to spend a boring evening at home is worth everything. There is so much pleasure to be gotten merely from the simple routines: getting coffee in the morning, reading the morning paper, planning the little errands of the day, so much pleasure to be derived from the most inconsequential type of things, from what some call a boring life. It comes from within."[37]

Dr. Victor sees euthanasia as antithetical to living a meaningful life in its end stage. "I am dreadfully offended by the whole notion," he says. "Euthanasia replaces the importance of life with an impersonal, crass discarding of sick people on the ash heap. It is anathema to true compassion and care."[38]

Let us wish the Missoula Project and its blend of hospice, community education and outreach well, and hope that it serves as a guide in transforming dying from the too often lonely and isolated experience it is now into an event centered in the love and involvement of the entire community, the way it should be.

We don't have to be part of the hospice movement or engaged in the euthanasia debate to make a real difference in the lives of suffering and dying people. We have that opportunity even with virtual strangers. I recall my former law partner, Jack A. Rameson III, of Woodland Hills, California, who many years ago taught me a lesson in compassion and dignity that I have never forgotten. Jack is an estate planner. We went out to a hospital to visit a woman who was dying of brain cancer, so she could sign her will.

As Rameson was explaining the will-signing process to her, she suddenly became ill. Now, there are those who would say that throwing up in front of strangers is undignified. But dignity depends, does it not, on how others react to the afflicted person? In this case, Rameson transformed what could have been a disturbing and perhaps humiliating moment for our client into one overflowing with *ubuntu*. He immediately ran to her side and gently held her head as she was in the act of being sick, so she would not soil her bedclothes. When she was finished, he took a damp cloth, wiped her face and brow, and gave her a cup of water. Then, when she felt better, we went on with our business as if nothing had happened.

That kind of outreaching love is the essence of community. It erases indignity. It welcomes those in need of assistance as vital parts of the community's life, as people of inherent value and worth.

Then there is the kind and loving care shown by my friend Tom Lorentzen as he participated intimately in his mother's death, not by mixing her a poison brew and hastening her end, but by acting as a loving and caring son who valued and welcomed her in each moment of her natural life. And in that caring he found himself comforted and transformed:

In July of 1990, my mother was diagnosed with early-stage kidney failure. I said, "Mom, I hope you will be okay." She responded by saying, "If I need you, I know you will know what to do." This statement was different from anything she had ever said to me before. I sensed change and I shed a tear.

In November 1991, Mom's condition worsened and she was placed in the hospital. I left Washington, D.C., my job, my girlfriend, and my dog behind, and rushed to her side. I sensed that my life had taken a dramatically different path, that I would not be soon in returning.

During the next seven months, I took care of my mother at home, cooking her meals, doing laundry, cleaning house, working at a job I was fortunate to obtain in San Francisco during the day. Leaving home at six in the morning, I would call her during the day to make sure she was all right.

She was in and out of the hospital until June of 1992, when the doctor told me she was dying. Together we informed her as I sat on the bed holding her hand. I watched her eyes change as the message was received. She looked at me with an expression that only Shakespeare could adequately describe. She then turned to the doctor, and with her New York sense of humor, said, "Thanks a lot!"

We revisited the possibility of kidney dialysis with the doctor. She asked two questions: Would it hurt? The doctor said there would be some discomfort and explained why. She then asked, "Will it give me strength?" The doctor explained that it would for a day or so, and then she would have to undergo another treatment.

With that, she gently shook her head and said, "No." I saw tears form in the doctor's eyes.

For ten days I stayed in the hospital room with her, leaving only to shave, shower and change clothes. At night I would sleep on the bed with her, holding her in my arms. During that time I smelled the aroma of her hair and daydreamed about what her life had been like from the time she was born. A strange and comforting sense of peace dominated my essence, as I held her like a child in my arms.

As my mother was traveling through the dying process, the intimacy of death became shared between us. She shared her love with others who visited the room.

As the end grew very near, gangrene began to set in, caused by her kidney failure. Mom required morphine to ease the pain, which she received during the last two to three days. At one point, I said to the doctor, "I can't believe I am saying this, but I hope she dies sooner rather than later." He and I agreed that we would do nothing to prolong her dying and that no treatment would be given to keep her going. We also agreed that she would receive sufficient pain medication to ensure that she felt no discomfort. I told him that I hoped she would die in my arms.

On the tenth day of her hospitalization, I awoke at four A.M. and noticed my mom fixing her hair. I moved to the reclining chair and awoke at six-thirty. Mom was lying quietly in bed. As I stirred, she asked, "Tom, are you still here?" I said, "Yes, Mom. Don't worry. Everything is all right." "Okay," she said—her last words.

A little while later I looked down at her as the morning sun was beginning to illuminate the room. Her breathing was barely observable. I lay on the bed and took her in my arms. As I did, her breathing gently stopped.

Tears immediately covered my face. In addition, two feelings simultaneously dominated my being. The most powerful was a sense of loss. Immediately overriding it, however, was a sense of enrichment. We had done everything we could to save her life. I had done everything I could to take care of her and give her life value, and to make sure that she was cared for and loved during her dying, temporarily giving up on my life to take care of her when she needed me most. My wish had been granted that she die in my arms.

My reward was a deepening of our love and a tightening of our friendship. I knew that I had gained the greatest wealth that can be achieved in life. By participating in the natural dying process with a loved one in the most intimate, loving, and caring manner possible, I had become enriched beyond anything I ever expected in life. What I am now, what I will always be, will stem from this experience. I am a very fortunate and lucky person.[39]

A Time to Choose

As we enter a new millennium, we are at a crossroads that forces us to choose between two mutually exclusive value systems. Will we remain on the trail that leads ultimately to the full realization of the equality-of-human-life ethic, and with it, the tremendous potential for the creation of a true community? Or do we take a hard turn down the slippery slope toward a coarsening of our views of the afflicted, the dying, the chronically ill, the disabled and those in pain or depression to the point where we feel they have a duty to die and get out of the way? To put it more bluntly: Will we choose the road of inclusion and caregiving for all, including the weakest and most vulnerable among us, or that of exclusion and ever-expanding killing opportunities? More simply yet: Will we choose to love each other or abandon each other? The bottom line: Will we keep or lose our *ubuntu*?

Appendix

IN THE COURSE OF THEIR LONG ADVOCACY, proponents of assisted suicide/euthanasia have developed certain standard arguments that they use in making their case. I have alluded, sometimes elliptically, to some of these arguments in the text of *Final Exit*. But I thought the reader might find it useful to see these talking points summarized along with a systematic response to them on my part.

1. Guidelines can prevent abuse.

Proponents of legalization will often acknowledge the possibility that weak and vulnerable persons will be pressured into a premature death, but they assure us that "guidelines will protect against abuse." This is a fantasy. Once killing is deemed an acceptable way to alleviate suffering in one case, it quickly becomes acceptable for one hundred cases.

- The Netherlands began allowing euthanasia in 1973 and has since fallen off an ethical vertical cliff. Not only are nondying patients euthanized, but so are people who have not asked to be killed.
- Dutch doctors now practice infanticide. According to two medical studies, about 8 percent of all infants who die each year are killed by doctors.
- Belgium has fallen off the same cliff in only a few years. The *very first* legal euthanasia did not follow the guidelines, yet nothing was done about it. A recent study found that 8 percent of infant deaths in Flanders are caused by euthanasia.

- Abuses are also occurring in Oregon, including the case of Kate Cheney, who had Alzheimer's disease and still received a lethal prescription—even though a psychiatrist said she was being pressured by her daughter and did not understand what she was asking for.
- In the United States, removing food and fluids from the cognitively disabled has, in a few short years, expanded from those in PVS to people who are conscious.

2. Euthanasia would be restricted to the "hard cases."

Euthanasia is sold as a way to prevent unbearable suffering when nothing else can be done to alleviate pain. But this is just spin.

- Pain can almost always be significantly alleviated with proper medical care.
- In Oregon, most people who have committed assisted suicide were not in untreatable pain.
- In Oregon, most people ask for assisted suicide because they are worried about losing control or the ability to do enjoyable activities. These are important issues, but they can be addressed and overcome by proper hospice care.
- Proper hospice care, including suicide prevention, can overcome the desire for assisted suicide.
- For those few cases in which pain or severe agitation cannot be eased, palliative sedation can alleviate suffering without killing the patient. (In palliative sedation, the patient dies from his or her disease, not the sedation or the intentional withdrawal of food and fluids.)

3. We put suffering animals to sleep, so why not people?

This argument can be seductive. But it misses the point that there is a crucial moral difference between animals and human beings. Society permits animals to be euthanized precisely because it recognizes that animals are not people. Indeed, the primary reasons most animals are euthanized underscore how dangerous it would be to permit the mercy killing of humans.

- We properly treat animals in ways we would never do people. We eat them, for example, experiment on them in medical research, and own them as pets. And sometimes, for humane reasons, we put them down.

- Dogs and cats are most often euthanized not because they are sick, but because they are abandoned.
- Thousands of pets are euthanized each year because they are no longer wanted.
- We put animals down because they are incontinent or because their veterinary treatment would be too expensive.
- We put animals down because we are not equipped to give them the kind of medical care we provide to dying, disabled or chronically ill humans.

4. There is no difference between "choice" in abortion and "choice" in euthanasia.

When abortion was first being legalized, opponents warned that it would lead directly to allowing euthanasia. Abortion rights proponents ridiculed the notion. Yet today's euthanasia advocates often try to identify their cause with the legalization of abortion. There are, however, crucial differences.

- Many people who support abortion rights oppose assisted suicide/euthanasia. These include almost all disability rights activists, medical and nursing professionals, "pro-choice" politicians such as former president Bill Clinton, and public policy activists like Ralph Nader.
- One reason why abortion is legal is that it is not deemed in law as the taking of a human life because a fetus is not deemed a "person." Once born, all human beings are legal persons.
- Infanticide is considered murder in every country (although this law is not enforced in the Netherlands if a doctor kills a dying or disabled baby).
- Restrictions are permitted for late-term abortions precisely because viable fetuses are deemed to be human lives under *Roe v. Wade*.
- Euthanasia should be decided on its own merits or demerits, regardless of one's position on abortion.

5. Polls show that most people support legalization.

It is true that many polls support legalization, at least for people who are terminally ill. But this means little.

- The answers obtained in polls often depend on how the questions are asked.
- Many polls find that the majority of people do not support legalization. For example, an August 2005 Pew Poll found that only 44 percent favor making it legal for doctors to "assist in suicide."
- The best polls are elections. Since 1991, there have been five statewide referendums to legalize euthanasia and/or assisted suicide. All polls found support in the high 60 or low 70 percent range. But when the votes were counted, four of the five referendums failed to pass. Michigan defeated legalization in 1998 by a stunning 71–29 percent.
- If assisted suicide were so popular, legislatures would legalize it. Yet politicians rarely run on the plank of assisted suicide.
- Many state legislatures have repeatedly refused to legalize assisted suicide in the last ten years, while several states, including, Michigan, Rhode Island, Iowa and Louisiana, have explicitly outlawed it.

6. Assisted suicide is needed as a "safety valve" to prevent doctors from keeping sick patients alive for too long.

Many people worry that doctors will "hook them up to machines" against their will, rather than allow them to die in peace. But this is no reason to legalize assisted suicide/euthanasia.

- The economics of medicine have changed. Today, in the era of "futile care theory," being denied the high-tech care you *want* is a bigger problem than being forced to receive care you don't want.
- Advance directives now allow people to instruct their doctors that they don't want high-tech care if they are dying or profoundly disabled.
- Hospice care permits people to refuse all life-sustaining treatment without losing the right to pain and symptom control.

7. Assisted suicide is the same as refusing unwanted life-sustaining treatment.

This is a prime example of how assisted suicide advocates try to confuse and blur vital distinctions.

- The United States Supreme Court ruled unanimously that there is a crucial difference between assisting suicide and removing unwanted treatment.
- When a patient dies by assisted suicide, death is caused by poison or some other form of induced death. When treatment is withdrawn, death is natural.
- When someone is overdosed or lethally injected, death is virtually certain. When treatment is withdrawn (other than food and fluids), the patient may not die for years.
- Studies show that many terminally ill people who at some point want assisted suicide later change their minds. Thus, suicide prevention is the compassionate approach.

8. Assisted suicide is the same as pain control.

Because pain control may require strong drugs, which can cause death, assisted suicide advocates often claim that palliation and euthanasia are ethically the same. But this is all wrong.

- Any legitimate medical treatment, including pain alleviation, can unintentionally lead to death. In assisted suicide, by contrast, death is the *intended effect*.
- We would never say that a patient who died during open-heart surgery was euthanized. Similarly, a patient who dies from the side effects of pain control has not been assisted in suicide or euthanized.
- Pain-control experts state that aggressive pain control is more likely to lengthen life than shorten it.
- We should encourage aggressive pain control when it is needed. Linking it to assisted suicide/euthanasia is likely to dissuade patients and doctors from following that approach. And that would lead to more suffering.

9. The only basis for opposing euthanasia is religious belief.

There are many people who oppose euthanasia for religious reasons. But they are certainly not alone. Indeed, the secular case against euthanasia is more powerful than religious arguments.

- Traditional medical ethics, including the Hippocratic Oath that is more than two thousand years old and predates Christianity, has always opposed mercy killing because it is a betrayal of the purpose of medicine and puts too much power into the doctor's hands.
- Killing is not a medical procedure. Medicine is about curing, maintaining health and alleviating suffering. It is not about ending lives.
- I give you three letters: H, M and O. In our health care system, where strained resources are the order of the day, legalizing assisted suicide could easily transform mercy killing into a form of cost control.
- Some of the most effective opponents of euthanasia are distinctly secular, particularly the disability rights movement, which is almost unanimous in its opposition to assisted suicide. Other secular opponents include medical professional organizations, hospice organizations and advocates for the poor.
- The many reasons for opposing euthanasia are not dependent on religion, but center on the various ways in which euthanasia would lead to the victimization of the dying, the elderly, the disabled and the depressed.

10. Only conservatives oppose assisted suicide.

The point of this misstatement is to attempt to transform assisted suicide advocacy from a relatively fringe phenomenon into a major liberal political cause. This, too, is all wet.

- Opposition to assisted suicide cuts across all political persuasions.
- Disability rights activists—who overwhelmingly are liberal politically—are among the world's most effective opponents of assisted suicide/euthanasia.
- The nation's oldest and largest Hispanic civil rights organization, League of United Latin American Citizens (LULAC), strongly opposes assisted suicide.

- Some of the country's most notable liberal leaders oppose assisted suicide/euthanasia, including consumer advocate Ralph Nader and civil libertarian (and atheist) Nat Hentoff.

RESOURCES

Sources of Information about Euthanasia From an Opposition Standpoint

International Task Force on Euthanasia and Assisted Suicide

PO Box 760
Steubenville, OH 43952
740-282-3810
www.iaetf.org
800-958-5678 for ordering materials such as the PMDD, the video *Euthanasia: False Light* and the book *Power Over Pain: How to Get the Pain Control You Need*, by Eric M. Chevlen, M.D., and Wesley J. Smith.

The Task Force is the primary international source of information and background material on euthanasia, assisted suicide, and related health-care issues. Among its activities, the Task Force:
- Provides information for radio, television, and print journalists
- Maintains an extensive and up-to-date library devoted solely to the issues surrounding euthanasia
- Upon request, prepares analyses of pending legislation
- Analyzes the probable impact of policies considered and/or adopted by medical, legal, and social work organizations
- Provides speakers for local and national radio and television programs, and for major international bioethical conferences
- Files amicus curiae briefs in major "right to die" cases

- Publishes position papers and fact sheets on euthanasia and related issues
- Prepares and provides specialized materials for health-care professionals, attorneys, ethicists, and for students ranging from middle school through graduate school
- Conducts training in effective communication of issues related to euthanasia, assisted suicide, death, and dying
- Provides information and assistance to individuals and groups regarding resources for medically vulnerable individuals and caregivers
- Publishes the bimonthly *Update* and maintains an informative Web site.
- Networks with individuals and organizations on five continents

Individuals and groups who network with the Task Force have a common concern about the threat of euthanasia but hold differing views on other public policy issues.

Physicians for Compassionate Care

Physicians for Compassionate Care is an association of physicians and other health professionals dedicated to preserving the traditional relation of the physician and patient as one in which the physician's primary task is to heal the patient and to minimize pain. The association promotes the health and well-being of patients by encouraging physicians to comfort patients and to assist those who are dying by support systems, minimizing pain, and treating depression. The association affirms the health restoring role of the physician and works to educate the profession and the public to the dangers of euthanasia and physician-assisted suicide and the inherent value of human life.

PCC
PO Box 6042
Portland, OR 97228-6042
Phone: 503-533-8154
Fax: 503-533-0429
www.pccef.org

Not Dead Yet

Not Dead Yet is a national disability rights group in the United States that actively opposes legalization of assisted suicide and euthanasia. Although ten other national disability rights groups also oppose legalization, NDY is the acknowledged leader of this community's opposition. NDY has also been involved in fighting against the starvation deaths of people with cognitive disabilities. In addition to traditional forms of political advocacy work, NDY uses nonviolent confrontation and civil disobedience when the organization considers it necessary.

Not Dead Yet
7521 Madison Street
Forest Park, IL 60130
Phone: 708-209-1500
Fax: 708-209-1735
E-mail: ndyet@aol.com
www.notdeadyet.org

Euthanasia Prevention Coalition (Canada)

The Euthanasia Prevention Coalition was established to prepare a well-informed, broadly based network of groups and individuals who support measures that will create an effective social barrier to euthanasia and assisted suicide.

The EPC provides research, information, and speakers; advocates on behalf of the vulnerable; and works to maintain the current legal prohibitions against euthanasia and assisted suicide.

Euthanasia Prevention Coalition
Box 25033
London ON N6C 6A8
Canada
Phone: 519-439-3348
Toll Free: 1-877-439-3348
Fax: 519-439-7053
E-mail: info@epcc.ca
www.epcc.ca

Compassionate Healthcare Network (Canada)

The Compassionate Healthcare Network (CHN) is a not-for-profit international anti-euthanasia network formed in 1992. CHN consists of health professionals and laypeople concerned about the crisis in medicine and health care. CHN opposes euthanasia by actively defending the inherent value of all human life. CHN involves a network of people who provide speakers and lead workshops; conduct research pertaining to euthanasia, assisted suicide and palliative care; and provide information to professionals, churches, government offices, lay organizations, students and other individuals.

CHN
11563 Bailey Cres
Surrey, BC V3V 2V4
Canada
Phone: 604-582-3844
Fax: 604-582-3844
E-mail: chn@intergate.ca
www.chninternational.com

ALERT (Great Britain)

ALERT was founded in 1991 to provide well-documented information on euthanasia, assisted suicide, and related issues, and to defend the lives and rights of the medically vulnerable.

ALERT
27 Walpole Street
London, SW3 4QS
Great Britain
Phone: 020-7730-2800
Fax: 020-7730-0710
E-mail: alert@donoharm.org.uk
www.donoharm.org.uk/alert

National Conference of Catholic Bishops
Attn: Richard Doerflinger,
Deputy Director of the Secretariat for Pro-Life Activities
3211 4th Street, NE
Washington, DC 20017
202-541-3000
www.nccbuscc.org/prolife/index.htm

New York State Task Force on Life and the Law
5 Penn Plaza
New York, NY 10001-1803
212-613-4303
www.health.state.ny.us

Hospice, Pain Control and Palliation

Agency for Health Care Policy and Research (AHCPR)
PO Box 8547
Silver Springs, MD 20907-8547
800-358-9295

This agency of the Department of Health and Human Services publishes many patient guides on topics of pain control and palliation that are available free of charge.

The National Hospice and Palliative Care Organization
1700 Diagonal Road, Suite 300
Alexandria, VA 22314
Phone: 800-658-8898
E-mail: info@nhpco.org
www.nhpco.org

Helpline phone number, helps the general public locate a hospice anywhere in the country at no charge. Can also e-mail for general questions about hospice or location of a hospice.

American Academy of Hospice and Palliative Medicine
4700 W. Lake Avenue
Glenview, IL 60025-1485
Phone: 847-375-4712
Fax: 847-375-6312
E-mail: aahpm@aahpm.org
www.aahpm.org

Originally organized as the Academy of Hospice Physicians in 1988, the American Academy of Hospice and Palliative Medicine (AAHPM) is the only organization in the United States for physicians dedicated to the advancement of hospice/palliative medicine, its practice, research and education.

American Chronic Pain Association
PO Box 850
Rocklin, CA 95677
916-632-0922
www.theacpa.org

The ACPA offers support and information for people with chronic pain.

American Pain Foundation
201 N. Charles Street, Suite 710
Baltimore, MD 21201
www.painfoundation.com

A nonprofit organization dedicated to providing information, advocacy, and education about the treatment of pain.

Disability Issues

Amyotrophic Lateral Sclerosis (ALS) Association
21021 Ventura Blvd., Suite 321
Woodland Hills, CA 91364
800-782-4747
www.alsa.org

The ALS Association is the only national nonprofit voluntary health organization dedicated solely to the fight against amyotrophic lateral sclerosis. Its mission is to find a cure for ALS and improve living with ALS.

Independent Living Resource Utilization Training Center
2323 S. Shepherd Street, Suite 1000
Houston, TX 77019
713-520-0232
www.ilru.org

The ILRU offers information about the independent-living movement, and provides the addresses and phone numbers of an independent-living center near you or one you love.

National Multiple Sclerosis Association
706 Haddonfield Road
Cherry Hill, NJ 08002
800-532-7667
www.nmsa.com

Offers information for patients and families about MS.

National Spinal Cord Injury Association
6701 Democracy Blvd., Suite 300
Bethesda, MD 20817
800-962-9629
www.spinalcord.org

The NSCIA offers information about spinal cord injury and referral services and access to support groups.

United Cerebral Palsy Foundation
1660 L Street NW, Suite 700
Washington DC 20036
800-872-5827
www.ucp.org

UCP offers a referral service and information about interventions, patient and family support, assistance technology, and employment.

Books

These books are excellent sources for those who wish to learn more about the topics discussed in this book.

Ira Byock, M.D., *Dying Well: The Prospect for Growth at the End of Life* (New York, Riverdale Books, 1997).
This moving and important book, written by the past president of the American Academy of Hospice and Palliative Medicine, illustrates the beneficence of hospice and the quality of life available for dying people when they are properly cared for and valued. If all dying persons were as well cared for as were the patients whose stories are recounted in this book, the assisted suicide movement would wither on the vine.

Kathleen Foley and Herbert Hendin, eds., *The Case Against Assisted Suicide: For the Right to End-of-Life Care* (Baltimore: Johns Hopkins University Press, 2002).
This book of essays, written by some of the world's most eminent secular opponents of assisted suicide and experts in end-of-life and palliative care, makes a compelling case against the euthanasia movement and in favor of hospice and palliative care. An excellent resource for persons involved in advocacy on the issues addressed.

Herbert Hendin, M.D., *Seduced by Death: Doctors, Patients and the Dutch Cure* (New York: W.W. Norton, 1997).
The noted psychiatrist may be the world's foremost expert on Dutch euthanasia. Hendin provides a detailed and disturbing account about what has gone wrong with Dutch medical ethics and the horrors that have resulted from that nation's acceptance of euthanasia.

Eric Chevlen, M.D., and Wesley J. Smith, *Power Over Pain: How to Get the Pain Control You Need* (Steubenville, Ohio: International Task Force on Euthanasia and Assisted Suicide, 2002).
Written by a noted pain-control specialist physician and the author of *Forced Exit, Power Over Pain* is designed as a readable and understandable tool to help patients and their families obtain optimal pain control.

Wesley J. Smith, *Culture of Death: The Assault on Medical Ethics in America* (San Francisco: Encounter Books, 2001).
The author of *Forced Exit* looks deeply into the bioethics movement

and discovers that assisted suicide is just the tip of the iceberg. *Culture of Death* was named Best Health Book of the Year at the 2001 Independent Publisher's Book Awards.

Jack Kevorkian, M.D., *Prescription Medicide: The Goodness of a Planned Death* (Buffalo, N.Y.: Prometheus Books, 1991).
Jack Kevorkian is not and never was a "retired physician who helped terminally ill people commit suicide," as he is often described in the media. Learn the truth about his chilling and macabre agenda in his own words.

Robert Jay Lifton, *The Nazi Doctors: Medical Killing and the Psychology of Genocide* (New York: Basic Books, 1996).
An excellent source for learning about the participation of German doctors in the Holocaust and how the values that led to the killing of hundreds of thousands of disabled persons between 1939 and 1945 are alive and well in the contemporary euthanasia movement.

Rita Marker, *Deadly Compassion: The Death of Ann Humphry and the Truth about Euthanasia* (New York: William Morrow, 1993).
This book, by the executive director of the International Task Force on Euthanasia and Assisted Suicide, had a tremendous influence on my decision to advocate against euthanasia and assisted suicide. Marker recounts the tragic story of the Hemlock Society's cofounder Ann Wicket; how she was abandoned by her husband, Derek Humphry, when she was diagnosed with breast cancer; and the reasons Wicket turned against the death culture before committing suicide.

Joseph P. Shapiro, *No Pity: People with Disabilities Forging a New Civil Rights Movement* (New York: Times Books, 1993).
An excellent account of the prejudice faced by people with disabilities and the empowering potential of the independent-living movement.

Peter Singer, *Rethinking Life and Death: The Collapse of Our Traditional Ethics* (New York: St. Martin's Press, 1994).
Singer, an icon of the bioethics movement, is more candid than most euthanasia advocates about where the death culture would take us. He promotes the destruction of the "sanctity of life" ethic in favor of

a "quality of life" approach in which euthanasia, assisted suicide, and infanticide would play vital parts.

Derek Humphry and Mary Clement, *Freedom to Die: People, Politics, and the Right-to-Die Movement* **(New York: St. Martin's Press, 1998).**
Humphry and Clement give the euthanasia movement's perspective about the so-called right to die. The book isn't noteworthy except for its admission that in the end, euthanasia and assisted suicide will be about money.

Advance Medical Directives

The American Medical Association, the American Bar Association, and the American Association of Retired Persons worked together to create a very detailed power of attorney that covers just about all circumstances, including whether you want food and fluids under specified conditions. To obtain the AMA/ABA/AARP Durable Power of Attorney for Health Care, contact:

AARP
601 E Street, NW
Washington, DC 20049
800-424-3410
www.aarp.org

The International Task Force on Euthanasia and Assisted Suicide publishes a power of attorney for health care that is often state-specific, called the Protective Medical Decision Document (PMDD). The PMDD empowers a health care proxy to make treatment and nontreatment decisions while prohibiting the proxy from agreeing to medical actions that are directly intended to cause death. The proxy you name in your PMDD has the authority to make the same medical decisions you could make if you were able to do so. Your proxy may also approve a DNR ("do not resuscitate") order or a "no aggressive treatment" order. He or she may determine that surgery, ventilator support, or other interventions should be provided, withheld, or withdrawn. However, the PMDD specifically denies your proxy the authority to approve of any *direct and intentional* ending of your life.

For more information on the PMDD, contact the International Task Force at the address and phone number provided earlier in this resource section.

Like a will or a trust, an advance directive is a legal document and should be treated as such. The laws of each state regarding their preparation and contents differ. A few states require specific language not used in the forms mentioned here. It is a good idea to have your attorney review any advance directive you sign, or prepare yours on the basis of your instructions and desires.

To find an attorney who knows the ins and outs of the laws concerning advance directives, contact your local bar association and ask for a lawyer who specializes in "elder law." Or contact:

National Academy of Elder Law Attorneys (NAELA)
1604 N. Country Club Road
Tucson, AZ 85716
520-881-4005
www.naela.com

ACKNOWLEDGMENTS

THE CREATION OF THIS BOOK WOULD LITERALLY have been impossible without the active assistance of so many people who freely shared their feelings, knowledge, attitudes and opinions with me, including: Peter Admiraal, M.D.; Dr. William S. Andereck; Patricia Anderson; Dan Avila; Robin Bernhoft, M.D.; James Bopp; William Burke, M.D.; Ira R. Byock, M.D.; Dana Cody; Diane Coleman; Matthew E. Conolly, M.D.; Yeates Cornwell, M.D.; Paul Corrao, M.D.; E. J. Dionne; Richard Doerflinger; Ljubisa J. Dragovic, M.D.; Beth Roney Drennan; Vincent Fortanasce, M.D.; Michael J. Franzblau, M.D.; Cheryl Eckstein, M.D.; Carol Gill; K F. Gunning, M.D.; Jacqulyn Hall; Herbert Hendin, M.D.; Nat Hentoff; Professor Dianne Irving; Larry Johnson; Melanie Zdan and Cara Elrod; Professor Yale Kamisar; Evan J. Kemp Jr.; W. C. M. Klijn; Dr. Gerald (Chip) Klooster and Mary Klooster; Charles Krauthammer; Madelaine Lawrence; Gary Lee, M.D.; Paul Longmore; Tom Lorentzen; Tom Marzen; Ginny McKibben; Steven H. Miles, M.D.; Donald Murphy, M.D.; Fr. Richard Neuhaus; Mark O'Brien; Timothy Quill, M.D.; Harvey Rosenfield; Matthew Rothschild; Daniel P. Sulmasy, M.D.; Dame Cicely Saunders, M.D.; Randolph Schiffer, M.D.; Bob, Mary and Bobby Schindler; Janie Hickock Siess; Lonny Shavelson, M.D.; Elizabeth Skoglund; Beverly Sloane; William Stothers; Eugene Sutorius; W. Russell Van Camp; Teri Van Camp; Terry Stimpson; William F. Stone; I. van der Sluis, M.D.; Dr. Maurice Victor; Nancy Valco; Richard Vigilante; Rebekah Vinson; Kathy Weaver; Jos V. M. Wellie; James Wirth; Kathy Wolfe; and Jessica Yu.

A hearty appreciation to my wonderful friends and colleagues who do such good and important work combating assisted suicide with the International Task Force on Euthanasia and Assisted Suicide: Rita Marker, Mike Marker, Kathi Hamlon, John Hamlon, Robert Hiltner and Nancy Minto. A hearty *muchas gracias* to all my pals at the Discovery Institute, with deep appreciation for the faith shown in my work by Bruce Chapman, Jay Richards, Steve Meyer, Mark Ryland and the rest of the gang. Ditto to the Center for Bioethics and Culture, especially to Jennifer Lahl (she who walks through walls) and Nigel Cameron.

I want to thank everyone at Times Books, the publisher of the first edition of this book, especially my editors Peter Smith and Betsy Rapoport. Also, to Mitch Muncy and Thomas Spence, who published the first revised edition of this book for Spence Publishing. My deep appreciation and respect to everyone who performs with such excellence at this edition's publisher, Encounter Books, particularly my stellar editor, Peter Collier, and Judy Hardin and Amy Packard.

Finally, my deep appreciation to and love for all of my friends and family who have put up with my many years of activism with such patience, good cheer, encouragement and affection, especially: Mark Pickup, Arthur Cribbs, Pastors Daniel Severson and Jim Brun, David Prentice, Pal Steve and Allison Hayward, Colin and Julia Smith, Peter and Lexie Demeralie. My special thanks to Bradford William Short for his assistance and support of my work. And my love to the Saunders family, Georgia, Connecticut and Rhode Island Branches; Jerry, Barbara, Jim, Vickie, Jennifer, Jeremiah, Sara, Stephen, Leslie, Rebecca, Eric and Joshua; to my dear mother, Leona; and most of all, to Debra J., my wife and total sweetheart.

NOTES

Introduction

1 "A Peaceful Passing," *Hemlock Quarterly*, no. 30 (January 1988).
2 Ibid., p. 7.
3 Ibid., p. 6.
4 Ibid., pp. 4–5.
5 Derek Humphry, "Self-Deliverance with Certainty," *Hemlock Quarterly*, no. 30 (January 1988).
6 Ibid., p. 4.
7 "Suicide Rate among the Elderly."
8 Wesley J. Smith, "The Whispers of Strangers," *Newsweek*, June 28, 1993.
9 Ibid.
10 Personal correspondence, June 24, 1993.
11 Personal correspondence, June 30, 1993.
12 Personal correspondence, June 29, 1993.
13 Personal correspondence, June 24, 1993.
14 Personal correspondence, August 23, 1993.
15 Personal correspondence, June 29, 1993.
16 Personal correspondence, June 23, 1993.
17 Personal correspondence, July 7, 1993.
18 Personal correspondence, July 7, 1993.
19 Personal correspondence, June 24, 1993.
20 Smith, "Whispers of Strangers."
21 Ann Landers, "One Eighty-Five-Year-Old's Old-Age Solution," *St. Louis Post Dispatch*, October 3, 1993.

Chapter 1: Death Fundamentalism

1 Stephanie Gutmann, "Death and the Maiden," *New Republic*, January 24, 1996, p. 24.
2 "Kevorkian Patient Was on Halcyon," *Detroit News*, November 3, 1991.

273

[3] Wes Allison, "Study: Kevorkian Patients Weren't Dying," *St. Petersberg Times*, December 8, 2000.

[4] "Attitudes toward Euthanasia Sharply Divided, Survey Finds," Reuters, June 29, 1996.

[5] Andrew Coyne, "The Slippery Slope That Leads to Death," *Globe and Mail* (Toronto), November 21, 1994.

[6] As of this writing there are four exceptions to this general rule: Oregon, which legalized assisted suicide in 1994; the Netherlands and Belgium, which have legalized euthanasia by doctors; and Switzerland, which permits nonphysicians to assist suicides, so long as the motive for doing so isn't "selfish."

[7] Derek Humphry, Letters to the Editor, *New York Times Magazine*, August 11, 1996.

[8] James L. Werth, "Using Rational Suicide as an Intervention to Prevent Irrational Suicide," *Crisis*, vol. 19, no. 4 (1998).

[9] Elliot D. Cohen, Ph.D., "Permitted Suicide: Model Rules for Mental Health Counseling," *Journal of Mental Health Counseling*, vol. 23, no. 4 (October 2001), pp. 279–94.

[10] Arthur Caplan, "System Messed Up, Hands Down," *Oakland Tribune*, May 31, 1996.

[11] For example, according to the Open Society's Web site, in recent years it gave hundreds of thousands of dollars to the Compassion in Dying Federation of America and the Death with Dignity National Center, among other grants.

[12] Jack Lessenberry, "Physician Assisted Suicide Is a Constitutional Right," in *Euthanasia: Opposing Viewpoints*, ed. Carol Wekesser (San Diego: Greenhaven Press, 1995), p. 91.

[13] Matthew Rothschild, interview with author, June 6, 1996.

[14] Dr. I. van der Sluis, interview with author, October 14, 1995.

[15] Paul Longmore, interview with author, July 13, 1996.

[16] Michael Vitez, "Right-to-Die Activists Study New Methods," *Philadelphia Inquirer*, November 12, 1999.

[17] Advertisement published by the Right to Die Network of Canada.

[18] "Euthanasia Sets Sail," interview with Philip Nitschke, *National Review Online*, June 5, 2001.

[19] "They Go to War, They Can Vote, So Why Can't Teenagers Read about Suicide Pill? Asks Nitschke," *Sydney Morning Herald*, August 11, 2001.

[20] Mark Hosenball, "The Real Jack Kevorkian," *Newsweek*, December 6, 1993.

[21] Jack Lessenberry, "Death Becomes Him," *Vanity Fair*, July 1994, p. 106.

[22] Hosenball, "The Real Jack Kevorkian."

[23] Jack Kevorkian, M.D., *Prescription Medicide: The Goodness of a Planned Death* (Buffalo, N.Y.: Prometheus Books, 1991), p. 211.

[24] Ibid., p. 243.

[25] Ibid., p. 214.

[26] *Report of the University of Rochester Medical Center Task Force on Physician-Assisted Suicide* (Rochester, N.Y.: University of Rochester, 1993), p. 5.

[27] Derek Humphry and Mary Clement, *Freedom to Die: People, Politics and the Right to Die Movement* (New York: St. Martin's Press, 1998), p. 333.

[28] Robert J. Lifton, *The Nazi Doctors: Medical Killing and the Psychology of Genocide* (New York: Basic Books, 1986), p. 49.

[29] Steve Drake, "Dangerous Times," *The Ragged Edge,* January 11, 2005.

[30] Andrew Solomon, "A Death of One's Own," *New Yorker,* May 22, 1995.

[31] Dr. Eric Chevlen, interview with author, September 6, 1996.

[32] Lonny Shavelson, *A Chosen Death: The Dying Confront Assisted Suicide* (New York: Simon & Schuster, 1995).

[33] Ibid., p. 75.

[34] Ibid., p. 92.

[35] Ibid., p. 93.

[36] Ibid., p. 94.

[37] Ibid., pp. 93–94.

[38] Lonny Shavelson, personal communication, at the studio of KQED-FM, San Francisco, March 14, 1996.

[39] Lonny Shavelson, interview with author, June 19, 1996.

[40] Shavelson, *A Chosen Death,* p. 94

[41] Shavelson interview.

[42] Peter Singer, *Rethinking Life and Death: The Collapse of Our Traditional Ethics* (New York: St. Martin's Press, 1995).

[43] Wesley J. Smith, *Culture of Death: The Assault on Medical Ethics in America* (San Francisco: Encounter Books, 2000).

[44] Singer, *Rethinking Life and Death,* pp. 213–14.

[45] Daniel J. Kevles, "We All Must Die: Who Can Tell Us When?" *New York Times,* May 7, 1995.

[46] Scott Judd, review of *Rethinking Life and Death* by Peter Singer, in *Hemock Timelines,* May-June 1995, p. 10.

[47] Ralph Mero, "Executive Director's Report," *Compassion in Dying Newsletter,* no. 4 (1995), p. 2.

[48] Lisa Belkin, "There's No Such Thing As a Simple Suicide," *New York Times Magazine,* November 14, 1993.

[49] Ann Landers, "When Taking Your Own Life Makes Sense," *San Francisco Examiner,* February 6, 1994.

[50] Belkin, "No Simple Suicide," p. 53.

[51] Harvey Max Chochinov et al., "Will to Live in the Terminally Ill," *Lancet,* vol. 354 (September 4, 1999), pp. 816–19.

[52] Herbert Hendin, "Selling Death and Dignity," *Hastings Center Report,* May-June 1995, p. 22.

[53] Ibid.

[54] Belkin, "No Simple Suicide," p. 75.

[55] Ibid., pp. 63, 74.

[56] Ibid., p. 50.

[57] Hendin, "Selling Death and Dignity," p. 22.

[58] On June 10, 1996, I telephoned the Washington State office of Compassion in Dying seeking comment from Ralph Mero. I was informed by Barbara Coombs Lee, now the executive director of the Compassion in Dying Federation, that Mero was no longer with the organization. She refused to tell me where I could reach Mero but promised to pass on the message to him along with my phone number. I never heard from Mero thereafter.

[59] "Crick Forced to Die: Campaigner," *The Australian*, May 24, 2002.

[60] Darren Gray, "Doctor Poses Doubts on Crick Suicide," *The Age*, May 27, 2002.

[61] Australian Associated Press, "Nitschke: Right-to-Die Civil Disobedience Has Begun," as published in *The Age*, May 23, 2002.

[62] "Diary Records Cancer Doubt," *Herald Sun* (Melbourne), May 27, 2002.

[63] "Australia Euthanasia Doctor Rejects Cancer Doubts," Reuters, May 25, 2002; Chris Griffith, Paula Doneman and Hedley Thomas, "Crick Told She Wasn't Dying," *Herald Sun* (Melbourne), May 29, 2002.

[64] "Crick Forced to Die: Campaigner."

Chapter 2: Creating a Caste of Disposable People

[1] Sharon S. Orr, interview with author, April 2, 1996.

[2] Richard John Neuhaus, "The Return of Eugenics," *Commentary*, April 1988, p. 19.

[3] For a more detailed description of the threat posed to the equality-of-life ethic by the bioethics movement, see: Wesley J. Smith, *Culture of Death: The Assault on Medical Ethics in America* (San Francisco Encounter Books, 2001).

[4] At this point, it is important to make a crucial distinction between cognitively disabled patients receiving tube-supplied food and fluids, and actively dying people. The cases I write about in this chapter concern the former, people who are profoundly cognitively disabled and whose tube-supplied food and fluids are removed for subjective, nonmedical "quality of life" considerations. There are other patients, however, who as part of the dying process quit eating as their organs shut down. This is a natural process. It would be medically inappropriate—not to mention pointless and cruel—to force nutrition and hydration into these actively dying patients.

[5] American Medical Association Council on Ethical and Judicial Affairs, "Opinion 2.15," 1986.

[6] See, for example, Geoffrey E. Pence, *Classic Cases in Medical Ethics*, 2nd ed. (New York: McGraw Hill, 1995), p. 17.

[7] *Cruzan v. Harmon and Lampkins*, Case No. CV384-9, Circuit Court of Jasper County, Missouri, transcript for March 9, 1988.

[8] *Nancy Beth Cruzan v. Robert Harmo et al.*, 760 SW 2d 408, November 1988.

[9] *Cruzan v. Director, Missouri Department of Health*, 110 Supreme Court 2841, 1990.

[10] Scott Canon, "New Right to Die Case Goes to Court," *Kansas City Star,* January 6, 1991.

[11] Ibid.

[12] Sharon Orr interview.

[13] Theresa Tighe, "State Releases Videotape of Busalacchi, Patient Appears to Be Responsive," *St. Louis Post Dispatch,* February 5, 1991.

[14] American Medical Association Council on Ethics and Judicial Affairs, "Opinion 2:20," 1994.

[15] Dr. William Burke, interview with author, 1996.

[16] *In re Conservatorship of Robert Wendland* (Case No. 65669, Superior Court of California, County of San Joaquin), trial testimony of Dr. Ronald Cranford.

[17] Kate Adamson, *Kate's Journey: Triumph over Adversity* (Redondo Beach, Calif.: Nosmada Press, 2004), p. xxiii.

[18] E-mail interview with Kate Adamson, April 9, 2005.

[19] Ibid.

[20] Fox News Network, *The O'Reilly Factor,* November 9, 2003.

[21] Wesley J. Smith, "A Painless Death?" *Daily Standard,* November 12, 2003.

[22] *Wendland* (Superior Court), Cranford trial testimony.

[23] *Wendland* (Superior Court), transcript of Cranford Deposition, May 7, 1996.

[24] *Wendland* (Superior Court), Cranford trial testimony.

[25] Dr. Vincent Fortanasce, interview with author, January 9, 1995.

[26] Fortanasce interview.

[27] *In re Correan Salter,* Case No. CV-94-160, Circuit Court, Baldwin County, Alabama.

[28] Medical Records of Michael Martin, New Medico Neurological Center of Michigan, Speech-Language Pathology Daily Treatment Notes, December 7, 1992.

[29] Ibid.

[30] Medical Records of Michael Martin, New Medico Neurological Center of Michigan, Augmentation Evaluation Summary, April 19, 1992.

[31] *In re Michael Martin,* Michigan Court of Appeals, Docket No. 161431, Judge Grieg's Observations of Michael Martin, attached to the appeal brief, court transcript, pp. 12–16.

[32] John H. Hess, J.D., "Looking for Traction on the Slippery Slope," *Issues of Law and Medicine,* vol. 11, no. 2, pp. 105–22. Hess and his brother were the lawyers for Michael Martin's mother and sister.

[33] Butterworth Hospital Ethics Committee, correspondence to Mary Martin, January 15, 1992.

[34] Hess, "Looking for Traction," pp. 107–8.

[35] *In re Michael Martin,* 504 NW 2d, 917 (Michigan Appellate, April 1993).

[36] "Mary, Mary, Quite Contrary, How Was I to Know? Michael Martin, Absolute Prescience, and the Right to Die in Michigan," *University of Detroit Mercy Law Review,* vol. 27 (1996), pp. 828, 832.

[37] Medical records of Robert Wendland, a nurse's note to the chart dated July 25, 1995.

[38] *In re Conservatorship of Robert Wendland* (Case No. 65669, Superior Court of California, County of San Joaquin), testimony of Rose Wendland, September 5, 1995.

[39] Jon Dann, Producer, "A Matter of Life and Death," KRON-TV (San Francisco) News, aired November 6, 1995.

[40] *In re Wendland* (Superior Court), testimony of various witnesses.

[41] *Wendland* (Superior Court), Declaration of Florence Wendland, July 12, 2001.

[42] Margaret Goodman, San Joaquin County Ombudsman assigned to Robert Wendland, interview with author, September 5, 1995.

[43] *Wendland* (Superior Court), testimony of Margaret Goodman, September 5, 1995.

[44] Janie Hickock Siess, interview with author, June 23, 1995.

[45] *Wendland* (Superior Court), testimony of Dr. Ronald Kass, September 5, 1995.

[46] Much was made of this aspect of the case by the California Supreme Court, where the case was ultimately decided. See *Conservatorship of Wendland*, 26 Cal. 4th 519 (2001).

[47] *In re Conservatorship of Wendland*, 78 Cal. App. 4th 517.

[48] *Wendland* (Superior Court) trial testimony of Dr. Ronald Cranford.

[49] *Wendland* (Superior Court) trial testimony of Dr. Ernest Bryant.

[50] *In re the Conservatorship of Robert Wendland*, Court of Appeals, Third Appellate District, Case No. Civil C-029439, "Appellant Robert Wendland's Opening Brief," p. 30.

[51] *Conservatorship of Robert Wendland*, "Respondent's Opening Brief on the Merits," in the Supreme Court of California, Case No. S 087265, p. 29.

[52] In the Circuit Court of Pinellas County, Florida, Probate Division, *In re Guardianship of Theresa Schiavo, an Incapacitated Person*, Case No. 90-2908BGD-003, Report of Guardian *ad litem* (hereafter, "Trial Court Case"). The Report of Alan Wolfson stated that the rehabilitation continued into 1994, but that may have been mistaken. Pat Anderson, the primary attorney for the Schindlers, who had access to the medical records—which I did not—told me that there are no records indicating the provision of any rehabilitation after 1992.

[53] Trial Court Case, Report of Guardian *ad litem* Richard L. Pearse, December 29, 1998.

[54] Ibid., Order of Judge George W. Greer, February 11, 2000.

[55] Ibid., Report of Jay Wolfson, Guardian *ad litem* for Theresea Marie Schiavo, to Governor Jeb Bush, December 1, 2003.

[56] Trial Court Case, Order of Court, February 11, 2000, "The court is mystified as to how these present tense verbs would have been used some six years after the death of Karen Ann Quinlan."

[57] Trial Court Case, Order of Court, February 11, 2000.

[58] Trial Court Case, Order of Court, February 25, 2005, in which Judge George W. Greer ordered the guardian Michael Schiavo to "cause the removal of nutrition and hydration from the ward, Theresa Schiavo," with no mention of the feeding tube.

[59] This has been repeatedly reported by me and other observers, and to my knowledge has never been denied by Michael Schiavo. For example, see: Wesley J. Smith, "The Interview That Wasn't," *Daily Standard*, October 28, 2003. Moreover, I confirmed these facts with attorney Patricia Anderson, who had read the record of the medical malpractice trial.

[60] Ibid.

[61] Trial Court Case, Report of Guardian *ad litem*.

[62] Ibid.

[63] Ibid.

[64] Arian Campo-Flores, "Who Has the Right to Die?" *Newsweek*, November 3, 2003.

[65] "Scorning the Courts in Florida," editorial, *New York Times*, October 23, 2003.

[66] Trial Court Case, Report of Guardian *ad litem*.

[67] I interviewed Anderson for: Wesley J. Smith, "The Rule of Terri's Case Strikes Again," *Daily Standard*, January 30, 2004.

[68] Florida Statutes, Chapter 2003-418.

[69] There is a widespread impression that Governor Jeb Bush appointed Wolfson as Terri's guardian. He did not. Under Terri's Law, the guardian was to be court-appointed.

[70] Florida H.B. 35-E.

[71] *Bush v. Schiavo*, Supreme Court of Florida, Case No. SC04-925

[72] Sworn Affidavit of Carla Sauer Iyer, R.N.

[73] For example, Affidavit of William Pope Cheshire Jr., M.D. (neurologist), dated March 23, 2005, testifying that there is "reasonable doubt" as to PVS diagnosis.

[74] Trial Court Case, denial of petition for immediate therapy and order to remove feeding tube, September 17, 2003.

[75] United States Senate Compromise Bill S-686.

[76] *Theresa Marie Schiavo v. Michael Schiavo*, U.S. District Court, Middle District of Florida, Tampa Division, Case No. 8:05 CV-530-T-27-TBM, Order Denying Plaintiff's First Amended Request for Temporary Restraining Order, March 25, 2005.

[77] Florida Statutes: Section 744.3675.

[78] Florida Statutes: Section 744.3685.

[79] Florida Statutes: Section 744.369 (4).

[80] Smith, "The Rule of Terri's Case."

[81] Daniel Callahan, "On Feeding the Dying," *Hastings Center Report*, October 1983, p. 22. During the debate within bioethics about the propriety of

withholding tube-supplied food and water during the early 1980s, preceding Cruzan, Callahan used the term "biologically tenacious" to describe profoundly disabled patients who do not die, stating, "Given the increasingly large pool of superannuated, chronically ill, physically marginalized elderly it [a denial of nutrition] could well become the non treatment of choice."

Chapter 3: Everything Old Is New Again

[1] This thought is generally attributed to Mahatma Gandhi. The late Senator Hubert Humphrey (D-MI) restated this noble idea in 1976: "The moral test of a government is how it treats those who are at the dawn of life, the children; those who are in the twilight of life, the aged; and those who are in the shadow of life, the sick, the needy, and the handicapped."

[2] "A New Ethic for Medicine and Society," editorial, *California Medicine,* vol. 113, no. 3 (September 1970), pp. 67–68.

[3] Peter Singer, *Rethinking Life and Death: The Collapse of Our Traditional Ethics* (New York: St. Martin's Press, 1995). For a detailed description of these attitudes in modern bioethics, see Wesley J. Smith, *Culture of Death: The Assault on Medical Ethics in America* (San Francisco: Encounter Books, 2001).

[4] Robert Jay Lifton, *The Nazi Doctors: Medical Killing and the Psychology of Genocide* (New York: Basic Books, 1986), p. 14.

[5] Michael Burleigh, *Death and Deliverance: Euthanasia in Germany, 1940–1945* (New York: Basic Books, 1986), p. 4.

[6] Lifton, *Nazi Doctors,* p. 48.

[7] Ibid., p. 46.

[8] Quoted in Burleigh, *Death and Deliverance,* p. 13.

[9] Ibid., pp. 13–14.

[10] Ibid., p. 14.

[11] Ibid., p. 15.

[12] Karl Binding and Alfred Hoche, M.D., *Permitting the Destruction of Life Not Worthy of Life: Its Extent and Form* (Leipzig: Felix Meiner Verlag, 1920), reprinted in *Issues in Law and Medicine,* vol. 8, no. 2 (1992), pp. 231–65.

[13] Lifton, *Nazi Doctors,* p. 46.

[14] Binding and Hoche, *Permitting the Destruction,* p. 247.

[15] Ibid., pp. 260–61.

[16] Ibid., p. 249.

[17] Ibid., p. 252.

[18] Burleigh, *Death and Deliverance,* p. 15.

[19] For a thoroughly detailed account of the American eugenics movement, see Edwin Black, *War Against the Weak: Eugenics and America's Campaign to Create a Master Race* (New York: Four Walls, Eight Windows, 2003). See also, Daniel J. Kevles, *In the Name of Eugenics* (Cambridge, Mass.: Harvard University Press, 1935).

[20] Adolf Hitler, *Mein Kampf,* quoted in Lifton, *Nazi Doctors,* p. 257.

[21] Lifton, *Nazi Doctors,* p. 27.

[22] Burleigh, *Death and Deliverance,* pp. 22–23.

[23] *New York Times,* October 8, 1933, as cited in Hugh Gregory Gallagher, *By Trust Betrayed: Patients, Physicians, and the License to Kill in the Third Reich* (Arlington, Va.: Vandamere Press, 1995), p. xiv.

[24] Dick Sobsey, Anne Donnellan and Gregor Wolbring, "Reflection on the Holocaust: Where Did It Begin and Has It Really Ended?" *Developmental Disabilities Journal,* vol. 22, no. 2 (1994).

[25] Richard Sobsey, interview with author, January 27, 1999.

[26] Ibid.

[27] As described in Lifton, *Nazi Doctors,* p. 49.

[28] As quoted in Sobsey et al., "Reflection on the Holocaust."

[29] Lifton, *Nazi Doctors,* p. 50.

[30] Burleigh, *Death and Deliverance,* pp. 95–96; Lifton, *Nazi Doctors,* pp. 50–51; Gallagher, *By Trust Betrayed,* pp. 95–96.

[31] Quoted in Burleigh, *Death and Deliverance,* p. 100.

[32] Ibid., p. 125.

[33] Ibid.

[34] Lifton, *Nazi Doctors,* p. 77.

[35] Hugh Gregory Gallagher, interview with author, May 21, 1996. When this interview took place, Gallagher was an opponent of assisted suicide. He later changed his position.

[36] Ibid.

[37] Quoted in Burleigh, *Death and Deliverance,* p. 178.

[38] Ibid.

[39] Michael Franzblau, M.D., "Investigate Nazi Ties of German Doctors," *San Francisco Chronicle,* December 29, 1993.

[40] *Buck v. Bell,* 274 U.S. 200.

[41] Ibid.

[42] "Three Generations of Imbeciles," editorial, *Detroit News,* December 16, 1992.

[43] Edwin Black, *War Against the Weak,* p. 247.

[44] Ian Dowbiggin, *A Merciful End: The Euthanasia Movement in Modern America* (Oxford: Oxford University Press, 2003), p. 44.

[45] Rita L. Marker et al., "Euthanasia: A Historical Overview," *Maryland Journal of Contemporary Issues,* Summer 1991, p. 276.

[46] Ibid.

[47] Cited in Rita Marker, *Deadly Compassion* (New York: William Morrow, 1993), p. 39.

[48] Dowbiggin, *A Merciful End,* p. 32.

[49] Arthur Caplan, "The Relevance of the Holocaust in Bioethics Today," in, *Medicine, Ethics, and the Third Reich: Historical and Contemporary Issues,* ed. John J. Michalczyk (London: Sheed & Ward, 1994), pp. 10–11.

[50] Lifton, *Nazi Doctors*, p. 17.

[51] Michael J. Franzblau, interview with author, February 27, 2002.

[52] Binding and Hoche, *Permitting the Destruction*, p. 241.

[53] *Compassion in Dying v. Washington*, 79 F. 3d. 790.

[54] Binding and Hoche, *Permitting the Destruction*, p. 241.

[55] *Compassion in Dying v. Washington*.

[56] Binding and Hoche, *Permitting the Destruction*, p. 241.

[57] *Compassion in Dying v. Washington*.

[58] Binding and Hoche, *Permitting the Destruction*, p. 241.

[59] *Compassion in Dying v. Washington*.

[60] Binding and Hoche, *Permitting the Destruction*, p. 242.

[61] *Compassion in Dying v. Washington*.

[62] Binding and Hoche, *Permitting the Destruction*, p. 265.

[63] *Compassion in Dying v. Washington*.

[64] Binding and Hoche, *Permitting the Destruction*, p. 261.

[65] *Compassion in Dying v. Washington*.

[66] Carol J. Gill, interview with author, December 4, 1995.

[67] Diane Coleman, interview with author, February 16, 1999.

[68] Gill interview.

[69] Leo Alexander, M.D., "Medical Science under Dictatorship," *New England Journal of Medicine*, vol. 241 (July 14, 1949); reprint, p. 8.

[70] Ibid., p. 11.

Chapter 4: Dutch Treat

[1] Leo Alexander, M.D., "Medical Science under Dictatorship," *New England Journal of Medicine*, vol. 241 (July 14, 1949); reprint, p. 9.

[2] Dr. I van der Sluis, interview with author, October 13, 1995.

[3] "Euthanasia Case Leeuwarden—1973" (excerpts from court's decision), trans. Walter Lagerway, *Issues in Law and Medicine*, vol. 3 (1988), pp. 429, 439–42.

[4] "Implications of Mercy," *Time,* March 5, 1973, p. 70.

[5] Ibid.

[6] Ibid.

[7] "Dutch Parliament Approves Law Permitting Euthanasia," *New York Times*, February 10, 1993.

[8] Carlos Gomez, "Regulating Death," (New York: The Free Press, 1991), p. 32.

[9] Timothy Quill, M.D., "Physician Assisted Death: Progress or Peril?" *Suicide and Life-Threatening Behavior*, vol. 24, no. 4, pp. 315–25, 318.

[10] K. F. Gunning, interview with author, October 18, 1995.

[11] Ibid.

[12] J. Remmelink et al., *Medical Decisions about the End of Life*, 2 vols., *Report of the Committee to Study the Medical Practice Concerning Euthanasia: The Study for the Committee on the Medical Practice Concerning Euthanasia* (The Hague, 1991). Cited hereafter as Remmelink Report I or II.

[13] Remmelink Report I, p. 14, n. 2.

[14] Richard Fenigsen, M.D., "The Report of the Dutch Government Committee on Euthanasia," *Issues in Law and Medicine*, vol. 7, no. 3 (November 1991), p. 340.

[15] Remmelink Report I, p. 13.

[16] Ibid., p. 15.

[17] Remmelink Report II, p. 49, Table 6.4.

[18] Ibid., p. 50, Table 6.6.

[19] Ibid., p. 58, Table 7.2.

[20] This figure was arrived at by calculating 8.5 percent (the approximate percentage of all Dutch deaths that resulted from killing by physicians) of the total number of yearly U.S. deaths, which in 1985 was a little over two million (*New York Public Library Desk Reference*, 1989, p. 613).

[21] "Dutch GPs Report Euthanasia as Death by Natural Causes," *British Medical Journal*, vol. 304 (February 1992).

[22] P. J. van der Maas, "Euthanasia and Other Medical Decisions Concerning the End of Life," *Health Policy Monographs*, vol. 2 (1992), p. 49.

[23] Fenigsen, "Report of the Dutch Government Committee on Euthanasia," p. 239; and "Special Report from the Netherlands," *New England Journal of Medicine*, November 1996, pp. 1699–711.

[24] Bregie D. Onwuteaka-Phillipsen et al., "Euthanasia and Other End-of-Life Decisions in the Netherlands in 1990, 1995, and 2001," *Lancet*, vol. 302, August 2, 2003.

[25] Henk Jochemsen and John Keown, *Journal of Medical Ethics*, vol. 25 (1999), pp. 16–21.

[26] Raphael Cohen-Almagor, *Euthanasia in the Netherlands: The Policy and Practice of Mercy Killing* (Boston: Kluwer Academic Publishers, 2004), p. 176.

[27] Ibid., p. 180.

[28] "Dutch Court Rejects Nurse's Defense in Euthanasia Case," Reuters, March 23, 1995.

[29] Tony Sheldon, "Dutch GP Found Guilty of Murder Faces No Penalty," *British Medical Journal*, March 3, 2001.

[30] Gunning interview.

[31] Herbert Hendin, M.D., "Assisted Suicide, Euthanasia, and Suicide Prevention: The Implications of the Dutch Experience," *Suicide and Life Threatening Behavior*, vol. 25, no. 1 (Spring 1995), p. 202.

[32] Ibid., pp. 202–3.

[33] Herbert Hendin, M.D., "Seduced by Death: Doctors, Patients, and the Dutch Cure," *Issues in Law and Medicine*, vol. 10, no. 2 (Fall 1994), p. 137.

[34] Ibid., p. 139.

[35] "Choosing Death," *Healthcare Quarterly*, WGBH-Boston, aired March 23, 1993.

[36] Ibid.

[37] Ibid.

[38] Hendin, "Assisted Suicide, Euthanasia, and Suicide Prevention," p. 197.

[39] "Choosing Death," *Healthcare Quarterly*.

[40] Ibid.

[41] Ibid.

[42] Mark O'Keefe, "The Dutch Way of Doctoring," *Oregonian*, January 9, 1995.

[43] Herbert Hendin, "Dying of Resentment," *New York Times*, January 9, 1995.

[44] Ibid.

[45] Gunning interview.

[46] Bert Keizer, *Dancing with Mr. D: Notes on Life and Death* (New York: Doubleday, 1996), p. 37.

[47] Ibid., p. 39.

[48] Ibid., p. 94.

[49] "CQ Interview: Arlene Juditch Klotzko and Dr. Boudewijn Chabot Discuss Assisted Suicide in the Absence of Somatic Illness," *Cambridge Quarterly of Healthcare Ethics*, vol. 4, no. 2 (Spring 1995), p. 243.

[50] Gene Kaufman, "State v. Chabot: A Euthanasia Case Note," *Ohio Northern University Law Review*, vol. 20, no. 3 (1994), pp. 816–17.

[51] Ibid., p. 817.

[52] Eugene Sutorius interview.

[53] Ibid.

[54] "Choosing Death," *Healthcare Quarterly*.

[55] "Dutch Court Says Baby's Euthanasia Justifiable," Reuters, April 26, 1995.

[56] Agnes van der Heide et al., "Medical End-of-Life Decisions Made for Neonates and Infants in the Netherlands," *Lancet*, vol. 350 (July 26, 1997), pp. 251–55.

[57] Astrid M. Vrakiing et al., "Medical End-of-Life Decisions Made for Neonates and Infants in the Netherlands, 1995–2001," *Lancet*, vol. 365 (April 9, 2005).

[58] "No Prosecution for Dutch Baby Euthanasia," Reuters, January 22, 2005.

[59] Eduard Verhagen and Peter J. J. Sauer, "The Groningen Protocol—Euthansia in Severely Ill Newborns," *New England Journal of Medicine*, March 10, 2005.

[60] "Netherlands Hospital Euthanizes Babies," Associated Press, November 30, 2004.

[61] "Report of the Dutch Royal Society of Medicine: Life-Terminating Actions with Incompetent Patients," Part I, "Severely Handicapped Newborns," *Issues in Law and Medicine*, vol. 8, no. 2 (1992).

[62] "Choosing Death," *Healthcare Quarterly*.

[63] G. G. Humphrey, Letters to the Editor, *Journal of American Medicine*, vol. 260 (1988), p. 788.

[64] Royal Dutch Medical Association, *Vision of Euthanasia* (The Hague: Royal Dutch Medical Association, 1986), p. 14.

[65] Dutch Minister Favors Suicide Pill," CNN.com, May 2001.

[66] Tony Shelton, "Dutch GP Cleared after Helping to End Man's 'Hopeless Existence,'" *British Medical Journal*, vol. 321 (2000), p. 1174.

[67] "Call to Allow 'Suffering from Life' Mercy Killings," Expatia News, December 16, 2004.

[68] Tony Sheldon, "Dutch Euthanasia Law Should Apply to Patients 'Suffering through Living,'" *British Medical Journal*, January 8, 2005.

[69] Dr. Pieter Admiraal, interview with author, September 14, 1995.

[70] H. Jack Gleiger, M.D., editorial, "Race and Health Care—An American Dilemma," *New England Journal of Medicine*, vol. 335, no. 11 (1996).

[71] W. C. M. Klijn, interview with author, September 14, 1995.

[72] Van der Sluis interview.

[73] Admiraal interview.

[74] Hendin, "Seduced by Death," pp. 158–59.

[75] Ibid.

[76] Ibid.

[77] Ibid.

[78] "Helping a Man Kill Himself Shown on Dutch TV," *New York Times*, November 13, 1994.

[79] Andrew Kelly (Reuters), "Audience Plays Solomon on Dutch TV," *Chicago Tribune*, October 28, 1993.

[80] Sarah Lambert, "Dutch Stand Idly By as Child Drowns," *San Francisco Examiner*, August 28, 1993.

[81] Ibid.

[82] *Levenswens-Verklaring* (Declaration on the Value of Life), wallet card, distributed by Stichting Schuilplaats, Veenendaal, Netherlands.

[83] "Doctors Help Kill One in Ten Belgians," BBC News, November 24, 2000.

[84] Wesley J. Smith, "Now They Want to Euthanize Children," *Daily Standard*, September 13, 2004.

[85] Veerle Provoost et al., "Medical End-of-Life Decisions in Neonates and Infants in Flanders," *Lancet*, vol. 365 (April 9, 2005).

[86] Samia A. Hurst and Alex Mauron, "Assisted Suicide and Euthanasia in Switzerland: Allowing a Role for Non-Physicians," *British Medical Journal*, February 1, 2003.

[87] For example, see: "UK Couple Die at Suicide Clinic," BBC News, April 15, 2003.

Chapter 5: Inventing the Right to Die

[1] Jack Kevorkian, M.D., "Fail-Safe Model for Justifiable Medically Assisted Suicide ('Medicide')," *American Journal of Forensic Psychiatry*, vol. 13, no. 1 (1992), pp. 11–12.

[2] Ibid., p. 22.

[3] Transcript of "Yes on 16" advertisement aired on various stations, beginning October 24, 1994.

[4] Transcript of "Yes on 16" advertisement aired on various stations, beginning October 12, 1994.

[5] Oregon Death with Dignity Act, Section 2.01.

[6] Ibid., Section 3.01.

[7] Gary L. Lee, M.D., interview with author, November 30, 1995.

[8] See, for example, Report of the New York State Task Force on Life and the Law, *When Death Is Sought: Assisted Suicide and Euthanasia in the Medical Context* (New York, 1994).

[9] Oregon Death with Dignity Act, Section 1.01.

[10] Ibid.

[11] Oregon Department of Human Services, *Seventh Annual Report on Oregon's Death with Dignity Act,* issued March 10, 2005.

[12] *Lee v. Harcleroad,* Case No. 94-6467:TC, U.S. District Court, District of Oregon, 1994, Complaint for Declaratory and Injunctive Relief.

[13] *Lee v. State of Oregon,* 891 F. Supp., 1995, pp. 1421, 1438.

[14] Ibid., p. 1439.

[15] "Federal Judge Refuses to Enforce Assisted Suicide Law," Associated Press, May 10, 1996.

[16] *Lee v. Oregon,* 107 F. 3d 1382; 1997.

[17] Correspondence from Attorney General Janet Reno to Representative Henry Hyde, June 5, 1998.

[18] "Memorandum for the Attorney General, U.S. Department of Justice, Washington, D.C., from Sheldon Bradshaw, Deputy Assistant Attorney General, and Robert J. Delahunty, Special Counsel," dated June 27, 2001, in *Issues in Law and Medicine,* vol. 17, p. 269.

[19] Ibid.

[20] *United States v. Oakland Cannabis Buyers' Cooperative,* 532 U.S. 483.

[21] Interpretive Rule, U.S. Department of Justice, "Dispensing Controlled Substances to Assist Suicide," 66 *FR* 56607 (November 2002).

[22] *Oregon v. Ashcroft,* U.S. District Court for the District of Oregon, Court Civil No. 01-1647-JO, Opinion and Order, April 17, 2002.

[23] *Oregon v. Ashcroft,* U.S.Court of Appeals for the Ninth Circuit, Case No. CV-01-0657-JO, May 26, 2004, opinion by Judge Richard C. Tallman, joined by Judge Donald P. Lay.

[24] Ibid., dissent by Judge J. Clifford Wallace.

[25] *Gonzales v. Oregon,* Case No. 04-623, Granted, February 22, 2005.

[26] Interview with Gregory Hamilton, M.D., March 8, 2002.

[27] Oregon Department of Human Services, *Seventh Annual Report,* Table 4.

[28] Timothy E. Quill, M.D., *Death and Dignity: Making Choices and Taking Charge* (New York: W.W. Norton & Co., 1994).

[29] Ibid.

[30] Kim Murphy, "Death Called 1st under Oregon's New Suicide Law," *Los Angeles Times,* March 26, 1998.

[31] Herbert Hendin et al., "Physician-Assisted Suicide: Reflections on Oregon's First Case," *Issues in Law and Medicine,* vol. 14, no. 3 (1998).

[32] Erin Hoover Barnett, "Is Mom Capable of Choosing to Die?" *Oregonian,* October 17, 1999.

[33] N. Gregory Hamilton and Catherine Hamilton, "Competing Paradigms of Responding to Assisted-Suicide Requests in Oregon: Case Report," presented at the American Psychiatric Association Annual Meeting, Symposium on Ethics and End of Life Care: New Insights and Challenges, May 6, 2004.

[34] Ibid.

[35] Bill Hewitt, "Last Wish: Defending Oregon's Assisted Suicide Law," *People*, November 26, 2001.

[36] Hamilton, "Competing Paradigms."

[37] Ibid.

[38] Ibid.

[39] Quill, *Death and Dignity*, p. 162.

[40] Oregon Health Department, *Seventh Annual Report*.

[41] Robert A. Pearlman et al., "Motivations for Physician-Assisted Suicide," *Journal of Internal Medicine*, vol. 20, no. 3 (2005), pp 234–39.

[42] Ibid.

[43] Robert Salamanca, "I Don't Want a Choice to Die," *San Francisco Chronicle*, February 19, 1997.

[44] *Compassion in Dying v. Washington*, U.S. Court of Appeals for the Ninth Circuit, 79 F. 3d. 790 (1996).

[45] Ira R. Byock, M.D., interview with author, June 18, 1996.

[46] Howard Mintz, "Dissenters Rip Right-to-Die Vote," *Recorder*, June 13, 1996.

[47] *Quill v. Dennis C. Vacco*, U.S. Court of Appeals for the Second Circuit, 80 F. 3d 716 (1996).

[48] Ibid.

[49] *In re Quinlan*, Supreme Court of New Jersey, 70 NJ 10.

[50] Diane Gianelli, "Karen Ann Quinlan's Family Remembers," *American Medical News*, December 15, 1989, pp. 49–50.

[51] Ronald Comeau's medical records, deposited with the Bennington Probate Court; Joseph Schaaf, interview with author, January 11, 1994; and interviews with most other participants in the case.

[52] *Washington v. Glucksberg*, 521 U. S. 702 (1997); *Vacco v. Quill*, 521 U. S. 793 (1997).

[53] *Washington v. Glucksburg*, p. 728.

[54] Ibid.

[55] Ibid., pp. 730–31.

[56] Ibid., p. 731.

[57] Ibid., pp. 732–32.

[58] Ibid., p. 732.

[59] Ibid.

[60] *Vacco v. Quill*, pp. 801–2.

[61] *People of Michigan v. Jack Kevorian*, 447 Mich. 436 (1994).

[62] *Krischer v. McIver*, 697 So. 2d 97 (1997).

[63] *Sampson v. State*, 31 P.3d 88 (2001).

[64] Rita Marker, "Dying for the Cause," *Philanthropy*, January-February 2001.

[65] The *Chronicle of Philanthropy*, September 20, 2001, reported that OSI had given both CIDF, the Death With Dignity National Center $100,000, while granting $75,000 to Oregon Death With Dignity Legal Defense and Education Fund.

[66] Rita Marker, interview with author, March 21, 2002.

Chapter 6: Euthanasia's Betrayal of Medicine

[1] New York State Task Force on Life and the Law, *When Death Is Sought: Assisted Suicide and Euthanasia in the Medical Context* (Albany, New York, 1994).

[2] Ibid., p. ix.

[3] Ibid., p. xiii.

[4] Ibid.

[5] Ibid.

[6] Ibid.

[7] Ibid.

[8] *Report of the University of Rochester Medical Center Task Force on Physician-Assisted Suicide* (Rochester, N.Y.: University of Rochester, 1993), p. 4.

[9] "When Will Adequate Pain Treatment Be the Norm?" editorial, *Journal of the American Medical Association*, vol. 274, no. 23 (December 20, 1995).

[10] "Painfully Clear," editorial, *American Medical News*, September 26, 1994.

[11] Ada Jacob, R.N., Ph.D., et al., "Special Report: New Clinical-Practice Guideline for the Management of Pain in Patients with Cancer," *New England Journal of Medicine*, vol. 330, no. 9 (March 3, 1994).

[12] Eric M. Chevlen, M.D., and Wesley J. Smith, *Power over Pain: How to Get the Pain Control You Need* (Steubenville, Ohio: International Task Force on Euthanasia and Assisted Suicide, 2002).

[13] Bruce Hilton, "Hospital Chains Are on a Buying Binge," *San Francisco Examiner*, August 23, 1996.

[14] Jeff Wong, "Woman Says She Would Seek Kevorkian's Help Days before Death," Associated Press, July 10, 1996.

[15] Dr. Ljubisa J. Dragovic, interview with author, August 21, 1996.

[16] Richard Leiby, "Just How Sick Was Rebecca Badger?" *Washington Post*, July 29, 1996.

[17] Robert Pear, "Many Doctors Shun Patients with Medicare," *New York Times*, March 17, 2002.

[18] Daniel P. Sulmasy, M.D., "Managed Care and Managed Death," *Archives of Internal Medicine*, January 23, 1995, p. 134.

[19] "When Doctors Become Subcontractors of Medical Care," *USA Today*, January 22, 1996.

[20] *In the Matter of the Accusation of the Commissioner of Corporations of the State of California v. TakeCare Health Plan, Inc.*, hearing before the Department of Corporations of the State of California, November 17, 1994, File No. 933-0290.

[21] Ibid., p. 7.

[22] Ibid., p. 4.

[23] Ibid., p. 6.

[24] Ibid., p. 12.

[25] Janet Price, "Subject: Oregaon Death with Dignity Act: Physician Participation," internal memo, August 6, 2002.

[26] Derek Humphry and Mary Clement, *Freedom to Die: People, Politics, and the Right to Die Movement* (New York: St. Martin's Press, 1998), p. 333.

[27] Ibid., p. 334.

[28] Harvey Rosenfield, *Silent Violence, Silent Death: The Hidden Epidemic of Medical Malpractice* (Washington, D.C.: Essential Books, 1994).

[29] Charles B. Inlander, Lowell S. Levin and Ed Weiner, *Medicine on Trial: The Appalling Story of Ineptitude, Malfeasance, Neglect, and Arrogance* (New York: Prentice Hall, 1994).

[30] T. A. Bremmam et al., *Patients, Doctors and Lawyers: Medical Injury, Malpractice Litigation, and Patient Compensation in New York,* Report of the Harvard Medical Practice Study to the State of New York (Cambridge, Mass.: Harvard University, 1990).

[31] Elizabeth Weise, "Medical Errors Still Claiming Many Lives," *USA Today,* May 18, 2005.

[32] Inlander, Levin and Weiner, *Medicine on Trial,* p. 178.

[33] I interviewed several people in the spring and summer of 1996 who were close to the administrative and civil cases that resulted from this incident. Although several spoke freely about what happened and all were in substantial agreement about them, none would permit me to use their names nor would they disclose the names of the principals.

[34] Sarah Henry, "The Battle over Assisted Suicide," *California Lawyer,* January 1996, p. 34.

[35] O'Neill, "Suicide Aid Worries Oregon Doctors."

[36] "Physicians 'Polarized' about Ethics of Helping Patients Die," *Physician's Management Newsline,* October 1994.

[37] Diane E. Meier, "A Change of Heart on Assisted Suicide," *New York Times,* April 24, 1998.

[38] Allen J. Bennett, M.D., "When Is Medical Treatment Futile?" *Issues in Law and Medicine,* vol. 9, no. 1 (1993), pp. 40, 43.

[39] Correspondence to California State Senator Ray Haynes, March 12, 2002, signed by Matt Moretti, Legislative Advocate, California Healthcare Association.

[40] Marcia Angell, M.D., "After Quinlan: The Dilemma of the Vegetative State," *New England Journal of Medicine,* vol. 330, no. 21 (May 1994), p. 1524.

[41] See: Wesley J. Smith, *Culture of Death: The Assault on Medical Ethics in America* (San Francisco: Encounter Books, 2001).

[42] Charles B. Clayman, ed., *The American Medical Association Encyclopedia of Medicine* (New York: Random House, 1989).

[43] Thomas Marzen, Attorney at Law, interview with author, November 14, 1995.

[44] Madelaine Lawrence. R.N., Ph.D., "The Unconscious Experience," *American Journal of Critical Care*, vol. 4, no. 3 (May 1995).

[45] Jeremy Laurance, "Vegetative State Diagnosis Wrong in Many Patients," *Times* (London), July 5, 1996.

[46] Daniel Callahan, *The Troubled Dream of Life* (New York: Simon & Schuster, 1993), pp. 201–2.

[47] Steven Miles, interview with author, February 9, 1999.

[48] State of Minnesota District Court, Probate Division, County of Hennepin, *In re Helga Wanglie*, "Findings of Fact, Conclusions of Law, and Order, July 1, 1991.

[49] *In re Terry Achtabowski, Jr.*, Docket No. 93-1247-AV, Michigan Court of Appeals, 1994, Appellee's Brief, p. 2.

[50] Dominic Lawson, "The Death of Medicine," *Sunday Telegraph* (London), April 25, 1999.

[51] Lawrence J. Schneiderman and Alexander Morgan Capron, "How Can Hospital Futility Policies Contribute to Establishing Standards of Practice?" *Cambridge Quarterly of Health Care Ethics*, vol. 9 (Fall 2000), pp. 524–31.

[52] Ibid., p. 529.

[53] "Draft Guidelines Supported by CCMD," press release, May 17, 1996.

[54] Dr. Donald J. Murphy, interview with author, July 3, 1996.

[55] Dr. Murphy quoted in Nat Hentoff, "Death: The Ultimate in Managed Care," *Washington Post*, July 16, 1994.

[56] The tale of the demise of CCMD was first published in: Wesley J. Smith, "Philanthropy's Brave New World," *Philanthropy*, January-February 2001, pp. 20–24, from which this recounting is taken.

[57] Leigh Hopper, "Baby Dies after Hospital Removes Breathing Tube," *Houston Chronicle*, March 16, 2005.

[58] Nicole Foy, "Facility May Take Life Support Case," Express News, April 29, 2005.

[59] Ezekiel J. Emanuel, M.D., Ph.D., "Cost Savings at the End of Life: What Do the Data Show?" *Journal of the American Medical Association*, vol. 275, no. 24 (June 1996), pp. 1907–14.

[60] Senate Finance Committee Hearings, "Advance Directives and Care at the End of Life," testimony of Joanne Lynn, M.D., May 5, 1994.

[61] Ezekiel J. Emanuel, M.D., Ph.D., and Linda L. Emanuel, M.D., Ph.D., "The Economics of Dying," *New England Journal of Medicine*, vol. 330, no. 8 (February 1994), p. 543.

[62] Murphy interview.

[63] Ibid.

[64] John Hardwig, "Is There a Duty to Die?" *Hastings Center Report*, March-April 1997, pp. 37–38.

[65] John Hardwig, interview with author, October 22, 1998.

66 Margaret P. Battin, "Global Life Expectancies and the Duty to Die," in *Is There a Duty to Die?* ed. James M. Humber and Robert F. Almeder (Totowa, N.J.: Humana Press, 2000), p. 18.

67 Judith Lee Kissell, "Grandma, the GNP, and the Duty to Die," in *Is There a Duty to Die?* p. 193.

68 Ibid., p. 200.

69 "Jasper Gerard Meets Baroness Warnock," *Times* (London), December 12, 2004.

Chapter 7: Euthanasia as an Enemy of the Disabled

1 Paul Longmore, interview with author, July 13, 1996.

2 Evan Kemp, speech before Capitol Hill Club, Washington, D.C., October 10, 1995.

3 Diane Coleman, "Not Dead Yet," in *The Case Against Assisted Suicide: For the Right to End of Life Care,* ed. Kathleen Foley, M.D., and Herbert Hendin, M,D. (Baltimore: Johns Hopkins University Press, 2002), p. 221.

4 Carol J. Gill, interview with author, December 4, 1995.

5 "Disability Rights and Assisted Suicide," editorial, *One Step Ahead*, August 22, 1994.

6 Advanced Directives and Disability, *One Step Ahead's Second Opinion,* vol. 2, no. 1 (Winter 1995).

7 Diane Coleman, interview with author, July 9, 1996.

8 Ibid.

9 Denny Boyd, "Where Were the Doctors When Robert Latimer Needed Them?" *Vancouver Sun,* November 30, 1994.

10 Larry Johnson, personal correspondence, February 7, 1994.

11 Larry Johnson, interview with author, February 7, 1996.

12 Teague Johnson, "My Body Is Not My Enemy," *Vancouver Sun,* December 9, 1994.

13 Teague Johnson, CompuServe open letter, April 4, 1994.

14 Teague Johnson, CompuServe open letter, undated.

15 Longmore interview.

16 Larry Johnson interview.

17 Canadian Broadcasting Corporation, "Petition Demands Clemency for Jailed Robert Latimer," December 14, 2001.

18 As set forth in Euthanasia Prevention Coalition newsletter, Winter 2001, and confirmed with Dick Sobsey by author, May 15, 2002.

19 *Bouvia v. Superior Court* (California Court of Appeals, 1986) 179 *California Appellate Report* 30.

20 Mark O'Brien, interview with author, July 10, 1996.

21 Gregory E. Pence, *Classic Cases in Medical Ethics* (New York: McGraw Hill, 1995).

22 Paul Longmore, "Urging the Handicapped to Die," *Los Angeles Times,* April 25, 1986.

23 Paul Longmore interview.

[24] Joseph Shapiro, *No Pity: People with Disabilities Forging a New Civil Rights Movement* (New York: Times Books, 1993), p. 259.

[25] Ibid., p. 287.

[26] K. A. Gerhart et al., in *Annals of Emergency Medicine,* vol. 23 (1994), pp. 807–12.

[27] R. Stensman, in *Scandinavian Journal of Rehabilitation Medicine,* vol. 17 (1985), pp. 87–99.

[28] J. R. Bach and M. C. Tilton, in *Archives of Physical Medicine and Rehabilitation,* vol. 71 (1990), pp. 191–96.

[29] Betsy J. Miner, "Messenger Jury Selection to Begin," *Lansing State Journal,* January 10, 1995.

[30] Valeri Basheda, "Verdict's Message: Parents Have Rights," *Detroit News,* February 3, 1995.

[31] Peter Singer, *Rethinking Life and Death: The Collapse of Our Traditional Ethics* (New York: St. Martin's Press, 1995), pp. 213–14.

[32] Lucette Lagnado, "Mercy Living," *Wall Street Journal,* January 10, 1995.

[33] Mary Voboril, "The Assisted Suicide of Myrna Lebov," *Newsday,* January 16, 1996.

[34] "Writer Wanted Relief," *Charleston Daily Mail,* July 8, 1995.

[35] Lucette Lagnado, "How Lebov Bared Her Soul to Rabbis of Lincoln Square," *Forward,* November 3, 1996.

[36] Lucette Lagnado, "DA Stepping Up Inquiry in Death of Myrna Lebov," *Forward,* July 21, 1996.

[37] Beverly Sloane, interview with author, April 19, 1996.

[38] George Delury Diary, "Countdown: A Daily Log of Myrna's Mental State and View toward Death," dates February 27 to July 4, 1995.

[39] *Dateline,* NBC, aired September 27, 1996.

[40] Delury Diary

[41] Ibid.

[42] Ibid.

[43] Ibid.

[44] Ibid.

[45] *Dateline,* NBC, September 27, 1996.

[46] George Delury, *But What If She Wants to Die?* (Buffalo, N.Y.: Prometheus Books, 1997).

[47] Susan Cheever, "An Act of Mercy?" *New York Times Book Review,* July 20, 1997.

[48] Beverly Sloane, interview with author, August 3, 1999.

[49] *Sloane v. Delury et al.,* Supreme Court of the State of New York, County of New York, Index No. 111960/97, "Judgment," November 14, 2001.

[50] "Family Values," *60 Minutes,* CBS, February 25, 1996.

[51] *In the Matter of Gerald Klooster Sr.,* ALI, Case Summary, File No. 95-01060 GD.

[52] Sabin Russell and Henry K. Lee, "Custody Fight Father Hospitalized," *San Francisco Chronicle,* September 25, 1996.

[53] Transcript of taped conversation between Susan Reynolds and John Bement, July 31, 1996.

[54] Susan Randall, interview with author, July 30, 1999.

Chapter 8: Hospice or Hemlock—The Choice Is Ours

[1] Robert M. Arnold and Stuart J. Youngner, "The Dead Donor Rule," *Kennedy Institute of Ethics Journals*, June 1993, p. 271.

[2] Dr. Robin Bernhoft, interview with author, August 27, 1996.

[3] Physicians for Compassionate Care, "Per Capita Morphine Use Figures Debunk Chilling Effect Myth," November 2001, based on DEA figures tracking morphine use state by state.

[4] Judith S. Blanchard and Debra D. Seale, "Lessons from the First Year of a State Cancer Pain Initiative," *Journal of Oncology Management*, November-December 1993.

[5] Eric M. Chevlen, M.D., and Wesley J. Smith, *Power over Pain: How to Get the Pain Control You Need* (Steubenville, Ohio: International Task Force on Euthanasia and Assisted Suicide, 2002), p. 210.

[6] "A Guide to Hospice Care," *Harvard Health Letter*, April 1993.

[7] Dr. Ira Byock, interview with author, June 18, 1996.

[8] Lonny Shavelson, *A Chosen Death: The Dying Confront Assisted Suicide* (New York: Simon & Schuster, 1995).

[9] Cicely Saunders, "A Hospice Perspective," in *The Case Against Assisted Suicide: For the Right to End-of-Life Care*, ed. Kathleen Foley and Herbert Hendin (Baltimore: Johns Hopkins University Press, 2002), p. 291.

[10] House Subcommittee on the Constitution, testimony of Carlos M. Gomez, M.D., April 29, 1996.

[11] Ira Byock, M.D., "Consciously Walking the Fine Line: Thoughts on a Hospice Response to Assisted Suicide and Euthanasia," *Journal of Palliative Care*, vol. 9, no. 3 (September 1993), pp. 25–28.

[12] Dr. Gary Lee interview.

[13] For more details about the founding of the hospice movement, see Wesley J. Smith, *Culture of Death: The Assault on Medical Ethics in America* (San Francisco: Encounter Books, 2001), pp. 21–24.

[14] *Charles Grodin Show*, CNBC, aired August 6, 1996.

[15] Mark O'Brien, interview with author, August 5, 1996.

[16] Ibid.

[17] Beth Roney Drennan, interview with author, April 13, 1995.

[18] Beth Roney Drennan, interview with author, May 27, 2002.

[19] Beth Roney Drennan, 1995 interview.

[20] Beth Roney Drennan, 2002 interview.

[21] Ibid.

[22] Robert Salamanca, "I Don't Want a Choice to Die," *San Francisco Chronicle*, February 19, 1997.

[23] Ed Edelson, "Dying Cite Loss of Social Ties in Seeking Suicide," *Health-Scout*, August 4, 2001.

[24] Melissa Schorr, "Terminally Ill Patients Spend Too Much Time Alone," Reuters, November 12, 2001.

[25] Dennis Brace, interview with author, April 13, 1995.

[26] Senate Finance Committee Hearings, "Advanced Directives and Care at the End of Life," testimony of Joanne Lynn, M.D., M.A., May 5, 1994.

[27] Patrick T. Hill, "Treating the Dying Patient," *Archives of Internal Medicine*, June 1995, p. 23.

[28] Ibid.

[29] John Hess, interview with author, August 12, 1996.

[30] Joseph Brean, "900,000 in Ontario Have No G.P.: Report," *National Post* (Toronto), April 11, 2002.

[31] Jeff Wong, "Woman Said She Would Seek Kevorkian's Help Days before Death," Associated Press, July 10, 1996.

[32] Dr. Lance K. Stell, interview with author, September 28, 1995.

[33] Ibid.

[34] Rev. Peter A. Clark, S.J., Ph.D., and Catherine M. Mikus, "Time for Policy," *Health Progress*, July-August 2000.

[35] Ira Byock, M.D., interview with author, June 18, 1996.

[36] Ibid.

[37] Dr. Maurice Victor, interview with author, August 7, 1996.

[38] Ibid.

[39] Thomas Lorentzen, interviews with author, June 6 and August 8, 1996.

Index